Medical Terminology

A PROGRAMMED SYSTEMS APPROACH

Eighth Edition

Genevieve Love
Smith

Phyllis E.
Davis

Jean Tannis
Dennerll

Revised by Jean Tannis Dennerll, BS, CMA
Instructor/Coordinator of Medical Assistant and Related Health Career Programs
Jackson Community College, Jackson, Michigan

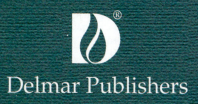

Delmar Publishers

an International Thomson Publishing company I(T)P®

Albany • Bonn ¥ Boston • Cincinnati • Detroit • London • Madrid
Melbourne • Mexico City • New York • Pacific Grove • Paris • San Francisco
Singapore • Tokyo • Toronto • Washington

NOTICE TO THE READER

Cover Design: Brucie Rosch

Delmar Staff

Publisher: Susan Simpfenderfer
Acquisitions Editor: Dawn Gerrain
Developmental Editor: Helen Yackel
Marketing Manager: Darryl Caron
Marketing Coordinator: Nina Lontrato
Editorial Assistant: Donna L. Leto

Team Assistant: Sandra Bruce
Production Manager: Linda Helfrich
Production Editor: Elizabeth LaManna
Production Coordinator: John Mickelbank
Art and Design Coordinator: Vincent S. Berger

For more information, contact Delmar, 3 Columbia Circle, PO Box 15015, Albany, NY 12212-0515; or find us on the World Wide Web at http://www.delmar.com

International Division List

Japan:
Thomson Learning
Palaceside Building 5F
1-1-1 Hitotsubashi, Chiyoda-ku
Tokyo 100 0003 Japan
Tel: 813 5218 6544
Fax: 813 5218 6551

Australia/New Zealand
Nelson/Thomson Learning
102 Dodds Street
South Melbourne, Victoria 3205
Australia
Tel: 61 39 685 4111
Fax: 61 39 685 4199

UK/Europe/Middle East:
Thomson Learning
Berkshire House
168-173 High Holborn
London
WC1V 7AA United Kingdom
Tel: 44 171 497 1422
Fax: 44 171 497 1426

Latin America:
Thomson Learning
Seneca, 53
Colonia Polanco
11560 Mexico D.F. Mexico
Tel: 525-281-2906
Fax: 525-281-2656

Canada:
Nelson/Thomson Learning
1120 Birchmount Road
Scarborough, Ontario
Canada M1K 5G4
Tel: 416-752-9100
Fax: 416-752-8102

Asia:
Thomson Learning
60 Albert Street, #15-01
Albert Complex
Singapore 189969
Tel: 65 336 6411
Fax: 65 336 7411

Spain:
Thomson Learning
Calle Magallanes, 25
28015-MADRID
ESPANA
Tel: 34 91 446 33 50
Fax: 34 91 445 62 18

Library of Congress Cataloging-in-Publication Data:
Smith, Genevieve Love.
   Medical terminology: a programmed systems approach / Genevieve Love Smith, Phyllis E. Davis, Jean Tannis Dennerll. — 8th ed. / revised by Jean Tannis Dennerll.
      p. cm.
   Includes indexes.
      ISBN: 0-7668-0063-6
   1. Medicine—Terminology—Programmed instruction. I. Davis, Phyllis E. II. Dennerll, Jean Tennis III. Title
   [DNLM: 1. Nomenclature programmed instruction. W. 18.2 S648m 1999]
R123.S6 1999
610'.1'4-dc21
DNLM/DLC for Library of Congress

98-24810
CIP

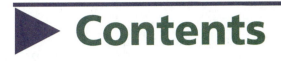

Contents

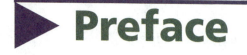

Preface

Medical Terminology: A Programmed Systems Approach, Eighth Edition, is a medical terminology text teaching a **word-building system** using a **programmed learning format.** Thousands of medical words may be built by learning the Latin and Greek prefixes, suffixes, and word roots from which our English medical words originate. Genevieve Smith and Phyllis Davis were the first to apply programmed learning to the teaching of medical terminology when they designed this text over 34 years ago, and this system has been refined through eight editions.

Medical Terminology: A Programmed Systems Approach, Eighth Edition, continues to be an accessible and successful way for individuals and groups to learn quickly and easily. In the 21 years I have been teaching medical terminology, I have been amazed by students' positive results using this text. Students with little or no previous study in the health care field can master this subject by using the materials in this text and supplement package.

Features of this edition

- **Programmed learning format** presents and reinforces word parts and word-building with over 1700 frames—more than any other medical terminology text. This format requires learners to actively participate in learning by writing in and confirming answers for every frame.

- **Unit divisions** revised into 15 units for easier semester assignment

- **New Student Practice Software** includes more than 1250 review exercises, activities and games with valuable feedback to make learning fun. See the *How to Use the Student Practice Software Section* on pages xiv and xv.

- **Full-color illustrations, diagrams, and photos** appear near their reference in text. Rather than flipping to an insert, art is immediately available for reference, making it even more useful for students. Color art stimulates interest and brings visual reality to the medical terms presented.

- **Word part color highlights,** such as **cyan** for prefixes, **magenta** for suffixes, and **bold** for word roots and combining forms, help facilitate student retention. Color provides a good memory tool for the student, while allowing for continual reinforcement of various word parts.

- **New frames** have been added and obsolete terms deleted to update the text, using the latest editions of International *Classification of Diseases, 9th edition, Clinical Modification* (ICD-9-CM), *and Current Procedural Terminology* (CPT) code books and other current references.

- **Four featured frames** to help students include:

  Information—present relevant and interesting facts to help student retention

  Spell Check—clues and special notes on troublesome spelling

  Take a Closer Look—analyzes similar terms

  Word Origins—help students learn Greek and Latin origins of medical terms to encourage memory retention through fascinating reference to mythology, legends and original language meanings. A Greek and Latin scholar, Dirk T. D. Held, PhD, Professor of Classics at Connecticut College, New London, Connecticut, reviewed these for accuracy of definitions and word origins.

- **New glossaries** at the end of each unit summarize terms and definitions in a format that can be used by students as a review tool.

- **Majority of answers in the frames align** with the blanks in the text column to allow easy use as the student reads across the page. The answer blank length also gives the student a visual clue in determining the answer length for single word answers.

- **Professional Profiles** describing a variety of Allied Health Professions along with color photos of the professional on the job. These profiles provide students with valuable information about possible career paths, while reinforcing the importance of knowing medical terminology to achieve career goals.

- **Abbreviation tables** have been updated with many new abbreviations associated with new medical terminology and diagnoses.

- **Review activities integrated after each unit.** Extensive review activities are integrated after each unit. Answers for all activities are included in Appendix (**purple** side tab)
  - **Circle and correct**
  - **Select and construct**
  - **Define and dissect**
  - **Matching abbreviations**
  - **Case study analysis**
  - **Crossword puzzles**

Comprehensive Supplements Package

- **Instructor's Manual** has been completely revised for use with this edition. It includes a correlation guide from the 7th to 8th edition, two sample course syllabi, quizzes, midterm and final exams, unit word part lists, additional case studies, and suggestions for course design using *Medical Terminology: A Programmed Systems Approach, Eighth Edition.*

- **Two 90-minute audiotapes** accompany this text and include specific frame references within the tapes. These tapes have been designed to allow students to listen to each term and repeat them aloud for pronunciation practice, as well as to hear term definitions and use in context. Students may also use the tapes to write the words and definitions, retesting spelling and definition comprehension.

- **Computerized Test Bank** includes over 1,250 questions with answers and is available in Windows format (3.5" disk) to easily create a variety of testing materials with your personal computer. You can even add your own questions to the question bank.

- **Text/Tape Package** is available for students to affordably have their own personal copy of the audiotapes to use where and when they wish.

- **Distance Learning Course Component** beginning January 1999 a distance learning web-based course complete with interface and lessons for each unit will be available through Delmar. Schools or training facilities may use the course to provide an on-line medical terminology course quickly and easily using our lessons as they are. Or they can customize lessons by adding, deleting and reorganizing components as they wish. Some of the components within each lesson will be lecture/presentation, pretest, exercises, testing and grading. A new Medical Terminology CD-ROM will also be available for use as a component of a distributed learning or traditional course.

It is our intent that *Medical Terminology: A Programmed Systems Approach, Eighth Edition,* be the best edition yet printed and that it continues to serve the needs of the students and teachers who use it. We maintain our commitment to the original philosophy and integrity of this classic text.

Jean Tannis Dennerll, BS, CMA

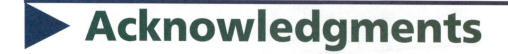

Acknowledgments

This valuable work, which is intended to accelerate and enhance student learning and instructor effectiveness, would not have been possible to create without the dedicated professional team at Delmar Publishers. I would like to thank Dawn Gerrain, Helen Yackel, Elizabeth LaManna, Vincent S. Berger, and John Mickelbank, who all played an important part in producing this work.

It is also impossible for me to function in a productive way without the support and encouragement of my husband and computer expert, Timothy J. Dennerll, PhD; my beautiful children, Diane and Raymond; my mother, Helen Tannis; and my colleagues at Jackson Community College.

I would also like to especially acknowledge several professionals from the health care community in Jackson, Michigan, who made a content contribution to this and to previous editions. They include:

Lynne Schrieber BS, RT(R), RDMS

Grant Brown, Pharm D, Ophon Care

Andrew J. Krapohl, MD, and Pat Krapohl, RN, MPH

Deanna Sioma, Doctor's Hospital

Foote Hospital:

    Shannon Griggs, RHIA

    Sally Mulnix, OT(R)

    Eva Maga ASCP, (MT)

    Maris Kalmbach, OT(R)

    Diane Jonas, CMT

    Cathy Rayl, RT(R)

    Mary Beth Reilly, Promotional Coordinator

Chip Smith, EMT-P, Jackson Emergency Services PC

Denise Brzozowski, COT, Mid Michigan Eye Center PC

Ann Blaxton, CCC-A, Professional Hearing Services

Sharon Rooney-Gandy, DO, General Surgery Board Certified

Shawn McKinney, COMT, The American College of Ophthalmic Technology, Hillsdale, MI

P. H. Ernest, MD, EyeCare Physicians

Noreen Calus, MS, RHIA

I would also like to thank the following reviewers:

Sandie Baillargeon, CMS
Career Canada College
Hamilton, Ontario

Lisa Carrigan, RN
Instructor, Health Occupations
Rock Hill Career Development Center
Rock Hill, SC

Maureen Donaldson
Bishop State Community College
Mobile, AL

Barbara Ensley, MS, RN, CMA-C
Haywood Community College
Clyde, NC

David J. Fitzpatrick, BBA, MS
Fisher College
Fall River, MA

Dirk T. D. Held, PhD
Professor of Classics
Connecticut College
New London, CT

Marty Hitchcock, CMA, MA
Gwinnett Technical Institute
Lawrenceville, GA

Charlotte A. Jensen, MA, BS
Cabrillo College
Aptos, CA

Kay Kavanaugh, MS, RT
Ivy Tech State College
Indianapolis, IN

Peggy Krueger, RN, BSN, MEd, CMA
Medical Assistant Program Coordinator
Linn-Benton Community College
Albany, OR

Thomas Longua
Denver Academy of Court Reporting
Denver, CO

Ruth Lorenson, EdD, RN
Aims Community College
Greeley, CO

Harriet D. Laronge, CMA
Program Director, Medical Assisting
    Medical Transcription/Coder Specialist
Sarasota County Vocational Technical Institute

Sue Moe
Health Division Instructor
Northwest Technical College
East Grand Forks, MN

Anita Pendo, BSN, RN
Nursing Department
Mohave Community College
Kingman, AZ

Donald C. Rizzo, PhD
Head: Mathematics and Science Academic Unit
Professor of Biology
Marygrove College
Detroit, MI

Molly F. Savage, BSN, RN
Central Piedmont Community College
Charlotte, NC

H. H. Skinner, Jr., MD
English/School of Nursing
Yakima Valley Community College
Yakima, WA

Ester Stovold
Instructor/Program Development
Medical Terminology and Transcription
    Programs
Selkirk College, Trail Campus
Trail, BC CANADA

List of Illustrations

About this Programmed System

*Medical Terminology: A Programmed Systems Approach,
Eighth Edition* is carefully designed to help you learn
medical terminology.

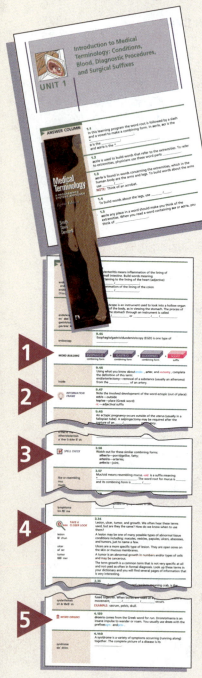

Objectives of the Learning System

Upon completion of this system,
the learner should be able to:

1. Build literally thousands of medical
   words from Greek and Latin prefixes, suffixes, word
   roots, and combining forms.
2. Define medical words by analyzing their Greek and Latin parts.
3. Spell medical words correctly.
4. Use a medical dictionary.
5. Pronounce medical words correctly.
6. Recall acceptable medical abbreviations that represent phrases and terms.

To maximize the benefits of this learning system, familiarize yourself with
the following features.

Programmed Learning Format

Information is presented and learned in small numbered sections called
frames. You will have an active part in learning medical terminology using
this successful programmed approach. The right column contains a state-
ment and an answer blank; the left column provides the answer. Cover the
answer column with a bookmark (two are provided as part of the back
cover). Read the right column of the frame and write your answer in the
blank. Pull down the bookmark to reveal the answer and confirm your
response. Then move on to the next frame. Learning one bit of information
at a time is part of programmed learning. Another part is continual
reinforcement of word parts and terms throughout the book.

Word-Building System and Word Parts

Word roots, combining forms, prefixes, suffixes are important building blocks in the word-building system. **Word roots** and **combining
forms** are highlight in bold, prefixes in blue with a hyphen after
each, and suffixes in magenta with a hyphen preceding each.

Featured Frames

Featured frames include:

Information—present interesting facts to
help retention

Spell check—clues and special notes on
troublesome spelling

 Take a Closer Look—analyzes similar
terms

Word Origins—help students learn
Greek and Latin origins of medical terms

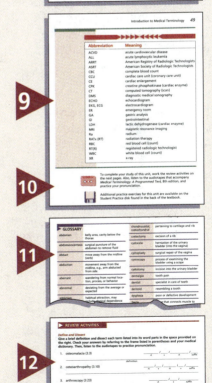

Full-Color Art
 6

Even more full color illustrations and photos included in this edition. Art and photos are placed near their reference—not in a separate color section. A complete list of all art is on pages x and xi.

Pronunciations
7

Pronunciations appear directly beneath each new term presented. The portion of the term receiving primary emphasis is bold. A pronunciation key including rules, symbols, and examples is on the inside front cover.

Professional Profiles
8

Vignettes and photos describing the function and credentials of many allied health professions are placed throughout the text. These profiles give information about various professions and possible career paths as well as reinforce the importance of medical terminology for all health professionals.

Abbreviations
9

Abbreviations are covered many ways. New frames have been added to work abbreviations, a list of abbreviations and meanings is included in each unit and several new activities were developed specifically to identify and test abbreviations. Appendix C (green side tab) includes a comprehensive list of abbreviations.

Audiotapes
 10

After completing each unit, you may want to listen to the audiotapes that accompany the text. You can use the tapes to listen to each term and repeat the term aloud for pronunciation practice. You may also write the term and its definition to check spelling and meaning comprehension.

Student Practice Software

Use the student practice software for a fun computerized review for each unit. Turn the page for the How to Use the Software section for more details.

Glossary
11

New to this edition are unit end glossaries that summarize terms and definitions in a frame-type format for easy study and review

Review Activities
12

Activities include a variety of exercises to reinforce terms learned within the frames Also included are *case study* excerpts from actual medical records featuring medical terms in context along with questions to test and reinforce spelling and definitions. *Crossword Puzzles* provide definition to term review in an easy, fun format.

► How to Use the Student Practice Software

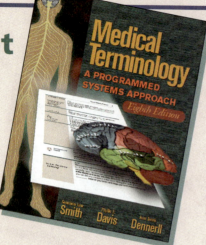

The Student Practice Software has been designed to accompany *Medical Terminology: A Programmed Systems Approach, Eighth Edition,* so you can learn even the toughest medical terms. By using these exercises and games, you'll challenge yourself to make your study of medical terms more effective, and have fun!

Getting started is easy. Follow the simple directions on the disk label to install the program on your computer. Then take advantage of the following features:

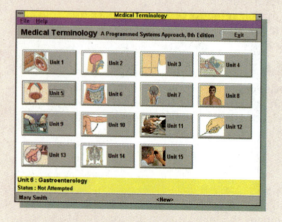

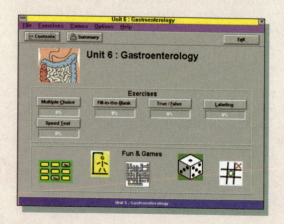

Main Menu

The main menu follows the unit organization of the text exactly—which makes it easy for you to find your way around. Just click on the button for the unit opening screen to select the exercises and games for that unit.

Tool Bar

As you navigate through the software, check the toolbar for other exercise, game, resetting and printing features. The button bar allows you to retrace your steps, while the *Exit* button gets you out of the program quickly and easily.

On-Line Help

If you get stuck, just press F1 or click *Help* on the toolbar for assistance. The on-line help includes instructions for all parts of the Student Practice Software.

Unit Screen

Here you have the opportunity to choose how you want to learn the material. Sleect one of the exercises for additional practice, review or self-testing. Or click on a game to practice unit terms in a fun format.

Exercises

The Software acts as your own private tutor. For each exercise, it chooses from a bank of over 1250 questions covering all 15 units. To start simply:

• Choose an exercise from those displayed such as multiple choice, fill-in, true/false, or labeling exercise, whichever appeals to you.

- Each exercise format includes a series of 10 questions randomly selected from that unit's bank of questions. Each question gives you two chances to answer correctly.
- Instant feedback tells whether your right or wrong. Plus rationales explain why an answer was correct and critical thinking hints are provided when first-choice answer is incorrect.
- The percentage of correct answers displays on the unit screen. An on-screen score sheet (which you can print) lets you track correct and incorrect answers.
- Review previous questions and answers of an exercise for more in-depth understanding. Or start an exercise over with a new, random set of questions.
- When you're ready for an additional challenge, try the timed Speed Test. Once you've finished, it displays your score and the time you took to complete the test, so you can see how much you've learned.

Games

To have fun while reinforcing your knowledge, enjoy each of the five simple games on this disk. You can play alone, with a partner, or on teams.

- **Concentration:** match terms or abbreviations to their corresponding definitions under the cards as the seconds tick by.
- **Hangman:** review your spelling and vocabulary by choosing the correct letters to spell medical terms before you're "hanged."
- **Crossword Puzzles:** using the definition clues provided, fill-in the medical terms to complete each puzzle. A click of the Check button highlights incorrect answers in blue.
- **Board Game:** challenge your classmates and increase your knowledge by playing this question-and-answer game.
- **Tic-Tac-Toe:** you or your team must correctly answer a medical question before placing an X or an O.

Minimum System Requirements:
Operating System: Windows® 3.1, Windows® 95 or newer, Windows NT™
Computer: 386 or newer
Memory: 8 MB RAM
Hard Drive Space: 2.5 MB RAM
Graphics: 16 Bit Color VGA
Floppy drive: 3-1/2 inch, high density
Mouse

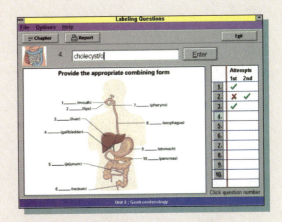

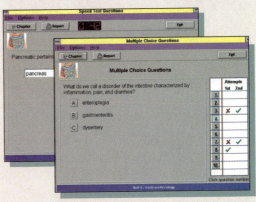

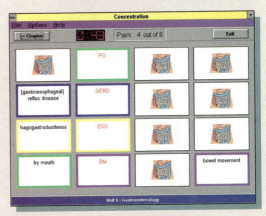

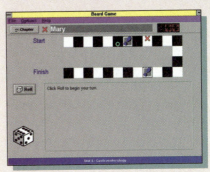

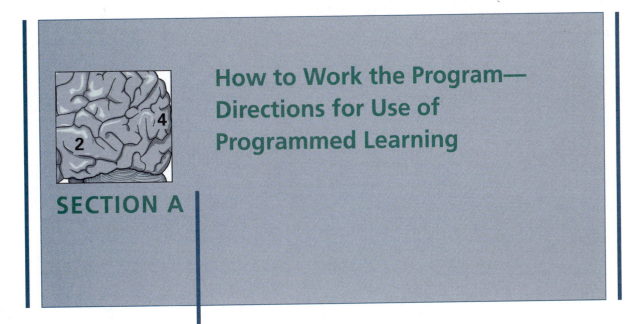

SECTION A

How to Work the Program—
Directions for Use of
Programmed Learning

ANSWER COLUMN	
	A.1 DIRECTIONS: Cover the answer column with the marker provided as part of the back cover. A frame is a piece of information, plus a blank (_____) in which you write. All this material following the number A.1 is a
frame Now go on to Frame A.2	_____. Check your answer by sliding down your cover paper.
correct Now go on to Frame A.3	**A.2** By checking your answer immediately, you know whether or not you are right. This immediate knowledge helps you to learn only what is (choose one) _____ (correct/incorrect). Check your answer by sliding down your cover paper.
program	**A.3** Programmed learning is a way of learning that gives you immediate feedback and allows you to work at your own speed. When you work a series of frames and are certain that you know the terms, you are learning from a _____. Check your answer by sliding down your cover paper.
check write	**A.4** Always _____ your answers immediately. Always _____ your answers in the blank or on a separate paper.

▶ **ANSWER COLUMN**

INFORMATION FRAME

A.5
When you write a new word and check your answer, you will usually find the pronunciation given. Pronounce the word *out loud* and listen to what you are saying. Practice proper pronunciation by listening to the audiotapes prepared to accompany *Medical Terminology: A Programmed Text*, 8th edition. Pronouncing words correctly assists in spelling correctly and speaking medical phrases correctly.

---

correctly

A.6
Practice saying each new word *out loud* several times. This helps you spell medical words _____ by becoming familiar with the sounds.

---

medical
one

A.7
When you see a blank space (_____), your answer will need only one word. In the sentence, "This is a program in _____ terminology," you know to use _____ word.

---

long

A.8
A single blank (_____) contains a clue. It is proportional to the length of the word needed. A short blank (_____) means one short word. A long blank (_____) means one _____ word.

---

one
length

A.9
Whenever you see a blank space (_____) you know to write (choose one) _____ (one/more than one) word. You also know something about the (choose one) _____ (length/complexity) of the word.

---

medical terminology
more than one word

A.10
Whenever you see an asterisk and a blank (*_____), your answer will require more than one word. In the sentence, "This is a programmed course in *_____," your answer requires *_____.

---

more than one word

A.11
In *_____, there is no clue to the length of the words. The important thing to remember is that an asterisk and a blank means *_____.

---

out loud

A.12
Use the Pronunciation Key on the inside back cover to aid in proper practice when saying words *_____.

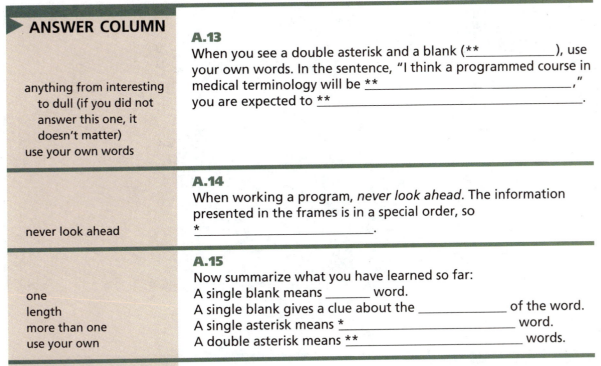

ANSWER COLUMN	**A.13** When you see a double asterisk and a blank (**_____), use your own words. In the sentence, "I think a programmed course in medical terminology will be **_____," you are expected to **_____.
anything from interesting to dull (if you did not answer this one, it doesn't matter) use your own words	

A.14
When working a program, *never look ahead*. The information presented in the frames is in a special order, so
*_____.

never look ahead

A.15
Now summarize what you have learned so far:
A single blank means _____ word.
A single blank gives a clue about the _____ of the word.
A single asterisk means *_____ word.
A double asterisk means **_____ words.

one
length
more than one
use your own

A.16
Saying, listening, seeing, writing, and *thinking* will do much for you. On the following drawing, find the parts of the brain used when saying, listening, seeing, writing, and thinking.

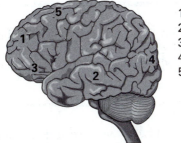

1. thinking area
2. hearing area
3. saying area
4. seeing area
5. writing area

INFORMATION FRAME

A.17
If you have five parts of the brain working for you at the same time, you will learn much faster. This is efficient learning. It makes sense to say a word, listen to it, look at it, write it, and think about it in one operation.

A.18
This programmed learning, word-building system encourages you to *read* (look and understand) about medical terms, *say* them aloud correctly, *listen* to them on audiotape, *write* the terms as answers in the blanks and review activities, and *think* about the terms as you use them to complete statements. Doing this uses at least _____ areas of your brain and helps you learn more efficiently.

Now, move on to the Word-Building System in the next section.

See how efficiently you are learning!

DERMAT
word root

The Word-Building System—Introduction to Word Parts Including Word Roots, Suffixes, Prefixes, Parts of Speech, Plural Formation

ANSWER COLUMN	
exceptions	**B.1** This is a word-building system. There are exceptions to all systems. This system of word-building also has _____.
System	**B.2** The Word-Building System is useful because it is impossible to memorize enough medical words! By using a few word parts, you can build thousands of words, if you know the Word-Building _____.
word root	**B.3** All words have a word root. Even ordinary, everyday words have a * _____.
word root	**B.4** The word root is the foundation of a word. Trans/**port**, ex/**port**, im/**port**, and sup/**port** have **port** as their * _____.
word root	**B.5** Suf/**fix**, pre/**fix**, af/**fix**, and **fix**/ation have **fix** as their * _____.
gastr	**B.6** The word root for stomach in **gastr**/itis, **gastr**/ectomy, and **gastr**/ic is _____.

4

ANSWER COLUMN	
word root	**B.7** The foundation of the word is the *_____.
	NOTE: A slash mark (diagonal) "/" is used to divide words into their word parts. EXAMPLE: **gastr/** **o/** **duoden/** **-ostomy** word root combining word root suffix vowel
combining form	**B.8** A *combining form* is a word root plus a vowel. In the word therm/o/meter, **therm/o** is the *_____.

WORD BUILDING

MICR	+	O	=	MICR/O
word root		vowel		combining form

INFORMATION FRAME

B.9
Adding a vowel (a, e, i, o, u, or y) to a word root to create a combining form allows two or more word roots to be joined to form a compound word. It also allows a word root to be joined with a suffix (ending of a word) to form a word. In addition, the vowel assists by making the term easier to pronounce.

vowel o	**B.10** In the word cyt/o/meter (instrument used to measure [count] cells), the *_____ allows **cyt** to be joined to **meter**.
combining form	**B.11** In the words micr/o/scope, micr/o/film, and micr/o/be, **micr/o** is the *_____.

INFORMATION FRAME

B.12
You will usually use a combining form when joining a word root to a suffix or other word root that begins with a *consonant* (for example, b, d, p, s, t, v).

WORD BUILDING

GASTR/O	+	DUODEN/O	+	SCOPY	=	GASTRODUODENOSCOPY
combining form		combining form		suffix		compound word

ANSWER COLUMN	
would neur/o/spasm	**B.13** You (choose one) _____ (would/would not) use a combining form to join the word roots **neur** and **spasm** to form _____ /_____ /_____.

INFORMATION FRAME

B.14
Use a word root, not a combining form, when joining a word root with a suffix or another word root that begins with a vowel (for example, a, e, i, o, u, y).

WORD BUILDING

DERMAT (word root) + ITIS (suffix) = DERMATITIS (word)

B.15
would not

lymph/adenopathy

You (choose one) _____ (would/would not) use a combining form to join the word parts **lymph** and **adenopathy** to form _____ /_____.

NOTE: Combining forms are never used as a suffix. They require an ending to complete a word. There are many exceptions to the rules about combining form usage stated above. Always consult your medical dictionary for correct spelling of new terms. That way you will know if the new word you created is actually a medical word.

B.16
compound words

Compound words can be formed when two or more word roots are used to build the word. Even in ordinary English, two or more word roots are used to form *_____ (for example, shorthand or download).

B.17
compound word

Sometimes word roots are words. Two or more word roots still form a compound word. Chickenpox is a
*_____.

WORD BUILDING

CHICKEN (word root) + POX (word root) = CHICKENPOX (compound word)

B.18
underage

Form a compound word using the word roots **under** and **age**.
_____

ANSWER COLUMN	
brainstem	**B.19** Form a compound word from the word roots **brain** and **stem**. _____
compound words	**B.20** Because they are formed by joining two or more word roots, therm/o/meter, cyt/o/meter, micr/o/scope, and micr/o/surgery are all *_____.
combining form whole word	**B.21** Compound words can also be formed from a combining form and a whole word. Thermometer is a compound word built from a combining form and a word. In the word therm/o/meter, **therm/o** is the *_____, meter is the *_____.

micr/o/scope
micr/o/surgery
micr/o/meter
	B.22
	Build a compound word from the combining form **micr/o** plus:
	    scope micr/o/_____ (instrument to see small things);
	    surgery micr/o/_____ (surgery using a microscope);
	    meter micr/o/_____ (measuring device for small things).

hydr/o/phobia
hydr/o/cele
hydr/o/therapy
	B.23
	Build a compound word from the combining form **hydr/o** plus:
	    phobia (fear of water) hydr/o/_____;
	    cele (fluid in a saclike cavity) hydr/o/_____;
	    therapy (water therapy) hydr/o/_____.

suffix	**B.24**
	-ic is an adjective suffix. In medical terminology, compound words are usually built from a combining form, a word root, and a suffix. In the word micr/o/scop/ic,
	    micr/o is the combining form;
	    scop is the word root;
	    -ic is the _____.

combining form suffix	**B.25** In medical terminology, compound words are usually built in the following order: combining form + word root + suffix. The word part coming first is usually a *_____. The word part that comes last is the _____.

ANSWER COLUMN

B.26

In the word therm/o/metr/ic,

    therm/o is the combining form;

word root

    metr   is the *_____;

suffix

    -ic   is the _____.

B.27

Build a word from:

    the combining form **electr/o**;

    the word root   **stat**;

    the suffix   **-ic**.

electr/o/stat/ic

_____ /_____ /_____ /_____

B.28

Build a word from:

    the combining form **hydr/o**;

    the word root   **chlor**;

    the suffix   **-ic**.

hydr/o/chlor/ic

hī drō **klor´** ik

_____ /_____ /_____ /_____

INFORMATION FRAME

B.29

If you missed either of the last two frames, rework the program starting with Frame B.24.

NOTE: The suffix is usually described first in the definition; for example, (1) pertaining to (-ic), (2) electricity—electric; or (1) inflammation (-itis) of the (2) bladder (**cyst**)—cystitis.

B.30

The ending that follows a word root is a suffix. You can change the meaning of a word by putting another part after it. This other

suffix

part is also called a _____ (highlighted in magenta).

NOTE: Notice in this book the suffixes are highlighted in magenta and proceded by a hyphen (-).

B.31

The suffix -er means one who or one which. The word root **port** (to carry) is changed by putting -er after it. In the word port/er

suffix

(one who carries), -er is a _____.

B.32

one who

A medical practitioner is *_____ practices medicine.

ANSWER COLUMN

suffix

B.33
In the word read/able, -able changes the meaning of **read**.
-able is a _____.

WORD BUILDING

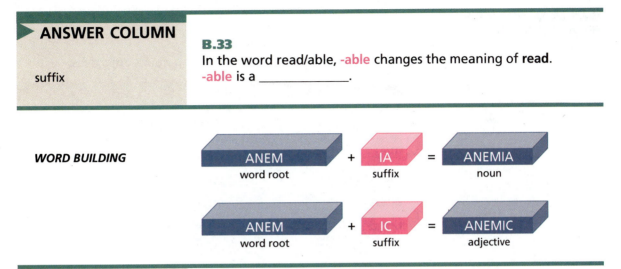

B.34
Suffixes also may change the part of speech of a word. For example, nouns (naming persons, places, or things) may be changed to adjectives (descriptors) such as:

Noun	Suffix	Adjective	Suffix
cyanosis	-osis	cyanotic	-otic
anemia	-ia	anemic	-ic
mucus	-us	mucous	-ous
ilium	-um	iliac	-ac
condyle	-e	condylar	-ar
carpus	-us	carpal	-al

B.35
In the words cyan/osis, anem/ia, and ili/um, the noun suffixes are _____, _____, and _____.

-osis
-ia
-um

► **ANSWER COLUMN**

B.36
List the suffixes that make the following nouns adjectives:

Adjective	Pertaining to
ili/ac	ilium
cyan/otic	cyanosis
anem/ic	anemia
duoden/al	duodenum
muc/ous	mucus
condyl/ar	condyle
man/iac	mania
arthr/itic	arthritis
eme/tic	emesis

-ac

-otic

-ic

-al

-ous

-ar

-iac

-itic

-tic

INFORMATION FRAME

B.37
Verbs are words that represent action or a state of being.
EXAMPLE: incise, ambulate, love.

B.38
The suffixes **-ed** or **-ing** added to the word vomit alter the tense of this verb (when the action takes place). Create the past tense by adding **-ed** to vomit: _____ , and the present participle by adding **-ing** to vomit: _____.

vomited
vomiting

B.39
Use the suffixes **-ed** and **-ing** with the word inject.
_____ past tense;
_____ present participle.

injected
injecting

► **ANSWER COLUMN**

Read and study this table. Then, move on to the next frame.

Noun Suffixes	Examples
-ism—condition, state, or theory	hyperthyroidism
-tion—condition	contraction, relaxation
-ist—specialist	psychiatrist
-er—one who	radiographer
-ity—quality	sensitivity

Adjectival Suffixes	Examples
-ous—possessing, having, full of	nervous, mucous
-able ⎫	injectable
-ible ⎭ —ability	edible

---

condition or state

B.40
Hyper/thyroid/ism is a _____ of too much secretion by the thyroid gland.

---

theory

B.41
Darwin/ism presents a theory of development. Mendel/ism presents a _____ of heredity.

---

condition
condition

B.42
Contrac/tion is a _____ of muscle shortening.
Relaxa/tion is the _____ of diminished tension.

---

nouns

B.43
Contraction and relaxation are (choose one) _____ (nouns/adjectives) because they name a condition.

---

a specialist
one who

B.44
A psychiatr/ist is *_____ who practices psychiatry. A medical practition/er is *_____ practices medicine.

► **ANSWER COLUMN**

noun	**B.45** The word practitioner is a (choose one) _____ (noun/adjective).
quality quality	**B.46** **-ity** indicates a quality. Conductiv/ity expresses the _____ of conducting nerve and muscle impulses. Sensitiv/ity expresses the _____ of nervous tissue excitability related to receiving stimuli.
noun	**B.47** Irritabil/ity is a (choose one) _____ (noun/adjective).
having a material (substance) having, possessing	**B.48** Mucus, a noun, is a watery secretion. Muc/ous, an adjective, refers to the nature of *_____ secreted by the mucous membrane. Ser/ous refers to the nature of _____ material lining closed body cavities such as the abdomen.
having, possessing nerve	**B.49** Nerv/ous refers to _____ too much stress, or having a type of tissue made of _____ cells.
adjectives	**B.50** Words ending in **-ous** are (choose one) _____ (nouns/adjectives).
ability ability	**B.51** **-ible** and **-able** indicate ability. To say a food is digestible is to say it has the _____ to be digested. To say a fracture is reducible is to say that it has the _____ to be reduced.
ability	**B.52** To say that lungs are inflatable is to say that they have the _____ to inflate.
adjectives	**B.53** Words ending in **-ible** or **-able** are (choose one) _____ (nouns/adjectives).

ANSWER COLUMN

🏛 *WORD ORIGINS*

B.54

Since most medical terms in English come from Greek and Latin words, the rules for forming plurals from singular nouns also often come from the Greek and Latin languages. We typically use "s" and "es" added to a singular noun to make it plural (i.e. chair [chairs], box [boxes]). Study the table indicating the proper plural ending associated with each singular noun ending.

Singular Suffixes	Plural Suffixes
Greek	
-on	-a
-ma	-mata
-sis	-ses
-nx	-ges
Latin	
-a	-ae
-us	-i
-um	-a
-is	-es
-ex	-ices
-ix	-ices
-ax	-aces

Now see if you are able to recognize the suffix patterns and write them in the blanks provided. Check you answers. Then look up each word in the medical dictionary.

Greek Singular Noun	Greek Plural Form
spermatozoon	spermatozoa
ganglion	ganglia
suffix _____	suffix _____
carcinoma	carcinomata
lipoma	lipomata
suffix _____	suffix _____
crisis	crises
prognosis	prognoses
suffix _____	suffix _____
larynx (laryng/o)	larynges
pharynx (pharyng/o)	pharynges
suffix _____	suffix _____

-on, -a

-ma, -mata

-is, -es

-nx, ges

Use what you just learned about Greek to form the plurals for the following terms.

protozoan _____

sarcoma _____

diagnosis _____

phalanx (phalang/o) _____

Great! Now go on to the Latin forms.

Latin Singular Noun	Latin Plural Form
vertebra	vertebrae
conjunctiva	conjunctivae

suffix _____ suffix _____

bacillus	bacilli
bronchus	bronchi

suffix _____ suffix _____

ilium	ilia
bacterium	bacteria

suffix _____ suffix _____

cortex (cortic/o) cortices

suffix _____ suffix _____

appendix (appendic/o) appendices

suffix _____ suffix _____

thorax (thorac/o) thoraces

suffix _____ suffix _____

Use what you just learned about Latin to form the plurals for the following terms.

coccus _____

calcaneum _____

vertex (**vertic/o**) _____

cervix (**cervic/o**) _____

thorax (**thorac/o**) _____

Great work! As you work through the text you may wish to refer back to this section to review the rules for plural formation. Plural forms will be included with many of the frames as you learn the singular noun form. When in doubt, consult your dictionary.

prefix

B.55

A prefix is a word part that goes in front of a word root. You can change the meaning of the word by putting another part in front of it. This other part is a _____.

NOTE: Notice in this book the prefixes are highlighted in blue and are followed by a hyphen.

Prefix	Word	New Word
ex-	tension	extension
ex-	press	express
dis-	please	displease
dis-	ease	disease

prefix

B.56

The prefix ex- means from or out from. The word press means to squeeze or push on. Placing ex- in front of press changes its meaning to "squeeze out." In the word ex/press, ex- is a _____.

prefix

B.57

In the word dis/ease, dis- changes the meaning of ease. dis- is a _____.

im-
sup-
trans-

B.58

In the words im/plant, sup/plant, and trans/plant, the prefixes are _____, _____, and _____.

word root

B.59

Before learning more, review what you have learned. The foundation of a word is a *_____.

prefix

B.60

The word part that is placed in front of a word root to change its meaning is a _____. In a later unit you will learn many prefixes.

suffix

B.61

The word part that follows a word root is a _____.

> ▶ **ANSWER COLUMN**

adjective verb	**B.62** A suffix may change a noun to an _____ or change the tense of a _____. Good!
combining form	**B.63** When a vowel is added to a word root, the word part that results is a *_____.
compound word	**B.64** When two or more word roots are used to form a word, the word formed is called a *_____.

Notice the diagrammed sentence below, which illustrates the use of adjectives, nouns, and verbs.

```
       adj    noun   verb        adj    noun      adj    noun
The medical assistant charted the patient's history of duodenal ulcer.
    |_____|         |_____|
          subject                          predicate
```

Notice the diagrammed words below indicating their word parts.

dysmenorrhea

dys-	men	o	-rrhea
prefix	word root		suffix
	combining form (vowel)		

acrodermatitis

acr	o	dermat	-itis
word root		word root	suffix
combining form (vowel)			

▶ **PRONUNCIATION NOTES**

Pronunciation symbols, descriptions, and rules are described on the inside front cover. They will also appear through the text below new terms and at other appropriate times. Refer to this Pronunciation Key or your medical dictionary when in doubt about how to say a word. Also, listen to the audiotapes to accompany *Medical Terminology: A Programmed Text,* 8th edition.

How do you know what to put where? Following, you will find material to assist you with word building. This is a system that you may have already figured out. If not, study these rules.

RULE I: Most of the time the definitions indicate the last part of the word first. The descriptive phrases usually start with the suffix and then indicate the body part.

EXAMPLES

1. Inflammation (1) of the bladder (2)

inflammation	/itis
(of the) bladder	**cyst/**
	cyst/itis
	(2) (1)

2. One who specializes (1) in skin disorders (2)

one who specializes (studies)	/ /logist
(in) skin (disorders)	**dermat/o/**
	dermat/o/logist
	(2) (1)

3. Pertaining to the abdomen (1) and bladder (2)

pertaining to	/ / /ic
(the) abdomen	**abdomin/o/ /**
(and) bladder	/ /**cyst/**
	abdomin/o/cyst/ic
	(2) (1)

RULE II: Where body systems are involved, words are usually built in the order that organs are studied in the system.

EXAMPLES

1. Inflammation of the stomach and small intestine

inflammation	/ / /itis
(of the) stomach	**gastr/o/ /**
(and) small intestine	/ /**enter/**
	gastr/o/enter/itis

2. Removal of the uterus, fallopian tubes, and ovaries

removal of	/ / / / /ectomy
(the) uterus	**hyster/o/ / / /**
fallopian tubes	/ /**salping/o/ /**
(and) ovaries	/ / / /**-oophor/**
	hyster/o/salping/o/-oophor/ectomy

RULE III: The body part usually comes first and the condition or procedure is the ending.

EXAMPLES

1. dermatomycosis
   (skin) (fungal condition)
2. cystoscopy
   (bladder) (process of examining the urinary bladder with a scope)

▶ REVIEW ACTIVITIES

Circle and Correct
Circle the correct answer for each question. Then, check your answers in Appendix A.

1. The base of the word is the
   a. prefix   b. combining form
   c. ending   d. word root

2. The _____ comes in front of the word root to change its meaning.
   a. prefix   b. combining form
   c. suffix   d. pronoun

3. The suffix may change
   a. part of speech   b. meaning
   c. plural/singular   d. a, b, and c

4. If two or more word roots are put together to make a word, it is a _____ word.
   a. combining form   b. compound
   c. complex   d. plural

5. The suffix -ity indicates
   a. singular form   b. ability
   c. quality   d. one who does

6. The suffix -ism indicates
   a. a verb ending   b. an adjective
   c. a condition   d. inflammation

7. When you want to join two word roots together you may use a(n)
   a. prefix   b. combining form
   c. adjective   d. consonant

8. The adjective suffix that indicates a material (substance) is
   a. -ia   b. -otic
   c. -us   d. -ous

Form the Plural
Using the rules you learned, form the plural of the following terms.

1. bursa   _____
2. coccus   _____
3. ovum   _____
4. sarcoma   _____
5. protozoan   _____
6. crisis   _____
7. appendix   _____

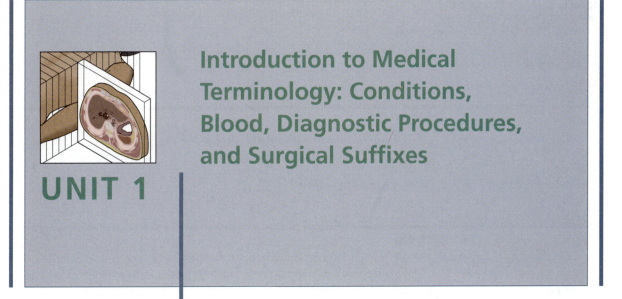

UNIT 1

Introduction to Medical Terminology: Conditions, Blood, Diagnostic Procedures, and Surgical Suffixes

ANSWER COLUMN	
	1.1 In this learning program the word root is followed by a slash and a vowel to make a combining form. In **acr/o**, **acr** is the
word root vowel combining form	*_____ ; **o** is the _____ ; and **acr/o** is the *_____ .
	1.2 **acr/o** is used to build words that refer to the *extremities*. To refer
acr/o or acr	to extremities, physicians use these word parts _____ .
	1.3 **acr/o** is found in words concerning the extremities, which in the human body are the arms and legs. To build words about the arms
acr/o	use _____ /____ . **NOTE:** Think of an acrobat.
	1.4
acr/o	To build words about the legs, use _____ /____ .
	1.5 **acr/o** any place in a word should make you think of the extremities. When you read a word containing **acr** or **acr/o**, you
extremities	think of _____ .

ANSWER COLUMN	
extremities	**1.6** In the word acr/o/paralysis (acroparalysis) **acr/o** refers to _____.
word root vowel combining form	**1.7** In **megal/o** (enlarged, large), **megal** is the *_____; **o** is the _____; and **megal/o** is the *_____.
extremities	**1.8** -megaly is used as a suffix for enlarged. The words acr/o/megaly (acromegaly), acr/o/cyan/osis (acrocyanosis), and acr/o/dermat/itis (acrodermatitis) all refer to the _____.
enlarged	**1.9** A word containing **megal/o** or -megaly will mean something is _____.

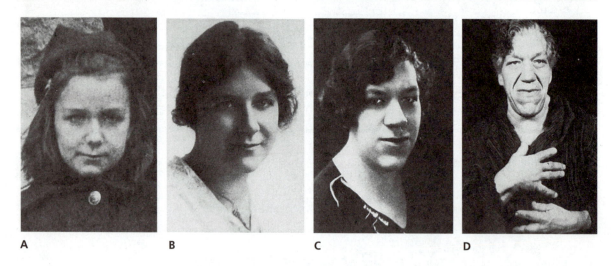

A   B   C   D

Advancing stages of acromegaly: A. age 9; B. age 16 with slight characteristics; C. age 33 with well-defined characteristics; D. age 52 with end-stage acromegaly (Reprinted from Clinical Pathological Conference, American Journal of Medicine, Vol. 20, p. 133 (1956) with permission from Excerpta Media Inc.)

ANSWER COLUMN	
acr/o/megaly ak rō **meg**′ ə lē	**1.10** Acr/o/megaly means enlargement of the extremities. The word that means a person has enlarged arms and legs, or hands and feet is _____ /_____ /_____.
acromegaly	**1.11** Acr/o/megal/ic gigantism is a specific disorder of the body. The signs are enlargement of the bones of the hands and feet as well as some of the bones of the head. The term describing these signs is _____.
noun	**1.12** -y is a suffix, meaning the process or condition, that makes a word a noun. Acromegaly is a _____.
skin	**1.13** **dermat/o** refers to the skin. When you see **dermat** or **dermat/o**, think immediately of _____.

skin
dermat/o/logy
dûr mə **tol**′ ō gē
	1.14
	-logy and -logist are suffixes:
	   -logos—Greek for study
	   -logy—noun, study of
	   -logist—noun, one who studies
	A dermat/o/logist (dermatologist) is a specialist in a field of medicine. This person specializes in diseases of the _____. The study of skin is _____ /_____ /_____.

acr/o/dermat/itis ak rō dûr mə **tī**′ tis	**1.15** Acr/o/dermat/itis (acrodermatitis) is a word that means inflammation of the skin of the extremities. A person with red, inflamed hands has _____ /_____ /_____ /_____.
inflammation	**1.16** Remembering the word acrodermatitis, which means inflammation of the skin of the extremities, draw a conclusion: -itis is a suffix that means _____.

▶ **ANSWER COLUMN**	**1.17** Paralysis is a word that means loss of movement. Form a compound word meaning paralysis of the extremities: _____ /_____ /_____.
acr/o/paralysis ak´ rō pə **ral**´ ə sis	
word root vowel combining form	**1.18** In **dermat/o, dermat** (skin) is the *_____; **o** is the _____; and **dermat/o** is the *_____ .

Contact dermatitis—poison oak (Courtesy of Timothy Berger, MD, Associate Clinical Professor, University of California, San Francisco)

skin	**1.19** Analyze the word dermat/itis. **-itis** means inflammation; **dermat** means of the _____.
-osis	**1.20** Dermat/osis means any skin condition. This word denotes an abnormal skin condition. The suffix that means condition, status, or process is _____.
acrodermatitis	**1.21** Signs of inflammation include redness, swelling, and heat. Acrodermatitis could result from stepping in a patch of poison ivy. A person with red, inflamed skin on his or her feet has _____.
-itis	**1.22** Dermat/itis means inflammation of the skin. There are many causes of inflammation, including infection, allergic reaction, and trauma. The suffix that means inflammation is _____.
dermat/itis dûr mə **tī**´ tis	**1.23** Bacterial, fungal, or parasitic infections may all cause red, inflamed skin called _____ /_____.

▶ **ANSWER COLUMN**

1.24
cyan/o is used in words to mean blue or blueness. When photographers want to say something about how a film reproduces the color blue, they use _____.

cyan/o or cyan

1.25
-osis: is a suffix
    forms a noun
    means disease, condition, status, or process
Build a word that means:
    condition of blueness _____ /_____;
    condition of the skin _____ /_____.

cyan/osis
sī ə **nō′** sis
dermat/osis
dûr mə **tō′** sis

1.26
-tic changes -osis from a noun to an adjective. Build the term that means pertaining to a condition of blueness: _____ /_____.

cyan/otic
sī ə **no′** tik

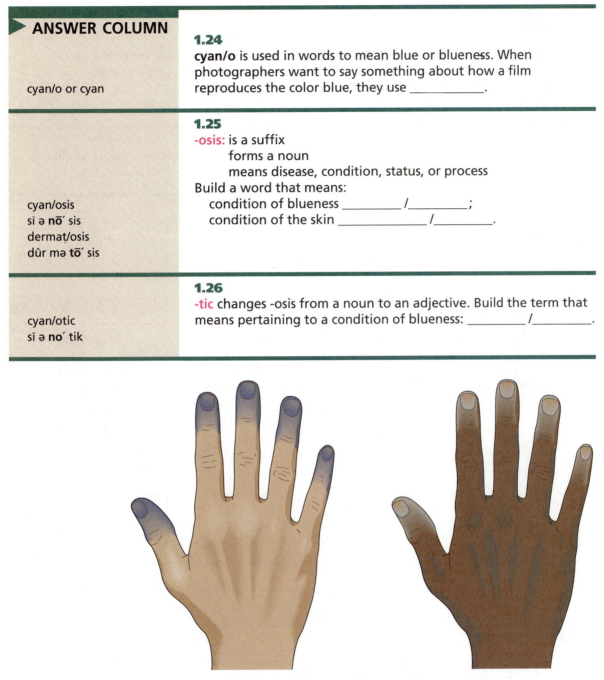

Acrocyanosis–Cyanosis (blueness of the extremities)

1.27
Acr/o/cyan/osis means blueness of the extremities. The part of the word that tells you that the color blue is involved is _____. The part of the word that tells you this is a condition is _____.

cyan
-osis

ANSWER COLUMN	
acr/o/cyan/osis ak rō sī ə **nō′** sis	**1.28** Acr/o/cyan/osis results from lack of oxygen. When the blood does not carry enough oxygen to the hands and feet, _____ /_____ /_____ /_____ results.
noun	**1.29** -osis is a suffix that makes a word a noun and means condition. Acrocyanosis is a (choose one) _____ (noun/verb).
tom	**1.30** The Greek word *tomos* means cutting. From this word we build many suffixes that refer to cutting: **-ectomy** (to cut out), **-tomy** (to cut into), **-tome** (an instrument that cuts), **-ostomy** (to form a new opening). The word root for cut is _____.

Suffix	Meaning	Example
-tome	cutting instrument	derm/a/tome
-tomy	to cut into (incise)	gastr/o/tomy
-ectomy	to cut out (excise)	duoden/ectomy
-ostomy	to form a new opening (surgical)	col/ostomy

cuts	**1.31** Remember to associate **tom** (**-tome**, **-ectomy**, **-ostomy**, and **-tomy**) with *cutting*. A tome is an instrument that _____.
derm/a/tome **dûr′** mə tōm	**1.32** A derm/a/tome is an instrument that cuts skin. When a physician wants a thin slice of a patient's skin for examination under a microscope, the physician will use a _____ /_____ /_____.
tom/o/gram **tō′** mō gram tom/o/graphy tō **mog′** ra fē	**1.33** -gram is a suffix from the Greek word *gramma*, meaning something written or drawn. -gram is used in medical terms to refer to a record or picture made by an instrument. A tom/o/graph makes an x-ray picture called a _____ /_____ /_____. The process of making such a picture is called _____ /_____ /_____.

▶ **ANSWER COLUMN**

---

tom/o/graph
tō′ mō graf

1.34
-graph is a suffix taken from the Greek verb *graphein*, meaning to write or record. In medical words, **-graph** refers to an *instrument* used to record data. A tom/o/graph is an x-ray instrument used to show tissue or organs in one plane (slice, so to speak). To obtain an x-ray of a slice of an organ, the radiographer would use a
_____ /_____ /_____.

NOTE: The word root for to cut is **tom**; the combining form is **tom/o.**

---

tom/o/graphy
tō **mog′** raf ē

tomograph

1.35
Adding a **-y** to **-graph** (as in biography) creates a suffix indicating the process of making a recording of data. The process of using a tomograph is called _____ /_____ /_____.
Computed tomography (CT) allows the radiologist to obtain a three-dimensional view of internal structures. A CT (or CAT) scanner is a type of _____.

💡 *INFORMATION FRAME*

1.36
Tomography is a radiographic procedure that uses x-rays to produce images of a slice or plane of the body. The following imaging procedures are all types of tomography:

　　MRI—magnetic resonance imaging
　　CT—computed tomography
　　PET—positron emission tomography
　　SPECT—single photon emission computed tomography

For more information use your medical dictionary or perform a library or Internet search of these topics.

1.37
Did you get it? If so, you are really learning medical terminology.

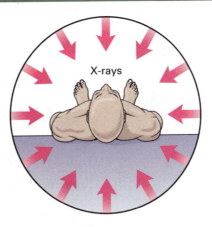

Direction of CT scan rays

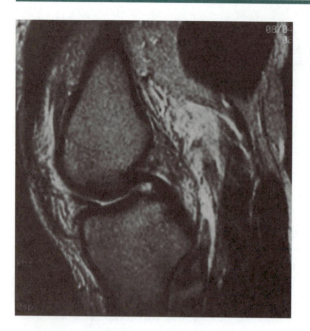

A. MRI (magnetic resonance imaging) of the knee acquired in the sagittal plane

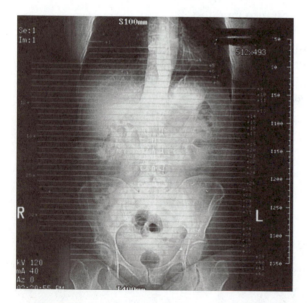

B. This scout view of the abdomen helps localize the scan parameters of a CT (computed tomography) scan. Each horizontal line indicates the level of one slice.

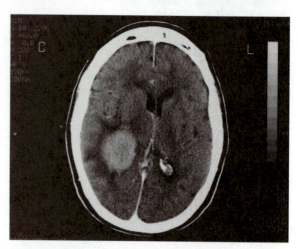

C. CAT (computed axial tomography) scan demonstrates a meningioma surrounded by edema.

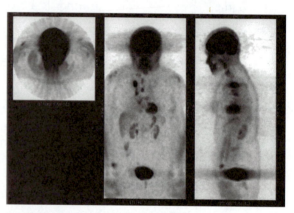

D. PET (positron emission tomography) scan demonstrating tumor in right lung

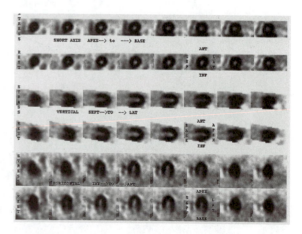

E. SPECT (single photon emission computed tomography)

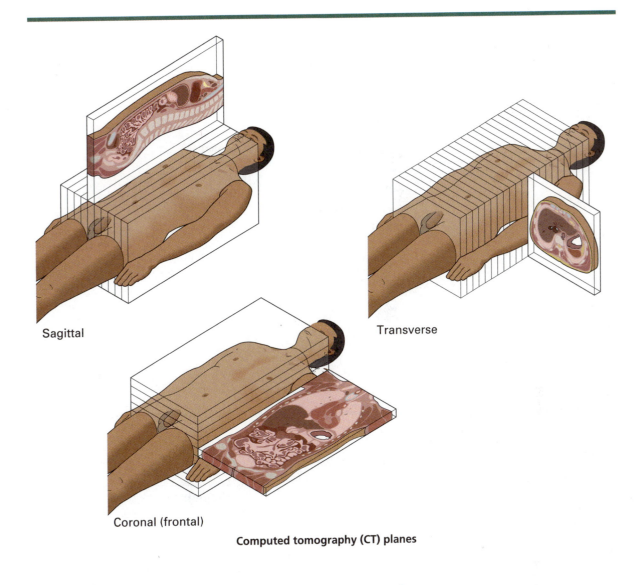

Sagittal

Transverse

Coronal (frontal)

Computed tomography (CT) planes

ANSWER COLUMN	
	1.38 **-pathy** is a suffix meaning disease. Dermat/o/pathy means a disease condition of the _____.
skin	
	1.39 Great! Now try this: **path/o** is a combining form meaning disease. Path/o/logy is the study of disease. A path/o/logist is a physician specializing in diagnosing (discovering) diseases. A pathologist usually works in the hospital laboratory department called _____ /_____ /_____.
path/o/logy path **ol′** ō gē	

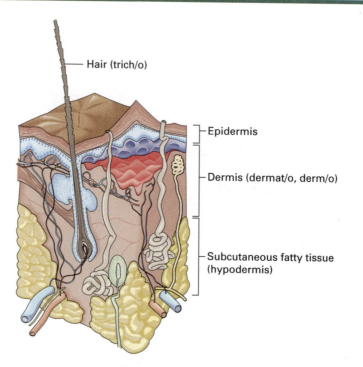

Structures of the skin

ANSWER COLUMN	
	1.40

► **ANSWER COLUMN**

blue skin or bluish
   discoloration of the skin
   (due to low O₂ levels)
noun

1.40
Derma is a word itself. It is a noun meaning skin. Cyan/o/derma is a
compound word. It means ** _____
and is a (choose one) _____ (noun/adjective).

NOTE: Most of these word parts are used as prefixes (e.g.,
leukocyte). An exception is **cyan/o**, which may be used either as a
prefix (cyanoderma) or as a word root within a word (acrocyanosis).

Use this information for building words involving color:
(Frames 1.41–1.71)

leuk/o	white
melan/o	black (dark pigment)
erythr/o	red
cyan/o	blue
chlor/o	green
xanth/o	yellow

erythr/o/derma
e rith´ rō **der´** mə
leuk/o/derma
lōō´ kō **der´** mə
xanth/o/derma
zan´ tho´ **der´** mə
melan/o/derma
mel´ an ō **der´** mə

1.41
Cyan/o/derma means blue skin. Build a word meaning:
    red skin _____ /_____ /_____;
    white skin (vitiligo) _____ /_____ /_____;
    yellow skin _____;
             (You draw the slashes)
    black (discolored) skin _____.
               (You draw the slashes)

melan/o/cyte
mel´ an ō sīt
leuk/o/cyte
lōō´ kō sīt
erythr/o/cyte
e **rith´** rō sīt

1.42
The suffix **-cyte** means cell. A chlor/o/cyte is a green cell (in plants). Build a word meaning:
    black cell (dark pigmented) _____ /_____ /_____;
    white (blood) cell _____ /_____ /_____;
    red (blood) cell _____ /_____ /_____.

melan/o/blast
erythr/o/blast
(You pronounce)

1.43
The suffix **-blast** means embryonic or immature cell. A leuk/o/blast is an embryonic white cell. Build a word meaning an embryonic cell of the following colors:
    black (dark pigment) _____ /_____ /_____;
    red _____ /_____ /_____.

xanth/emia
zan **thē'** mē ə
erythr/emia
e rith **rē'** mē ə
chlor/emia
klor **ē'** mē ə

1.44
-emia is a suffix from the Greek word *hema*, for blood. **-emia** means blood condition. An/emia is lack of blood. Build words involving the following colors when referring to blood conditions:
    yellow (jaundice) _____ /_____;
    red (polycythemia) _____ /_____;
    green (increased chlorine in the blood) _____ /_____.

NOTE: Chlorosis is a condition in which the skin takes on a greenish tinge due to anemia.

▶ ANSWER COLUMN

eeee *TAKE A CLOSER LOOK*

1.45
Look at the following terms that are very similar:
    erythema
    erythremia
    erythroderma.
From the word parts you have learned so far, see if you can analyze them without looking up the answers. Which one

erythremia
erythroderma

    is a blood condition? _____ ;
    is a skin condition? _____ .
Good! Now look up each term in the dictionary. You will find that they are similar in spelling but different in meaning and use. Write the definitions here:
    erythema _____ ;
    erythremia _____ ;
    erythroderma _____ .

---

green
yellow
red
white
black

1.46
chlor/o means _____ .
xanth/o means _____ .
erythr/o means _____ .
leuk/o means _____ .
melan/o means _____ .

---

cyan/o/derma
sī´ ə nō **dûr´** mə

1.47
Cyanoderma sometimes occurs when children swim too long in cold water. A person who has a bluish discoloration of the skin is described as having _____ /_____ /_____ .

---

leuk/o or leuk

1.48
leuk/o means *white*. Pay attention to the "eu" spelling. There are many words in medicine that refer to white. To say something is white, use _____ .

---

white skin, abnormally
  white skin, lack of
  pigment of the skin,
  vitiligo

1.49
Leuk/o/derma means *_____
_____ .

---

leuk/o/derma

1.50
A disease in which people have patchy white areas on their skin is called vitiligo (vit i lī´ gō). Sometimes these white areas are also called _____ /_____ /_____ .

▶ **ANSWER COLUMN**

☑ *SPELL CHECK*

1.51
You may notice that some medical terms are particularly unusual and difficult to spell correctly. From time to time in this program you will be given a Spell Check frame which includes spelling hints that may be of assistance. Notice the unusual diphthong (two vowels together) in the combining form leuk/o. The "eu" is pronounced like a long "u" sound, but do not forget the e first, even though it is silent. The correct spelling is l-e-u-k-o, as in leukocyte and leukoderma.

PRONUNCIATION NOTE: As a general rule in medical words, when two vowels are together, the second vowel's long sound is used, as in:
ea says ā;
ae says ē;
ie says ē;
ei says ī.

---

cyt/o

1.52
cyt/o refers to cells. A cell is the smallest structural unit of all living things. To refer to this smallest part of the body, the combining form _____ /_____ is used.

---

cyt/o
cells

1.53
Cytology is the study of cells. The part of cyt/o/logy that means cells is _____ /_____. A cyt/o/lo/gist studies _____.

---

cyt/o/logy

1.54
-logy is a suffix that means the study of. Build a word that means the study of cells. _____ /_____ /_____

---

path/o/logy
path **ol'** ō gē or
eti/o/logy
e tē **ol'** ō jē

1.55
Cyt/o/logists study the cause of diseases of the cell, like leukemia. The study of the cause of disease is _____ /_____ /_____ .

---

cyt/o/meter
sīt **om'** et er
cyt/o/metry
sīt **om'** et rē

1.56
-meter is a suffix meaning an instrument used to measure or count something. The instrument used to count cells is called a _____ /_____ /_____. **-metry** is a suffix meaning the process of measuring or counting something. The process of counting cells is called _____ /_____ /_____.

---

instrument

process

1.57
The word cyt/o/meter refers to the _____ used to measure or count. The word cyt/o/metry refers to the _____ of measuring or counting.

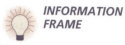
INFORMATION
FRAME

1.58
Cytotechnologists prepare and screen human tissue slides to detect abnormalities. They are usually supervised by pathologists, who are physicians that specialize in the study of disease.

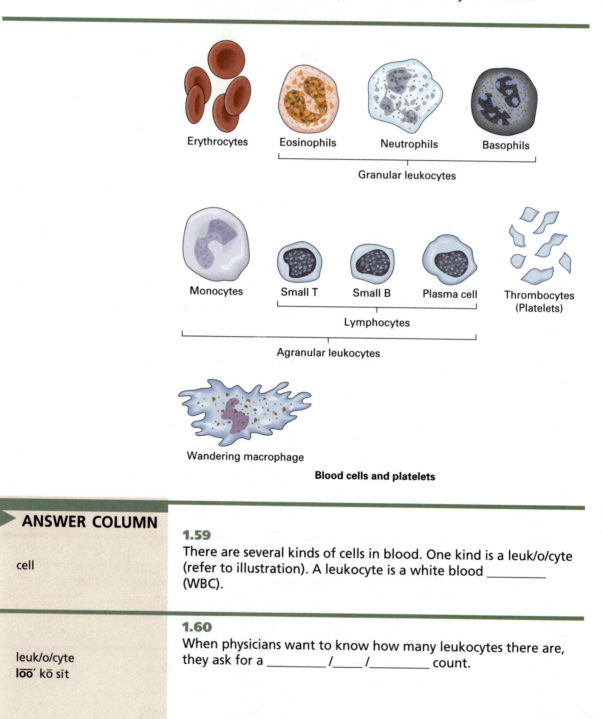

Erythrocytes   Eosinophils   Neutrophils   Basophils

Granular leukocytes

Monocytes   Small T   Small B   Plasma cell   Thrombocytes (Platelets)

Lymphocytes

Agranular leukocytes

Wandering macrophage

Blood cells and platelets

ANSWER COLUMN	
cell	**1.59** There are several kinds of cells in blood. One kind is a leuk/o/cyte (refer to illustration). A leukocyte is a white blood _____ (WBC).
leuk/o/cyte lōō′ kō sīt	**1.60** When physicians want to know how many leukocytes there are, they ask for a _____ /____ /_____ count.

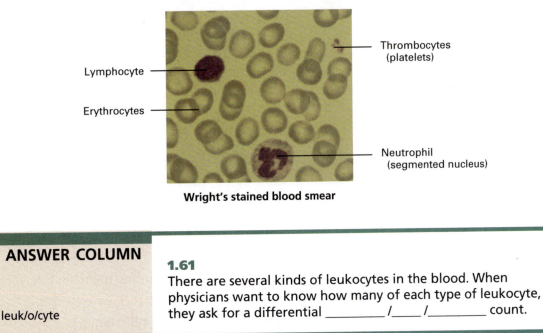

Lymphocyte

Erythrocytes

Thrombocytes
(platelets)

Neutrophil
(segmented nucleus)

Wright's stained blood smear

ANSWER COLUMN

leuk/o/cyte

1.61
There are several kinds of leukocytes in the blood. When physicians want to know how many of each type of leukocyte, they ask for a differential _____ /_____ /_____ count.

leuk/o/cyt/o/penia
lōō′ kō sĭ′ tō **pē**′ nē ə

1.62
-penia is the Greek word (suffix) for poverty. The word that means decrease in or not enough white blood cells is _____ /_____ /_____ /_____ /_____.

penia

1.63
Leuk/o/cyt/o/penia (leukopenia) means a decrease in white blood cells. The part of the word that means decrease in is _____.

leukocytopenia

1.64
If the body does not produce enough white blood cells, the patient suffers from _____.

leuk/emia
lōō **kē**′ mē ə

1.65
You have heard of leuk/emia, popularly called "blood cancer." -ia is a noun suffix meaning condition. em comes from the Greek word *hema*, meaning blood. A noun meaning, literally, a condition of white blood is _____ /_____.

leukemia

1.66
In leukemia the blood is not really white. A laboratory finding of this disease is the presence of too many immature white cells (leukocytes) in the blood. This finding was used to name the disease _____.

> ANSWER COLUMN

1.67
Look at the table of values that follows. A WBC of 25,000 would be abnormally high. -osis may be used to indicate an increase in numbers of blood cells. Build a word that means an increase in white blood cells _____ /____ /_____ /_____;
[red blood] cells _____ /____ /_____ /_____.

leuk/o/cyt/osis
loo′ kō sī tō′ sis
erythr/o/cyt/osis
e rith′ rō sī tō′ sis

> ▶▶▶◀◀◀

COMPLETE BLOOD COUNT (CBC)	
Test	**Normal Average Values**
Specimen: Whole blood	
Hgb (Hb)—Hemoglobin	12–16 grams/100 milliliters
Hct—Hematocrit	36–48% formed elements
RBC—Red blood cell count	4.2–6.2 million/mm³
WBC—White blood cell count	5,000–10,000/mm³
Platelet (thrombocyte) count	350,000–450,000/mm³

Diff—White blood cell differential count—Wright's stain smear analysis based on 100 WBCs:

Neutrophil bands: 3–5% Neutrophil (segs): 54–62%
Lymphocytes: 25–33% Monocytes: 3–7%
Eosinophils: 1–3% Basophils: 0–1%

1.68
lymph/o, from the Latin word *lympha*, meaning water or liquid, is used to refer to lymph/atic system structures. A lymph/o/cyte is a type of WBC produced by the _____ /_____ system.

lymph/atic
lim fa′ tik

1.69
A type of leukocyte produced by the lymphatic system is a _____ /____ /_____.

lymph/o/cyte
lim′ fō sīt

1.70
Acute lymphocytic leukemia (ALL) is a disease involving the _____ /____ /_____.

lymph/o/cytes

ANSWER COLUMN	
erythr/o/cytes e rith´ rō sīts	**1.71** **erythr/o** means red. Cells that contain a red substance (hemoglobin) are called red blood cells (RBCs) or _____ /_____ /_____.
erythr/o/cyt/o/penia e rith´ rō sīt ō pē´ nē ə	**1.72** Look at the CBC values in the table on page 34. An RBC of 2 million would be abnormally low. **-penia** is a suffix indicating deficiency in number. A patient who lacks red blood cells suffers from _____ /_____ /_____ /_____ /_____.
thromb/o/cyt/o/penia thromb´ ō sīt ō pē´ nē ə	**1.73** Another type of blood cell is the thromb/o/cyte. Thrombocytes prevent bleeding by allowing the blood to clot. An abnormal decrease in the number of these clot-forming cells is _____ /_____ /_____ /_____ /_____.
thrombocytes	**1.74** Blood-clotting cells (thrombocytes) are also called platelets. A platelet count would be done to obtain the number of _____.
thromb/o/cytes throm´ bō sīts or platelets plāt´ lets	**1.75** **thromb/o** means blood clot. The blood cells that help form blood clots are _____ /_____ /_____.
thromb/o/cyt/osis thromb´ ō sī tō´ sis erythr/o/cyt/osis e rith´ rō sī tō´ sis	**1.76** Recall that used as a suffix with blood cells, **-osis** indicates a condition characterized by increase in number. Build a term meaning increase in number of platelets (thrombocytes) _____ /_____ /_____ /_____; red blood cells (erythrocytes) _____ /_____ /_____ /_____.
blast/o	**1.77** A blast/o/cyte is an embryonic or immature cell. The combining form for embryonic or immature is _____ /_____. Think of this . . . when you have a "blast," you may act immature!

► **ANSWER COLUMN**

blast

1.78
A cell in its embryonic stage is called a _____.

cell
sel

1.79
-**cyte** may be used as a suffix to indicate a type of cell. A leuk/o/cyte is a term referring to a type of white blood _____.

immature or embryonic

1.80
-**blast** may be used at the end of a word to indicate an immature or embryonic cell. A hist/o/blast is a group of tissue cells that are * _____.

hist/o/blast
his′ tō blast
hist/o/logy
his **tol′** ō jē
hist/o/logist
his **tol′** ō jist
hist/o/cyte
his′ tō sīt

1.81
Hist/o means tissues. Build a word that means:
immature tissue _____ /_____/_____;
the study of tissues _____ /_____/_____;
one who studies tissues _____ /_____/_____;
a tissue cell _____ /_____/_____.

INFORMATION FRAME

1.82
Remember, your best friend is your medical dictionary. Look up the new terms you have learned for in-depth definitions.

megaly

1.83
In the word acr/o/megaly, the suffix for enlarged is _____.

megal/o

1.84
The combining form for enlarged is _____ /_____.

enlarged heart or enlargement of the heart

1.85
cardi/o is the combining form for words about the heart. Cardi/o/megaly is a noun that means * _____ _____.

megal/o/cardia
meg′ ə lō **kär′** dē ə

1.86
Megal/o/cardia also means enlargement or overdevelopment of the heart. When something causes increase in the size of the heart, _____ /_____ /_____ exists.

ANSWER COLUMN	
megal/o/cardia meg′ ə lō **kär**′ dē ə or cardi/o/megaly kär′ dē ō **meg**′ ə lē	**1.87** Megalocardia refers to heart muscle. When any muscle exercises, it gets larger. If the heart muscle has to overexercise, _____ /____ /_____ will probably occur.
megalocardia	**1.88** Cardiac enlargement (CE) may be caused by prolonged, severe asthma that can cut down the supply of oxygen to the body and make the heart work harder. A word for CE is _____.
gastr	**1.89** Megal/o/gastria means large or enlarged stomach. The word root for stomach is _____.
megal/o/gastria meg′ ə lō **gas**′ trē ə	**1.90** **megal/o** means large; **gastr**, from the Greek *gaster*, is the word root for stomach, and **-ia** is a noun suffix. Form a noun that means large or enlargement of the stomach: _____ /____ /_____.
gastr/o/megaly gas′ trō **meg**′ ə lē megal/o/gastria meg′ ə lō **gas**′ trē ə	**1.91** Another word for enlargement of the stomach is gastr/o/megaly. When the stomach is so large that it crowds other organs, _____ /____ /_____ or _____ /____ /_____ exists.
gastromegaly	**1.92** Enlargement of the stomach is called megalogastria or _____.
condition	**1.93** **-ia** is a noun suffix for condition. When megalogastria occurs, an undesirable _____ exists.
mania	**1.94** Mania is an English word that comes directly from the Greek word *mania*, which means madness. Many mental disorders are designated by compound words that end in this word, _____, meaning a condition of madness or excessive preoccupation.

▶ **ANSWER COLUMN**

1.95

Mania is a noun for condition. The condition is madness or, more properly, mental disorder. The suffix that tells you mania is a noun and shows a condition is _____.

-ia

1.96

Megal/o/mania is a symptom of a mental disorder in which the patient has delusions of grandeur. Patients who have greatly enlarged opinions of themselves suffer from

_____ / _____ / _____ .

megal/o/mania
meg´ ə lō **mā´** nē ə

1.97

People with megalomania are often treated in mental health centers. Many such centers have a patient who claims to be a king or president. These patients' are diagnosed with

_____ .

megalomania

1.98

Many people think Adolf Hitler, World War II Nazi leader, suffered from delusions of grandeur or _____ .

megalomania

INFORMATION FRAME

1.99

-ic and **-ac** are adjective suffixes that mean pertaining to. The following are adjectival forms of the words you have just learned:

leukemic	leukocytic
dermic	cyanotic
manic	melanic
gastric	xanthemic
cardiac	erythroblastic

1.100

Megal/o/cardia means *_____ .
cardi is the word root for _____ .

enlargement of the heart
heart

1.101

cardi/o (card/o) is used in building words that refer to the heart. Card/itis means *_____ .

NOTE: When the suffix being used begins with a vowel, the combining form is usually not required (i.e., card/itis, cardi/ectomy). When the suffix being used begins with a consonant, a combining form is usually required (i.e., cardi/o/dynia, cardi/o/logy).

inflammation of the heart

1.102

A cardi/o/logist is a specialist in the study of diseases of the _____ .

heart

ANSWER COLUMN	
	1.103 A cardi/o/logist diagnoses heart disease. The specialist who determines that a heart is diseased is a _____ /_____ /_____.
cardi/o/logist kär′ dē **ol**′ ō jist	
	1.104 A cardiologist discovers irregularities in the flow of the blood in the heart. The physician catheterizes the heart to view blood flow through the vessels of the heart. This heart specialist is a _____.
cardiologist	
	1.105 A person who reads electr/o/cardi/o/grams (records of electrical impulses given off by the heart) is also a _____.
cardiologist	
💡 *INFORMATION FRAME*	**1.106** When hospitalized, a patient with a severe heart condition is usually treated in a cardiac care unit (CCU). An electr/o/cardi/o/gram (EKG or ECG) may be performed to assess heart function.
	1.107 **-gram** is the suffix meaning record or a picture. **electr/o** is the combining form for *electrical*. Give the meaning of electr/o/cardi/o/gram. ** _____
record of electrical waves given off by the heart (or equivalent)	_____.

Conduction system of the heart showing the source of electrical impulses produced on an ECG (EKG)

ANSWER COLUMN	

▶ **ANSWER COLUMN**

1.108
You will recall that **graph** is a word root indicating an instrument used to make a recording or any pictorial device. Electr/o/cardi/o/gram is the record produced. Electr/o/cardi/o/graph is the instrument used to record the picture, or

electr/o/cardi/o/gram
e lek´ trō **kär´** dē ō gram

_____ /_____ /_____ /_____ /_____.

1.109
-**graphy** is a suffix for the *process* of making a recording (EKG or ECG). The electr/o/cardi/o/gram is a record obtained by the process of electr/o/cardi/o/graphy. A technologist can learn electrocardiography, but it takes a cardiologist to read the

electrocardiogram

_____.

NOTE: The suffix -**gram** refers to the actual paper readout or picture on a computer screen. Think of obtaining a telegram from a telegraph.

1.110
A physician can read a tracing that looks like this,

Ventricular fibrillation

Complete heart block (atrial rate, 107; ventricular rate, 43)

and learn something about a person's heart. The physician is a

cardiologist
electrocardiogram

_____ and is reading an _____.

1.111
son/o is a combining form taken from the Latin word *sonus,* meaning sound. A supersonic transport travels above the speed of sound. A son/o/gram is a picture made by a sonograph. The process of obtaining the sonogram is called

son/o/graphy
son **og´** ra fē

_____ /_____ /_____ (ultrasonography).

ANSWER COLUMN	
son/o/graph/er son **og**´ ra fer	**1.112** Recall that the suffix **-er** means one who. The person who (one who) performs sonography is called a _____ /_____ /_____ /_____.
ech/o/cardi/o/gram ek´ ō **kär**´ dē ō gram	**1.113** **ech/o** is a combining form meaning sound made by *reflected sound* waves. A record of sound waves reflected through the heart is an _____ /_____ /_____ /_____ /_____.
ech/o/cardi/o/graphy ek´ ō kär dē **og**´ ra fē	**1.114** The process of making the echocardiogram is called _____ /_____ /_____ /_____ /_____. NOTE: *Echo*cardiography uses sound waves; *electro*cardiography uses electricity.

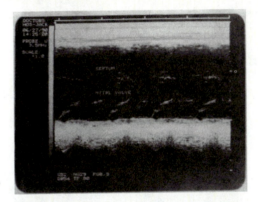 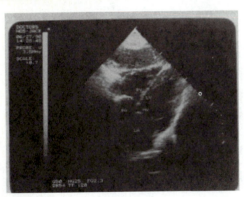

A.   B.

Echocardiogram (Prepared by Lynne Schreiber, BS, RDMS, RT[R])

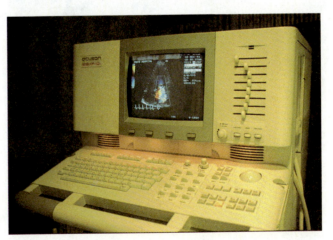

C.

Echocardiograph (Photo by Marcia Butterfield, courtesy of W. A. Foote Memorial Hospital, Jackson, MI)

radi/o/gram **rād**′ ē ō gram	**1.115** **radi/o** is a combining form from the Latin word *radius*, meaning a ray coming from a central point. **radi/o** is used to refer to radiation such as that used in x-rays. A picture made by using x-rays (XR) is called a _____ /_____ /_____. NOTE: In practice, this is usually called a radiograph.

radi/o/grapher
rād′ ē **og**′ ra fer
radi/o/logist
rād ē **ol**′ ō jist
	1.116
	Build words for the following meanings:
	    one who takes x-rays _____ /_____ /_____;
	    a physician specialist who studies (interprets) x-rays
	    _____ /_____ /_____.

radiologist	**1.117** Radiation therapists (RATx) use x-rays to irradiate a cancerous area. These treatments would be supervised by a physician specialist called a _____.

Professional Profiles ◄◄◄◄◄◄◄◄◄◄◄◄◄◄◄◄◄◄◄◄◄◄◄◄◄◄◄◄◄◄

Registered Radiologic Technologists (RT[R]) use ionizing radiation (x-rays) to create images for diagnostic interpretation by physicians called radiologists. Knowledge of positioning patients for exposure, operation of the x-ray equipment and developers, anatomy and pathology, and human relations is essential. Education may be hospital or college based ranging from certificates to advanced degrees. The American Society of Radiologic Technologists (ASRT) and the American Registry of Radiologic Technologists (ARRT) monitor education standards and registration in this profession.

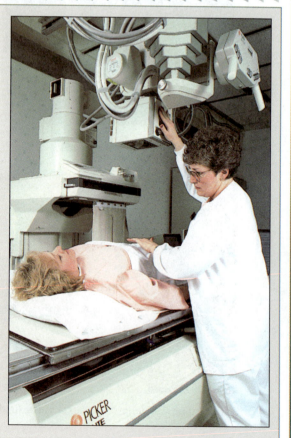

Radiographer positioning patient for x-ray (Photo by Marcia Butterfield, courtesy of W. A. Foote Memorial Hospital, Jackson, MI)

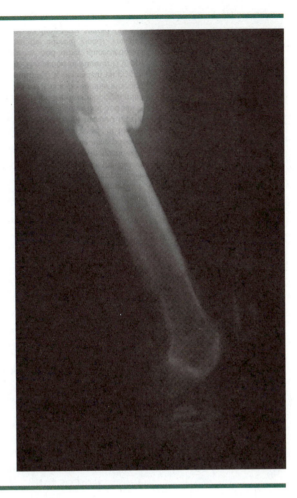

Radiograph: fractured femur (From Burke, *Human Anatomy & Physiology in Health and Disease,* 3rd ed., Albany, NY: Delmar Publishers Inc., 1992)

▶ **ANSWER COLUMN**

	1.118 -algia is one suffix that means pain. Form a word that means heart pain. (Since -algia is a suffix that begins with a vowel, you will use the word root rather than the combining form.)
cardi/algia kär′ de **al**′ jē ə	_____ /_____
	1.119 Gastr/algia means pain in the stomach. When a patient complains of pain in the heart, this symptom is known medically as
cardialgia	_____.
	1.120 One suffix for pain is _____. Stomach pain is
-algia gastr/algia gas **tral**′ jē ə	_____ /_____.

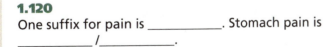

► **ANSWER COLUMN**

stomach

1.121
Recall -megaly is a suffix meaning *enlarged*. Gastromegaly is one word for enlarged stomach. **gastr/o** is the combining form for
_____.

excision or removal

1.122
Recall that tome referred to cutting or a cutting instrument. Gastr/ectomy means excision (removal) of all or part of the stomach. -ectomy is a suffix meaning _____. (Refer to Frame 1.30.)

INFORMATION FRAME

1.123
This is a free frame for those who are interested. Others may go on.

		meaning
ect/o	combining form	outside
tom/e	combining form	cut
-y	noun suffix	

Add **ect om y** = ectomy means excision

NOTE: One "t" is dropped when tome is preceded by "ect".

INFORMATION FRAME

1.124
Here's another free frame for those interested in -ostomy.

		meaning
os	combining form	mouth, opening
tom/e	combining form	cut
-y	noun suffix	

Add **os tom y** = ostomy means opening by cutting

gastr/ostomy
gas **tros´** tō mē

1.125
If a person is unable to swallow and tube feeding directly into the stomach is necessary, a new opening may be made through the stomach, called a _____ /_____.

gastr/o/duoden/ostomy
gas´ trō dōō´ ō də **nos´** tə mē

1.126
Gastr/o/duoden/o/stomy means forming a new opening between the stomach and duodenum. A surgeon who removes the natural connection between the duodenum and stomach and then forms a new connection is doing a
_____ /____ /_____ /_____.

gastroduodenostomy

1.127
A gastroduodenostomy is a surgical procedure. When the pyloric sphincter (a valve that controls the amount of food going from the stomach to the duodenum) no longer functions, a _____ may be done.

Gastroduodenostomy   Gastrostomy

► **ANSWER COLUMN**	
	1.128 When a portion of the first part of the small intestine is removed because of cancer, a new opening is formed by performing a
gastroduodenostomy	_____.
	1.129 **-tomy** is a suffix meaning incision into. A duoden/o/tomy is an incision into the _____ /_____.
duoden/um do͞o ō **dē´** nəm do͞o **od´** ə nəm	
	1.130 An incision into the duodenum is a _____ /____ /_____.
duoden/o/tomy do͞o´ ō də **not´** ə mē	
	1.131 A gastr/ectomy is a surgical procedure. When a stomach ulcer has perforated, a partial _____ /_____ may be indicated to remove part of the stomach. **NOTE:** The combining form is not used when the suffix begins with a vowel.
gastr/ectomy gas **trek´** tə mē	
gastrectomy	**1.132** Cancer of the stomach may be treated by a _____.

► ANSWER COLUMN

gastr/itis gas **trī′** tis	**1.133** Form a word that means inflammation of the stomach: _____ /_____ .
gastr/o/megaly megal/o/gastria	**1.134** Two words that mean enlargement of the stomach are _____ /_____ /_____ and _____ /_____ /_____.
duoden/o	**1.135** **duoden/o** is used in words that refer to the first part of the small intestine, the duoden/um. To build words about the duodenum, use _____ /_____. An outline of terms and illustration showing the digestive system may be found in Unit 6.
duoden/um	**1.136** The duoden/um is the first part of the small intestine that connects with the stomach. **duoden/o** is a combining form that refers to the _____ /_____.

WORD BUILDING

GASTR + O + DUODEN + OSTOMY
word root vowel word root suffix

forming an opening between the stomach and duodenum	**1.137** Gastr/o/duoden/ostomy means formation of a new opening between the stomach and duodenum. **-ostomy** is a combining form you can use as a suffix to mean forming an opening. Gastr/o/duoden/ostomy means *_____ _____.
duodenotomy	**1.138** A surgeon who incises the duodenum is performing a _____.
duodenitis	**1.139** Inflammation is characterized by redness and swelling of a body part. **-itis** is a suffix for inflammation. When physicians are listing conditions of the duodenum and they want to say it is inflamed, they use the word _____.

▶ ANSWER COLUMN	
-itis duoden/itis dōō′ ō də **nī**′ tis dōō od′ e **nī**′ tis	**1.140** The suffix for inflammation is _____. The word for inflammation of the duodenum is _____ /_____.
-al	**1.141** Duoden/al is an adjective. -al is an adjectival suffix meaning pertaining to (whatever the adjective modifies). One adjectival suffix is _____.
duoden/al dōō ō **dē**′ nəl dōō **od**′ ə nəl ulcer lesion	**1.142** In duoden/al ulcer and duoden/al lesion, the adjective is _____ /_____ and the nouns modified are _____ and _____.
duodenal	**1.143** In the sentence, "duodenal carcinoma was present," the adjective meaning pertaining to the duodenum is _____.
duodenal	**1.144** The adjectival form of duodenum is _____.
duoden/ostomy dōō′ ō də **nos**′ tə mē	**1.145** Recall that -ostomy means making a new opening. The word to form a new opening into the duodenum is _____ /_____.
gastr/o/duoden/ostomy gas′ trō dōō′ ō dēn **os**′ tō mē	**1.146** A duodenostomy can be formed in more than one manner. If it is formed with the stomach, it is called a _____ /_____ /_____ /_____.
-ectomy -tomy -ostomy	**1.147** The suffix for excision is _____. The suffix for incision is _____. The suffix for forming a new opening is _____.

► **ANSWER COLUMN**

Use the material in the following chart to work the next frame.

WORDS ARE FORMED BY
I.   Word root + suffix
(a) dermat/itis
(b) cyan/osis
(c) duoden/al
II.   Combining form + suffix
(this can be a word itself)
(a) acr/o/cyan/osis
(b) leuk/o/cyte
III.   Any number of combining forms + word root + suffix
(a) leuk/o/cyt/o/pen/ia
(b) electr/o/cardi/o/graphy

1.48

word root
suffix
word root
suffix
duoden
-al
combining form
word root
suffix
combining form
suffix
combining form
combining form
suffix
electr/o
cardi/o
-graphy

In I(a), **dermat** is the *_____;
          -itis   is the _____.
In I(b), **cyan** is the *_____;
          -osis is the _____.
In I(c), the word root is _____;
          the suffix is _____.
In II(a), **acr/o** is the *_____;
          cyan is the *_____;
          -osis is the _____.
In II(b), **leuk/o** is the *_____;
          -cyte   is the _____.
In III(a), **leuk/o** is a *_____;
          cyt/o   is a *_____;
          -penia is a _____.
In III(b), the first combining form is _____ /_____;
the second combining form is _____ /_____;
the suffix is _____.
Good job!

Take five minutes and study the list of abbreviations in the table that follows.

Abbreviation	Meaning
ACVD	acute cardiovascular disease
ALL	acute lymphocytic leukemia
ARRT	American Registry of Radiologic Technologists
ASRT	American Society of Radiologic Technologists
CBC	complete blood count
CCU	cardiac care unit (coronary care unit)
CE	cardiac enlargement
CPK	creatine phosphokinase (cardiac enzyme)
CT	computed tomography (scan)
DMS	diagnostic medical sonography
ECHO	echocardiogram
EKG, ECG	electrocardiogram
ER	emergency room
GA	gastric analysis
GI	gastrointestinal
LDH	lactic dehydrogenase (cardiac enzyme)
MRI	magnetic resonance imaging
Ra	radium
RATx (RT)	radiation therapy
RBC	red blood cell (count)
RT(R)	registered radiologic technologist
WBC	white blood cell (count)
XR	x-ray

To complete your study of this unit, work the review activities on the next pages. Also, listen to the audiotapes that accompany *Medical Terminology: A Programmed Text,* 8th edition, and practice your pronunciation.

Additional practice exercises for this unit are available on the Student Practice disk found in the back of the textbook.

► REVIEW ACTIVITIES

Circle and Correct
Circle the correct answer for each question. Then, check your answers in Appendix A.

1. Combining form for extremities:
   a. acr   b. acro
   c. arc   d. arco

2. Word root for stomach:
   a. gastro   b. gastric
   c. stomat   d. gastr

3. Compound word:
   a. duodenum   b. microscope
   c. dermatitis   d. subglossal

4. Suffix for incision:
   a. -ex   b. -de
   c. -tomy   d. -ectomy

5. Suffix for enlarged:
   a. -ex   b. -sub
   c. -megaly   d. -hyper

6. Noun for first part of the small intestine:
   a. colon   b. duodenal
   c. enteric   d. duodenum

7. Verb for removed:
   a. excision   b. excised
   c. ectomy   d. exeresis

8. Adjective for heart:
   a. cardiac   b. cardious
   c. cardium   d. cranial

9. Suffix for condition:
   a. es   b. ia
   c. itis   d. o

10. Pronunciation symbol for accent:
    a. –   b. ə
    c. ´   d. ^

11. Suffix meaning instrument used to cut slices:
    a. -tome   b. -tomy
    c. -meter   d. -graph

12. Adjective for condition of blueness:
    a. cyanosis   b. xanthotic
    c. cyanous   d. cyanotic

13. Word root for x-ray:
    a. tom   b. graph
    c. echo   d. radi

14. Suffix for making a new opening:
    a. -itis   b. -ectomy
    c. -ostomy   d. -tomy

15. Erythro means:
    a. green   b. red
    c. white   d. blue

▶ REVIEW ACTIVITIES

Select and Construct
Select the correct word parts from the list below and construct medical terms that represent the given meaning.

ac	acro	al	algia	blast	cardi(o)
chlor	cyano	cyt(e)(o)	derm(a)o	dermato	duodeno
echo	electro	emia	er	erythro	gastro(ia)
gram	graph	graphy	ia	ic	itis
leuko	logy	mania	megal(o)(y)	melano	osis
ostomy	paralysis	pathy	penia	radio	sono
thrombo	tom(e)(o)	tomy	um	xantho	

1. paralysis of the extremities _____

2. inflammation of the skin _____

3. blueness of the skin _____

4. disease condition of the skin _____

5. red blood cell _____

6. embryonic dark pigmented cell _____

7. decrease in the number of platelets _____

8. enlargement of the stomach _____

9. overenlarged opinion of self _____

10. instrument used to make a recording of heart activity _____

11. incision into the first part of the small intestine _____

12. adjectival form of the word for heart _____

13. the process of obtaining an image from reflected sound _____

14. the picture (record) of sound reflected through the heart _____

15. one who takes x-rays _____

16. increase in WBC _____

17. enlarged extremities _____

18. x-ray picture made through slices of the body _____

19. condition of yellow skin (jaundice) _____

20. the study of cells _____

▶ **REVIEW ACTIVITIES**

Define and Dissect
Give a brief definition and dissect each term listed into its word parts in the space provided on the right. Check your answers by referring to the frame listed in parentheses and your medical dictionary. Then, listen to the audiotapes to practice pronunciation.

Key: rt (word root), v (vowel)

1. acromegaly (1.10)

   _____ / ____ / _____
       rt   v   suffix

   _____
   definition

2. dermatologist (1.14)

   _____ / ____ / _____
       rt   v   suffix

3. acrocyanosis (1.2)

   _____ / ____ / _____ / _____
     rt   v   rt   suffix

4. cyanotic (1.26)

   _____ / ____ / _____
       rt   v   suffix

5. dermatome (1.32)

   _____ / ____ / _____
       rt   v   suffix

6. erythroderma (1.41)

   _____ / ____ / _____
       rt   v   suffix

7. melanocyte (1.42)

   _____ / ____ / _____
       rt   v   rt/suffix

8. echocardiography (1.114)

   ____ / ___ / _____ / ___ / _____
     rt   v   rt   v   suffix

9. leukocytopenia (1.62)

   _____ / ___ / _____ / ___ / _____
     rt   v   rt   v   suffix

10. thrombocytes (1.75)

    _____ / ____ / _____
        rt   v   suffix

11. cardiomegaly (1.87)

    _____ / ____ / _____
        rt   v   suffix

12. megalogastria (1.134)

    _____ / ____ / _____
        rt   v   rt/suffix

13. electrocardiograph (1.108)   _____ /__ /_____ /__ /_____
    rt   v   rt   v   suffix

14. radiologist (1.116)   _____ /____ /_____
    rt   v   suffix

15. gastrectomy (1.131)   _____ /_____
    rt   suffix

16. gastroduodenostomy (1.126)   _____ /__ /_____ /__ /_____
    rt   v   rt   v   suffix

17. erythrocytosis (1.76)   _____ /____ /_____ /_____
    rt   v   rt   suffix

18. sonographer (1.112)   _____ /____ /_____
    rt   v   suffix

19. radiographer (1.116)   _____ /____ /_____
    rt   v   suffix

20. acrodermatitis (1.15)   _____ /____ /_____ /_____
    rt   v   rt   suffix

21. erythremia (1.44)   _____ /_____
    rt   suffix

22. cardialgia (1.118)   _____ /_____
    rt   suffix

23. duodenotomy (1.130)   _____ /____ /_____
    rt   v   suffix

24. tomography (1.35)   _____ /____ /_____
    rt   v   suffix

25. cardiologist (1.103)   _____ /____ /_____
    rt   v   suffix

▶ **REVIEW ACTIVITIES**

Abbreviation Matching
Match the following abbreviations with their definition.

_____ 1. ALL	a. registered radiologic technologist
_____ 2. EKG	b. cardiac care unit
_____ 3. CT	c. echocardiogram
_____ 4. CCU	d. computed tomography
_____ 5. DMS	e. cardiac tomogram
_____ 6. GI	f. gastric contents
_____ 7. ACVD	g. gastrointestinal
_____ 8. GA	h. diagnostic medical sonography
_____ 9. Ra	i. radium
_____ 10. ECHO	j. cardiac block catheter
	k. electrocardiogram
	l. acute lymphocytic leukemia
	m. acute cardiovascular disease
	n. gastric analysis

Abbreviation Fill-in
Fill in the blanks with the correct abbreviation.

11. The WBC and RBC are part of the _____.

12. The CBC includes the _____ and the _____, which count the white and red blood cells.

13. Magnetic resonance imaging and radiography produce films of structures inside the body in a noninvasive way. The RT(R) with specialized training may perform either an _____ or an _____.

14. The _____ can assist the patient as they perform an MRI or x-ray.

15. Echocardiography is one type of sonography that is specifically used to view the heart. A _____ program can train individuals to perform _____ for diagnosis of heart disease.

16. A patient suffering from chest pain may be admitted to the _____. A cardiologist may order an _____ to understand the electrical changes in the heart and an _____ to see the efficiency of blood flow through the heart. LDH and CPK may also be performed as blood tests for cardiac enzymes.

17. When the heart muscle is damaged, the level of cardiac enzymes _____ and _____ could rise.

▶ **CASE STUDIES**

The following case study is taken from an actual medical record. The patient name has been changed to protect confidentiality. By reading the case in each unit and studying the medical terms, you will gain a deeper understanding of the meaning and especially of the use of these terms. You will notice that several words are in color. These are key medical terms that you may or may not have learned through the word-building system.

Write the term next to its meaning given below. Then, draw slashes to analyze the word parts. You will also note the use of medical abbreviations. Look these up in your dictionary or find them in Appendix B. If you have any questions about the answers, refer to your medical dictionary or check with your instructor for the answers in Appendix A.

CASE STUDY 1-1

DISCHARGE SUMMARY

Pt: age 76

Dx: 1. Acute chest pain—etiology unknown

Mr. Harry Hart, a 76-year-old Caucasian male, was admitted through the emergency room (ER) where he was presented via ambulance with substernal chest pain. Mr. Hart was also seen by Dr. Rick Cardio in cardiac consultation and a dictated note is available on his chart.

Serial electrocardiograms were obtained during the course of Mr. Hart's hospitalization. These failed to reveal any acute injury. An echocardiogram was performed and interpreted by Dr. Cardio and found to be within normal limits. The chest x-ray was performed revealing no active cardiopulmonary disease with aortic arteriosclerosis being present. Radionuclide (isotope) cardiac angiography was performed and read as negative. The laboratory results were normal with a slightly elevated LDH.

Mr. Hart was admitted to CCU on routine coronary care orders. Cardiac consultation was obtained and after we ruled out any acute cardiac event, he was transferred to Stepdown with continuous cardiac telemetry. By the 19th of June his condition was stable enough to warrant discharge.

1. severe and short term   _____

2. pertaining to the heart   _____

3. sonography of the heart   _____

4. below the sternum   _____

5. electronic data transmission   _____

6. hardening of the arteries   _____

7. x-ray of a vessel   _____

8. pertaining to heart and lungs   _____

9. transport vehicle   _____

10. study of cause   _____

11. EKG   _____

12. radiograph   _____

▶ CROSSWORD PUZZLE

Check your answers by going back through the frames or checking the solution in Appendix C.

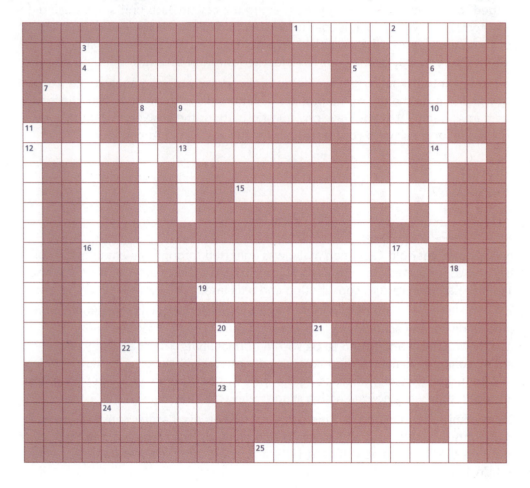

Across

1. blueness of the skin
4. extremities—loss of movement
7. diagnostic medical sonography (abbreviation)
9. enlarged extremities
10. suffix for incision into
12. sonography of the heart
14. magnetic resonance imaging (abbreviation)
15. physician x-ray specialist
16. instrument to picture heart function
19. embryonic melanocyte
22. high WBC
23. study of the skin
24. process of making a picture (suffix)
25. excision of the stomach

Down

2. inflammation of the skin
3. new opening of the stomach and duodenum
5. red skin
6. counting of cells
8. low platelet count
11. enlarged heart
13. suffix for inflammation
17. physician disease specialist
18. computed _____ (x-ray)
20. acute cardiovascular disease (abbreviation)
21. combining form for tissue

▶ GLOSSARY

acrodermatitis	inflammation of the skin on the extremities	duodenum	first part of the small intestine
acromegaly	enlargement of the extremities	echocardiography	sonography of the heart
acroparalysis	loss of movement of the extremities	electrocardiogram	picture (tracing) representing the electrical activity of the heart during the cardiac cycle
blastocyte	immature cell	electrocardiograph	instrument that produces the electrocardiogram
cardialgia	heart pain	electrocardiography	process of using the electrocardiograph
cardiologist	physician specialist in heart disease	erythrema	abnormally red blood due to too many erythrocytes
cardiomegaly	enlarged heart	erythroblast	immature red blood cell
cyanoderma	blueness of the skin	erythrocytes	red blood cells
cyanosis	condition of blueness	erythrocytopenia	low number of erythrocytes
cytologist	a physician or technologist who studies cellular disease	erythrocytosis	high number of erythrocytes
cytology	the science studying cells	erythrodermia	redness of the skin
cytometer	instrument used to count cells	etiology	the study of the origin of disease
cytometry	process of using a cytometer	gastralgia	stomach pain
dermatitis	inflammation of the skin	gastrectomy	excision of the stomach
dermatologist	a physician who specializes in skin disorders and health	gastric	pertaining to the stomach (adj.)
dermatology	the science studying the skin	gastroduodenostomy	making a new opening between the stomach and duodenum
dermatome	instrument used to cut slices of skin tissue	gastromegaly	enlarged stomach
duodenal	pertaining to the duodenum (adj.)	gastrostomy	making a new opening in the stomach
duodenotomy	incision into the duodenum	histoblast	immature tissue cells

► GLOSSARY

histology	the science of studying tissues
leukemia	blood cancer involving leukocytes
leukocyte	white blood cell
leukocytopenia	low number of leukocytes
leukocytosis	high number of leukocytes
leukoderma	abnormally white skin (vitiligo)
lymphatic	pertaining to the lymph system
lymphocyte	lymphatic system white blood cell
megalomania	abnormally enlarged self-image
melanoblast	immature melanocyte
melanocyte	pigment cell
melanoderma	dark patches of skin
pathologist	physician specialist in the study of disease
pathology	the science studying disease
radiogram	x-ray picture (film) (radiograph)
radiograph	instrument used to produce the radiogram or the x-ray film
radiography	process of producing radiograms (radiographs)
radiologist	physician specialist in the interpretation of radiograms and other diagnostic imaging modalities
sonogram	image of the body produced by computerized reflected sound
sonograph	instrument that reflects sound waves through the body, picks them up with a transducer, and uses a computer to create an image of body structures
sonographer	technologist that performs sonography
sonography	process of using a sonograph (ultrasonography)
thrombocytes	platelets, blood-clotting cell fragments
thrombocytopenia	low number of thrombocytes
thrombocytosis	high number of thrombocytes
tomogram	picture made by a tomograph
tomograph	instrument that uses x-ray to produce images through planes (slices) of the body
tomography	the process of using a tomograph
xanthemia	yellow condition of the blood (carotenemia)

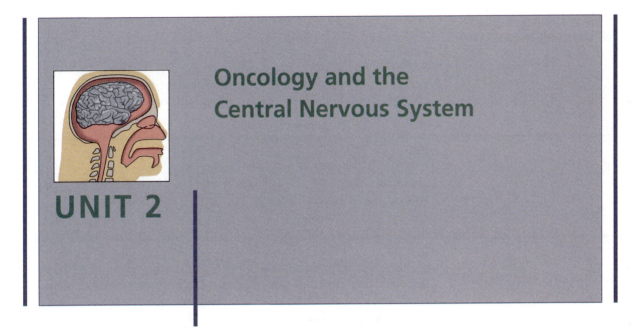

UNIT 2

Oncology and the Central Nervous System

ANSWER COLUMN	
	2.1 You can form words without even knowing the meaning. In the next three frames use what is needed from **encephal/o** + **-itis** to form a word: _____ /_____.
encephal/itis	

	2.2
	Use what is needed from **encephal/o**
	        malac/o
	        -ia
	_____ /_____ /_____ /____.

encephal/o/malac/ia en sef´ ə lō mal ā´ shə	

	2.3
	Use what is needed from **encephal/o**
	        mening/o
	        -itis
	_____ /_____ /_____ /_____.

encephal/o/mening/itis en sef´ ə lō men´ in **jī´** tis	

	2.4
	Use what is needed from **encephal/o**
	        myel/o
	        -pathy
	_____ /_____ /_____ /____ /_____.

encephal/o/myel/o/pathy en sef´ ə lō mī´ əl **op´** ath ē	

59

> **ANSWER COLUMN**

2.5

A prefix goes in front of a word to change its meaning. In the words hyper/trophy, hyper/emia, and hyper/emesis, **hyper-** changes the meaning of trophy, emia, and emesis. **hyper-** is a

prefix   _____.

2.6

hyper- is a prefix that means above or more than normal. In common slang, someone who is overactive is hyper. To say that a person is overly critical, you would use the word

hyper-   _____ /critic/al.

ℯeee *TAKE A CLOSER LOOK*

2.7

Our bodies do not work well when imbalanced by excesses. Look up the following conditions that are all caused by excesses. Write the substance or nature of the excess next to the term.

hyper-

hypercholesterolemia _____

hypertoxicity _____

hyperflexion _____

hyperactivity _____

hyperlipemia _____

hyperproteinuria _____

2.8

hypo- is a prefix that is just the opposite of **hyper-**. The prefix for below or less than normal is _____.

hypo-

ℯeee *TAKE A CLOSER LOOK*

2.9

Below normal levels of substances, sizes, or activity may also produce critical imbalance. Use your dictionary to discover the nature of each condition and write your answer next to the term.

hypo-

hypocalcemia _____

hypodactylia _____

hyposensitive _____

hypothermia _____

hypokalemia _____

hypothyroidism _____

hypodermic _____

2.10

Hypo/troph/y (atrophy) means progressive degeneration. When an organ or tissue that has developed properly wastes away or decreases in size, it is undergoing _____ /_____ /_____.

hypo/troph/y or
hī **pot´** rə fē
atrophy
a´ trō fē

Hypotrophy   Hypertrophy

ANSWER COLUMN	
	2.11 Hyperemesis gravidarum is a complication of pregnancy that can require hospitalization. The part of the disorder that tells you
hyperemesis	excessive vomiting occurs is _____.
	2.12 Gallbladder attacks can cause excessive vomiting. This, too, is
hyperemesis	called _____.
	2.13 Hypertrophy means overdevelopment. **-trophy** comes from the Greek word *trophe*, for nourishment. See the connection between nourishment and development? Overdevelopment is called
hyper/troph/y hī **pûr´** trə fē	_____ /_____ /_____.
	2.14 Many organs can hypertrophy. If the heart overdevelops, the
hypertrophy	condition is _____ of the heart.

ANSWER COLUMN	
hyper/tension hī pûr **ten´** shən	**2.15** Abnormally high blood pressure (BP) (tension) is called _____ /_____.
high blood pressure	**2.16** Essential hypertension and nonessential hypertension are both conditions of *_____.
hypo/tension hī pō **ten´** shun	**2.17** If hypertension is elevated BP, then hypo/tension indicates lowered BP. A blood pressure of 120/80 mmHg is a normal average. A BP of 90/60 mmHg may indicate _____ /_____. **NOTE:** mmHg means millimeters of mercury.
hypertension	**2.18** Diuretic medications may be prescribed to lower the blood pressure (BP) in patients with _____ by increasing excretion of fluids.
aden aden/o	**2.19** **aden/o** is used in words that refer to glands. The word root is _____. The combining form is _____ /_____.
aden/itis ad ə **nī´** tis	**2.20** Build a word that means inflammation of a gland (word root + suffix rule): _____ /_____.
-ectomy aden- aden/ectomy ad ə **nek´** tə mē	**2.21** Aden/ectomy means excision or removal of a gland. The part that means excision is _____. The part that means gland is _____. The word for removal of a gland is _____ /_____.
adenectomy	**2.22** An adenectomy is a surgical procedure. If a gland is tumorous, part or all of it can be excised. This operation is an _____.
aden/oma	**2.23** A tumor is an abnormal growth of cells, also referred to as a neoplasm. **-oma** is the suffix for tumor. Form a word that means tumor of a gland: _____ /_____

ANSWER COLUMN	
adenoma	**2.24** Sometimes the thyroid gland develops an adenoma. In this case, a patient's history might read, "… hyperthyroidism noted—due to presence of a thyroid _____."
adenoma adenectomy or thyroidectomy	**2.25** When a thyroid _____ (tumor of a gland) is found, a partial _____ (excision of gland) may be performed.
word root vowel aden/o/pathy ad ə **nop´** ə thē	**2.26** Recall -pathy is a suffix meaning disease. Aden/o/pathy means any disease of a gland. In this word you have a *_____ plus a _____ and suffix to form the word _____ /_____ /_____.
adenopathy	**2.27** Adenopathy means glandular disease in general. When the diagnosis is made of a diseased gland but the disease is not specifically known or stated, the word used is _____.
Adenopathy adenoma adenectomy	**2.28** _____ (glandular disease) could be diagnosed as an _____ (glandular tumor). If so, the surgeon may advise that an _____ (excision of a gland) be performed.
lymph/aden/o/pathy lim fad´ ə **nop´** ə thē	**2.29** Recall **lymph/o** refers to lymphatic tissue. Any disease of the lymph glands could be called _____ /_____ /_____ /_____.
adenitis adenectomy	**2.30** When a gland is found to have a mild _____ (inflammation), no _____ (surgery) is indicated.
tumor fat	**2.31** An adenoma is a glandular tumor. -oma is the suffix for _____. A lip/oma is a tumor containing fat. **lip/o** is the combining form for _____.
lip/oma lip **ō´** mə	**2.32** A lip/oma is usually benign (noncancerous). A fatty tumor is called a _____ /_____.

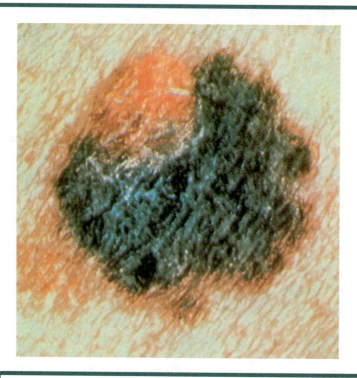

Melanoma (Courtesy of the American Academy of Dermatology)

▶ **ANSWER COLUMN**

lymph/oma
lim **fō´** mə

2.33
A tumor composed of lymph tissue is called a
_____ /_____.

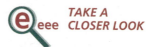 *TAKE A CLOSER LOOK*

2.34
Lesion, ulcer, tumor, and growth. We often hear these terms used, but are they the same? How do we know when to use them?

lesion
lē´ zhun

A lesion may be one of many possible types of abnormal tissue conditions including: macules, vesicles, papules, ulcers, abscesses, and tumors, just to name a few.

ulcer
ul´ ser

Ulcers are a more specific type of lesion. They are open sores on the skin or mucous membranes.

tumor
too´ mer

A tumor is an abnormal growth in numbers and/or types of cells and may be cancerous.

The term growth is a common term that is not very specific at all and not used as often in formal diagnosis. Look up these terms in your dictionary and you will find several pages of information that is very interesting.

2.35
carcin/o, from the Greek word *carcinos*, meaning crab, is the combining form for cancer (Ca, CA). A carcin/oma is a
*_____.

cancerous tumor or
malignant tumor

► ANSWER COLUMN	
carcinoma	**2.36** A carcinoma may occur in almost any part of the body. A stomach cancer is called gastric _____.
✓ SPELL CHECK	**2.37** Make sure you use and say the correct form: metastasis singular noun metastases plural noun metastatic adjective metastasize(d) verb
carcin/oma kär sin ō′ mə	**2.38** Metastasis is the transfer of a disease from one organ to another not connected to it. Carcinoma may metastasize (spread to other parts of the body) through the lymphatic system. The intestine has a rich blood supply. For this reason, intestinal _____ /_____ is extremely dangerous, as it may metastasize to the liver. **NOTE:** meta- means beyond and -stasis means in one place (staying). Metastasis (met., metas., mets.) means spreading beyond the original place.
meta/stasis me **ta**′ sta sis	**2.39** A carcinoma may spread to another body part. The piece that grows in a new location is called a _____ /_____.
carcinoma	**2.40** Carcinoma may be confined to the site (from the Latin *situs*; think of *situ*ation) of its origin. In this case, it is called _____ in situ.
aden/o/carcinoma ad′ ə nō kär sin ō′ mə	**2.41** Form a word that means cancer of glandular tissue: _____ /_____ /_____.
sarc/oma sär **kō**′ mə	**2.42** Carcinoma indicates the cancer originated from epithelial-type tissue. When cancer of connective-type tissue is found, it is called sarc/oma. Bone cancer is a type of _____ /_____.

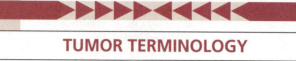

TUMOR TERMINOLOGY

Combining Form	Meaning	Tumor
Epithelial Tissue		
Benign	*Noncancerous*	
aden/o	gland	adenoma
melan/o	dark pigmented	melanoma
papill/o	small elevation of tissue	papilloma
fibr/o	fibrous tissue	fibroadenoma
Malignant	*Cancerous*	*Carcinoma*
aden/o	gland, glandular tissue	adenocarcinoma
melan/o	dark pigmented	melanocarcinoma (malignant melanoma)
		squamous cell carcinoma
		basal cell carcinoma
Connective-Hematopoietic-Nerve Tissue		
Benign		
oste/o	bone	osteoma
chondr/o	cartilage	chondroma
leiomy/o	smooth muscle	leiomyoma
lip/o	fat	lipoma
ather/o	fatty, porridgelike	atheroma
hem/angi/o	blood vessel	hemangioma
neur/o	nerve	neuroma
Malignant		
oste/o	bone	osteosarcoma
chondr/o	cartilage	chondrosarcoma
leiomy/o	smooth muscle	leiomyosarcoma
lip/o	fat	liposarcoma
angi/o	vessel	angiosarcoma
leuk/o	white	leukemia
myel/o	bone marrow	myeloma
lymph/o	lymphatic	lymphosarcoma
neur/o	nerve	neurosarcoma

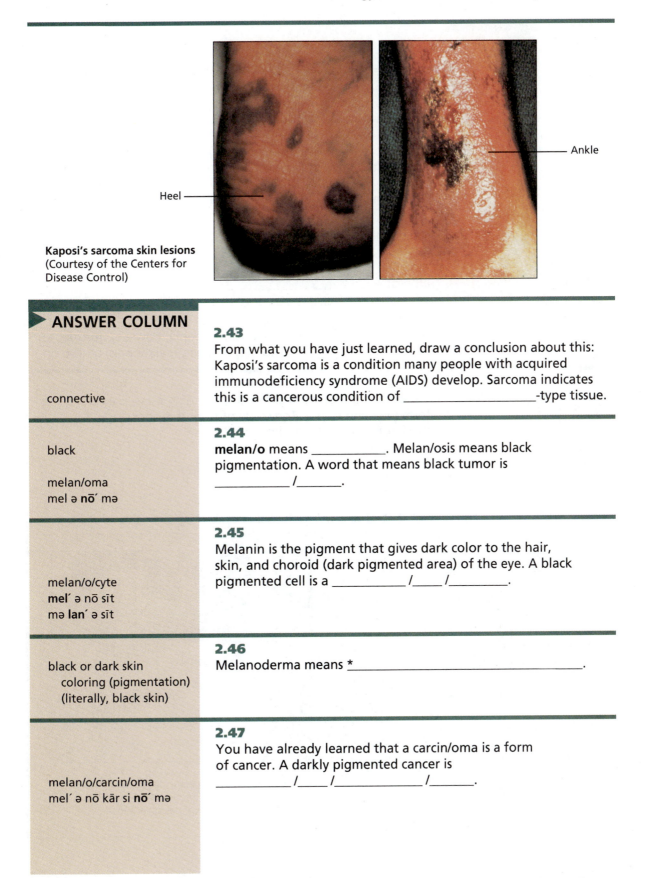

Heel ———

——— Ankle

Kaposi's sarcoma skin lesions
(Courtesy of the Centers for
Disease Control)

ANSWER COLUMN	
▶ **ANSWER COLUMN**	**2.43** From what you have just learned, draw a conclusion about this: Kaposi's sarcoma is a condition many people with acquired immunodeficiency syndrome (AIDS) develop. Sarcoma indicates
connective	this is a cancerous condition of _____-type tissue.
black melan/oma mel ə **nō´** mə	**2.44** **melan/o** means _____. Melan/osis means black pigmentation. A word that means black tumor is _____ /_____.
melan/o/cyte **mel´** ə nō sīt mə **lan´** ə sīt	**2.45** Melanin is the pigment that gives dark color to the hair, skin, and choroid (dark pigmented area) of the eye. A black pigmented cell is a _____ /____ /_____.

black or dark skin
    coloring (pigmentation)
    (literally, black skin)
	2.46
	Melanoderma means *_____.

melan/o/carcin/oma mel´ ə nō kär si **nō´** mə	**2.47** You have already learned that a carcin/oma is a form of cancer. A darkly pigmented cancer is _____ /____ /_____ /_____.

▶ ANSWER COLUMN

2.48

Whenever any hairless mole on the skin turns black and grows, a physician should be consulted for there is possible danger of black-mole cancer or _____.

melanocarcinoma

2.49

Plural Formation

Recall from the Word-Building section before Unit 1 that medical words often have special suffixes for plural formation. Words that end in **-oma** form a plural by using **-mata** as the suffix. In the list below, the first plural is done for you; *you* form the rest:

Singular	Plural
carcinoma	carcinomata
lipoma	_____
sarcoma	_____
atheroma	_____
adenoma	_____
melanoma	_____

lipomata
sarcomata
atheromata
adenomata
melanomata

NOTE: This is formal grammar. Most people, however, just put an "s" on the end, e.g., carcinomas, lipomas, melanomas, and so on.

2.50

onc/o from the Greek word *oncos*, meaning mass, is a combining form meaning tumor. The study of tumors is onc/o/logy. A specialist who studies tumors is called an

_____ / ____ / _____.

onc/o/logist
on **kol′** ō jist

Professional Profiles ◀◀◀◀◀◀◀◀◀◀◀◀◀◀◀◀◀◀◀◀◀◀◀◀◀◀◀◀◀◀◀◀◀◀◀◀◀

Medical technologists (MTs [ASCP]), medical laboratory technicians (MLTs), and certified laboratory assistants (CLAs) physically and chemically analyze as well as culture urine, blood, and other body fluids and tissues to determine the presence of all types of diseases. They work closely with physician specialists such as oncologists, pathologists, and hematologists. Knowledge of specimen collection, anatomy and physiology, biochemistry, laboratory equipment, asepsis, and quality control is essential. The American Society of Clinical Pathology (ASCP) is a professional organization that oversees credentialing and education in the medical laboratory professions.

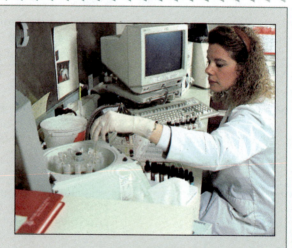

Medical technologist performing blood analysis
(Photo by Marcia Butterfield, courtesy of W. A. Foote Memorial Hospital, Jackson, MI)

ANSWER COLUMN	
onc/o/logy on **kol**′ ō jē	**2.51** A hospitalized patient with a disease caused by a tumor would be treated in the _____ /____ /_____ unit.
lip/o lip/oid **lip**′ oid	**2.52** The combining form for fat is _____ /____. **-oid** is a suffix that means like or resembling. Build a word that means fatlike or resembling fat: _____ /_____.
fat lipoid	**2.53** The word lipoid is used in chemistry or pathology. It describes a substance that looks like fat, dissolves like fat, but is not _____. A word that means resembling fat is _____.
lipoid	**2.54** In proper amounts cholesterol is essential to health, but too much may cause atherosclerosis (hardening of blood vessels due to fatty deposits). Cholesterol is an alcohol that resembles fat; therefore, it is _____.
ather/oma a ther **ō**′ mə ather/o/scler/osis a′ ther ō skler **ō**′ sis	**2.55** **ather/o** is the combining form for fatty or porridgelike. A tumorlike thickening and degeneration of the blood vessel walls that is caused by fatty deposits is called an _____ /_____. Hardening of vessel walls, due to fatty deposits is called _____ /____ /_____ /_____.
✔ SPELL CHECK	**2.56** Watch out for these similar combining forms: **ather/o**—porridgelike, fatty; **arteri/o**—arteries; **arthr/o**—joint.
like or resembling muc muc/o	**2.57** Muc/oid means resembling mucus. **-oid** is a suffix meaning *_____. The word root for mucus is _____ and its combining form is _____ /____.
muc/oid **myōō**′ koid	**2.58** Mucoid is an adjective that means resembling or like mucus. There is a substance in connective tissue that resembles mucus. This is a _____ /_____ substance.

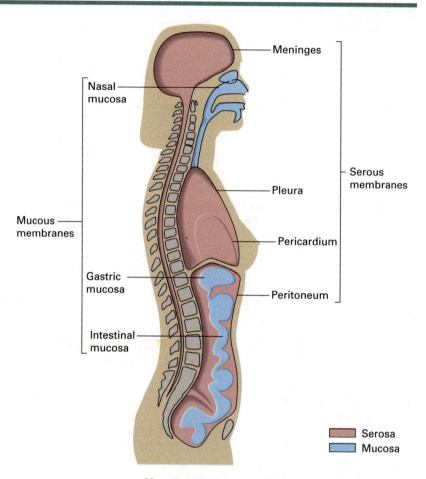

Mucous and serous membranes

ANSWER COLUMN	
	2.59 Muc/us is a secretion of the muc/ous membrane. **-us** is a noun suffix. **-ous** is an adjectival suffix. The muc/ous membrane secretes _____ /____.
muc/us **myōō′ kəs**	
	2.60 Mucus is secreted by cells in the nose. It traps dust and bacteria from the air. One of the body's protective devices is _____.
mucus	
mucus muc/ous **myōō′ kəs**	**2.61** The mucous membrane secretes _____. The tissue that secretes mucus is the_____ /_____ membrane or muc/osa.
mucus mucous	**2.62** The noun (the secretion) built from **muc/o** is _____. The adjective (pertaining to) built from muc/o is _____.

ANSWER COLUMN	
muc/osa myōō kō′ sə	**2.63** The mucous membrane or mucosa is found lining the open body cavities. This protective, mucous membrane also can be called the _____ /_____. **NOTE:** The digestive system is considered an open body cavity because it is essentially open from mouth to anus.
mucosa	**2.64** The stomach lining is the gastric _____.
mucus mucoid mucosa or mucous membrane	**2.65** The mucosa secretes _____. Anything that resembles mucus is _____. Mucoid substances are not mucus; therefore, they are not secreted by the *_____.
ser/osa se rō′ sə	**2.66** The serous membranes line the closed body cavities and cover the outside of organs such as the intestines. Serosa is the noun form. The intestinal _____ /_____ is a membrane that covers the intestine.
ser/ous ser′ us	**2.67** The mucous membranes line the open body cavities and the _____ /_____ (adjective) membranes line the closed cavities.
cephal	**2.68** At this stage of word building, students sometimes find that they have one big pain in the head. The word for pain in the head is cephal/algia (often shortened to cephalgia). The word root for head is _____.
algia	**2.69** One suffix for pain is _____.

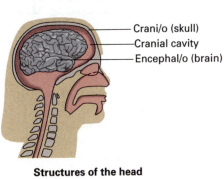

Cephal/o (head)

Crani/o (skull)
Cranial cavity
Encephal/o (brain)

Structures of the head

ANSWER COLUMN	
cephal/algia sef ə **lal**´ jē ə	**2.70** If you are suffering from cephal/algia, persevere, for later this gets to be fun. Any pain in the head may be called _____ /_____.
cephalalgia	**2.71** The combining form for head is **cephal/o**. The word for pain in the head is _____.
cephal/o/dynia sef ə lō **din**´ ē ə cephal/algia	**2.72** *Odyne* is a Greek word for pain. Another word for pain in the head is cephal/o/dynia. This word shows the combining form plus a suffix. If this seems a headache, relax. Either word, _____ /_____ /_____ or _____ /_____, will do for headache. **NOTE:** cephalgia is also correct spelling.
word root combining form	**2.73** Recall the suffixes -algia and -dynia. They are usually interchangeable. When -algia is used as a suffix it is preceded by a (choose one) *_____ (combining form/word root). When -dynia is used, it is preceded by a (choose one) *_____ (combining form/word root).
cephal/o/dynic sef ə lō **din**´ ik	**2.74** -dynia can take the adjectival form -dynic. An adjective that means pertaining to head pain is _____ /_____ /_____.
cephalodynic	**2.75** To say medically that headache (HA) discomfort exists, use the adjective _____ for headache.
cephalalgia cephalodynia cephalodynic	**2.76** Two nouns for head pain are _____ and _____. The adjective used for head pain is _____.
adjective ic	**2.77** Cephal/ic means pertaining to or toward the head. Cephal/ic is a(n) _____ (noun/adjective). This is evident because cephalic ends in _____.
cephal/ic sə **fal**´ ik	**2.78** Cephalic is an adjective. A case history reporting head cuts due to an accident might read, "_____ /_____ lacerations present."

ANSWER COLUMN	
cephalic	**2.79** In the phrase "lack of cephalic orientation," the adjective is _____.
encephal/itis en sef´ ə lī´ tis	**2.80** *In*side the head, *en*closed in bone, is the brain; **encephal/o** is used in words pertaining to the brain. Build a word meaning inflammation of the brain: _____ /_____.
-oma encephal/oma en sef ə lō´ mə	**2.81** The suffix for tumor is _____. Use what is necessary from **encephal/o** to build a word for brain tumor: _____ /_____.
brain	**2.82** The Greek word for hernia is *kele*, indicating an abnormal protrusion or swelling; the suffix is -cele. Encephal/o/cele is a word meaning herniation of _____ tissue.

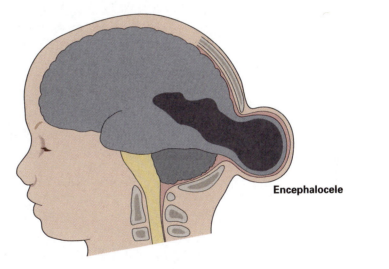

Encephalocele

encephal/o/cele en **sef**´ ə lō sēl	**2.83** An encephalocele occurs when some brain tissue protrudes through a cranial fissure (see illustration). The word for herniation of brain tissue is _____ /____ /_____.

ANSWER COLUMN	
encephalocele	**2.84** Any hernia is a projection of a part from its natural cavity. Herniation is indicated by **-cele**. A projection of brain tissue from its natural cavity is an _____.
encephalocele	**2.85** Brain herniation is sometimes a finding in hydrocephaly. This condition, in medical language, is called an _____.
softening of brain tissue	**2.86** Malacia is a word meaning softening of a tissue. Encephal/o/malac/ia means *_____.
encephal/o/tomy en sef′ ə **lot**′ ō mē	**2.87** **-tomy** is used as a suffix for making an *incision* or temporary opening. An incision into the brain is an _____ /_____ /_____.

Sagittal section of the brain

ANSWER COLUMN	
malac/o/tomy mal ə **kot´** ə mē	**2.88** Using what is necessary from **malac/o** with the suffix **-tomy**, form a word that means incision of soft areas: _____ /__ /_____.
encephal/o/malac/ia en sef´ ə lō mə **lā´** shə	**2.89** Encephal/o/malac/ia ends in **-ia**. **-ia** is a suffix that forms a noun and indicates a condition. A noun meaning softening of brain tissue is _____ /_____ /_____ /_____.
encephalomalacia	**2.90** An accident causing brain injury could result in the softening of some brain tissue, or _____.
electr/o/encephal/o/gram e lek´ trō en **sef´** ə lō gram	**2.91** From your knowledge of the word parts **electr/o**, **encephal/o**, and **-gram** build a term meaning picture of the electrical activity of the brain: _____ /_____ /_____ /_____ /_____ (EEG).
electr/o/encephal/o/graphy e lek´ trō en sef ə **log´** ra fē electr/o/encephal/o/graph e lek´ trō en **sef´** ə lō graf	**2.92** The process of recording electrical brain activity is called _____ /_____ /_____ /_____ /_____. The instrument used to record the EEG is an _____ /_____ /_____ /_____ /_____.
surgical repair of the skull or cranium	**2.93** **crani/o** is used in words referring to the crani/um or skull. **-plasty** is the suffix for surgical repair. Crani/o/plasty means *_____.
crani/o/malac/ia krā nē ō mə **lā´** shə	**2.94** The word for softening of the bones of the skull is _____ /_____ /_____ /_____.
crani/ectomy krā´ nē **ek´** tə mē	**2.95** The word meaning excision of part of the cranium is _____ /_____.
crani/o/tomy krā nē **ot´** ə mē	**2.96** The word for incision into the skull is _____ /__ /_____.

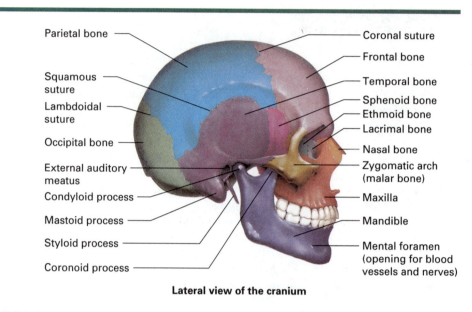

Parietal bone

Squamous
suture

Lambdoidal
suture

Occipital bone

External auditory
meatus

Condyloid process

Mastoid process

Styloid process

Coronoid process

Coronal suture

Frontal bone

Temporal bone

Sphenoid bone

Ethmoid bone

Lacrimal bone

Nasal bone

Zygomatic arch
(malar bone)

Maxilla

Mandible

Mental foramen
(opening for blood
vessels and nerves)

Lateral view of the cranium

ANSWER COLUMN	
	2.97 **-meter** is the suffix for instrument used to measure. An instrument used to measure the cranium is the _____ /____ /_____.
crani/o/meter krā′ nē **om**′ ə tər	
cranial cranial	**2.98** There are cranial bones. There are also _____ nerves. There are grooves and furrows called _____ fissures.
adjectival	**2.99** Crani/al is the (choose one) _____ (noun/adjectival) form of cranium.
cerebr/um **ser**′ ə brəm, sə **rē**′ brəm	**2.100** Crani/o/cerebr/al refers to the skull and the cerebr/um. The cerebr/um is a part of the brain. **Cerebr/o** is used to build words about the _____ /____.
cerebrum	**2.101** The cerebrum is the part of the brain in which thought occurs. When you think, you are using your _____.
cerebrum	**2.102** Feeling is interpreted in the cerebrum. Motor impulses also arise in the _____.

ANSWER COLUMN	
cerebrum	**2.103** Thinking, feeling, and movement are controlled by the gray matter of the _____. (Were you ever told to use your gray matter? This is why.)
cerebr/al **ser´** ə brəl, sə **rē´** brəl	**2.104** The adjectival form of cerebrum is _____ /____.
cerebral	**2.105** There is a cerebral reflex. There are cerebral fissures. You have probably heard of _____ hemorrhage (bleeding).
inflammation of the cerebrum	**2.106** Cerebr/itis means *_____.
a cerebral tumor	**2.107** A cerebr/oma is *_____.
cerebr/o/tomy ser ə **brot´** ə mē	**2.108** An incision into the cerebrum to drain an abscess is a _____ /____ /_____.
cerebrum (brain)	**2.109** The vascular system refers to the blood vessels. A cerebr/o/vascular accident (CVA; stroke) occurs because of a vascular lesion within the _____ that blocks blood flow or causes a hemorrhage.
cerebr/o/vascul/ar ser ē´ brō **vas´** kū lär	**2.110** People with hypertension are a high risk for CVA or _____ /____ /_____ /____ accident.
high blood pressure vessels of the heart abnormal function	**2.111** Use what you have learned to analyze the following condition by writing its meaning: hyper/tensive *_____ cardi/o/vascul/ar *_____ dis/ease *_____ Abbreviation: HCVD

ANSWER COLUMN	
	2.112 Cerebr/o/spin/al refers to the brain and spinal cord. There is fluid that bathes the cerebrum and spinal cord. It is _____ /_____ /_____ /_____ fluid (CSF).
cerebr/o/spin/al ser ē´ brō **spī**´ nəl	
cerebrospinal	**2.113** A spin/al puncture is sometimes done to remove _____ fluid.
cerebrospinal	**2.114** There is even a disease called _____ meningitis.
mening/es me **nin**´ jēz	**2.115** *Meninx* is a Greek word for membrane. **mening/o** is the combining form for the meninges, a three-layered membrane that covers the brain and spinal cord. These three layers are the pia mater, arachnoid, and dura mater. The protective covering of the brain and spinal cord is the _____ /_____.
mening/o/cele me **nin**´ gō sēl	**2.116** A herniation of the meninges is a _____ /_____ /_____.
meninges	**2.117** A mening/o/cele is a herniation of the _____.
meninges	**2.118** Mening/o/malac/ia means softening of the _____.
mening/itis men in **jī**´ tis	**2.119** Mening/itis can occur as cerebr/al meningitis, as spin/al meningitis, or as cerebr/o/spin/al _____ /_____.
meningitis	**2.120** There are many kinds of meningitis. The tubercle bacillus can cause tuberculous meningitis. Mening/o/cocci are bacteria that cause epidemic _____. **PRONUNCIATION NOTE:** When g is followed by e, i, y it is usually pronounced like a "j" (soft g) as in ginger. When g is followed by a, o, u it is pronounced like a hard "g" sound as in goat, gate, and gut. Practice: meningitis, meningocele j (soft g) (hard g)

Abbreviation	Meaning
AIDS	acquired immunodeficiency syndrome
ASCP	American Society of Clinical Pathology
BCC	basal cell carcinoma
BP	blood pressure
Ca, CA	cancer
CIS	carcinoma in situ
CLA	certified laboratory assistant
CP	cerebral palsy
CSF	cerebrospinal fluid
CV	cardiovascular
CVA	cerebrovascular accident (stroke)
EEG	electroencephalogram
HA	headache
HCVD	hypertensive cardiovascular disease
MBD	minimal brain dysfunction
met., metas., mets.	metastasis
MLT	medical laboratory technician
mmHg	millimeters of mercury (pressure)
MT	medical technologist
TIA	transient ischemic attack

To complete your study of this unit, work the review activities on the next pages. Also, listen to the audiotapes that accompany *Medical Terminology: A Programmed Text,* 8th edition, and practice your pronunciation.

Additional practice exercises for this unit are available on the Student Practice disk found in the back of the textbook.

▶ REVIEW ACTIVITIES

Circle and Correct
Circle the correct answer for each question. Then, check your answers in Appendix A.

1. Word root for development:
   a. troph   b. tropic
   c. tome   d. path

2. Combining form for gland:
   a. glandul   b. adreno
   c. adeno   d. glando

3. Prefix for below or less than normal:
   a. hyper-   b. hypo-
   c. ology-   d. en-

4. Suffix for disease condition:
   a. -pathy   b. -patho
   c. -tropho   d. -ic

5. Combining form for cancer:
   a. cancerous   b. situ
   c. carcino   d. neoplasm

6. Suffix for one who studies:
   a. -logy   b. -ist
   c. -logist   d. -er

7. Suffix for instrument that records:
   a. -phonogram   b. -graph
   c. -gram   d. -graphy

8. Word root for head:
   a. myel   b. cephal
   c. encephal   d. crani

9. Suffix for herniation:
   a. -itis   b. -malacia
   c. -cytes   d. -cele

10. Combining form for brain:
    a. myelo   b. encephalo
    c. cerebr   d. meningo

11. The membrane surrounding the closed cavities:
    a. mucosa   b. dermal
    c. serosa   d. meninges

12. Suffix for like or resembling:
    a. -oid   b. -oma
    c. -ous   d. -ible

13. Combining form for skull:
    a. cephal/o   b. occipital
    c. crani/o   d. oste/o

14. Word root for tumor:
    a. oma   b. onc
    c. sarc/o   d. carcin

15. Suffix for pain:
    a. -cele   b. -oid
    c. -alic   d. -dynia

▶ REVIEW ACTIVITIES

Select and Construct

Select the correct word parts from the list below and construct medical terms that represent the given meaning.

aden(o)	carcin(o)	cele	cephal(o)	cerebr(o)
crani(o)	ectomy	electr(o)	encephal(o)	epitheli(o)
graph	graphy	hyper	hypo	itis
lip(o)	logist	logy	lymph(o)	malac(ia)
mening(o)	muc(o)	mucosa	oid	oma
onc(o)	pathy	plasty	sarc(o)	spinal
tension	tomy	trophy		

1. herniation of the brain _____

2. instrument for recording brain function _____

3. surgical repair of the skull _____

4. brain and spinal cord (adjective) _____

5. malignant tumor of a gland _____

6. resembling mucus _____

7. fatty tumor _____

8. softening of the skull _____

9. incision into the cerebrum _____

10. inflammation of the meninges _____

11. one who studies tumors _____

12. connective tissue tumor _____

13. tumor involving lymph glands _____

14. overdevelopment _____

15. low blood pressure _____

Now, on your own, use the word parts list above to construct other medical terms.

16. _____   _____
          word   meaning

17. _____   _____
          word   meaning

18. _____   _____
          word   meaning

19. _____   _____
          word   meaning

20. _____   _____
          word   meaning

▶ **REVIEW ACTIVITIES**

Define and Dissect
Give a brief definition and dissect each term listed into its word parts in the space provided on the right. Check your answers by referring to the frame listed in parentheses and your medical dictionary. Then, listen to the audiotapes to practice pronunciation.

1. encephalomalacia (2.89)

    _____ /___ /_____ /____
    rt   v   rt   suffix

    _____
                 definition

2. hypertrophy (2.13)

    _____ /_____ /_____
      pre   rt   suffix

3. hyperemesis (2.11)

    _____ /_____
       pre   rt/suffix

4. adenectomy (2.21)

    _____ /_____
        rt   suffix

5. hypertension (2.15)

    _____ /_____
       pre   rt/suffix

6. carcinoma (2.38)

    _____ /_____
         rt   suffix

7. lipoid (2.52)

    _____ /_____
         rt   suffix

8. oncology (2.51)

    _____ /___ /_____
       rt   v   suffix

9. mucosa (2.63)

    _____ /_____
       rt   suffix

10. cephalalgia (2.70)

    _____ /_____
         rt   suffix

11. encephalocele (2.83)

    _____ /___ /_____
         rt   v   suffix

12. electroencephalogram (2.91)

_____ / __ / _____ / __ / _____
rt   v   rt   v   suffix

13. craniomalacia (2.94)

_____ / __ / _____
rt   v   rt/suffix

14. cerebrotomy (2.108)

_____ / __ / _____
rt   v   suffix

15. meningitis (2.119)

_____ / _____
rt   suffix

16. cerebrospinal (2.112)

_____ / __ / _____ / _____
rt   v   rt   suffix

17. hypotrophy (2.10)

_____ / _____ / _____
pre   rt   suffix

18. atheroma (2.55)

_____ / _____
rt   suffix

19. cerebrovascular (2.110)

_____ / __ / _____ / _____
rt   v   rt   suffix

20. metastasis (2.39)

_____ / _____ / _____
pre   rt   suffix

21. serous (2.65)

_____ / _____
rt   suffix

22. craniometer (2.97)

_____ / __ / _____
rt   v   suffix

23. lesion (2.34)

_____ / _____
rt   suffix

► REVIEW ACTIVITIES

Abbreviation Matching
Match the following abbreviations with their definition.

_____ 1. ASCP

_____ 2. EEG

_____ 3. MBD

_____ 4. met., metas., mets.

_____ 5. TIA

_____ 6. CP

_____ 7. CSF

_____ 8. CIS

_____ 9. HA

_____ 10. Ca

a. basal cell carcinoma

b. cancer

c. metastasis

d. American Society of Clinical Pathology

e. electrocardiogram

f. heart and chronic venereal disease

g. minimal brain dysfunction

h. cerebospinal fluid

i. carcinoma in situ

j. heart attack

k. cerebral palsy

l. electroencephalogram

m. headache

n. transient ischemia attack

Abbreviation Fill-ins
Fill in the blanks with the correct abbreviations.

11. The medical laboratory technician (_____) prepared the blood sample for testing.

12. Having blood pressure (_____) that is abnormally high (200/100 _____) and blood vessel disease is serious for the patient with _____.

13. The patient has experienced several episodes of blurred vision, dizziness, and fatigue brought on by a loss of blood flow to the brain. A _____ could be a precursor to a stroke or _____, which is followed by paralysis, loss of consciousness, and possibly death.

14. The biopsy indicated a basal cell carcinoma (_____).

▶ **CASE STUDIES**

Write the term next to its meaning given below. Then, draw slashes to analyze the word parts. Note the use of medical abbreviations. Look these up in your dictionary or find them in Appendix B. If you have any questions about the answers, refer to your medical dictionary or check with your instructor for the answers in Appendix A.

CASE STUDY 2-1
PRESENT ILLNESS FROM HISTORY AND PHYSICAL REPORT

Pt: female, age 45, grav IV, para IV

Dx: Carcinoma in situ, uterine cervix

Ms. Sally Pingo was seen on August 28th after approximately an eight-year absence from this gynecology office. She had a Pap smear done in Dr. Lapar's office on August 4th, which described squamous cell carcinoma in situ. Therefore, an in-office colposcopy was done on the same day and minimal abnormalities were noted by visualization of the cervix. Appropriate biopsies were taken, and the pathology report described severe dysplasia and/or squamous carcinoma in situ, possible poikilocytotic atypia from cervical biopsies. Also, the endocervical curettings had strips of squamous epithelium exhibiting severe dysplasia and/or carcinoma in situ with glandular atypia. Therefore, we decided to offer Ms. Pingo a D&C and LASER conization to further delineate the extent of the pathology. She accepted and was scheduled.

1. dilation and curettage   _____

2. inside the neck of the uterus   _____

3. different cell shapes   _____

4. abnormal (poor) development   _____

5. not typical   _____

6. fourth pregnancy, fourth birth   _____

7. cancerous tumor   _____

8. process of using a colposcope   _____

9. excision of a cone of tissue   _____

10. specialty—females   _____

11. Papanicolaou test   _____

12. excision of tissue for study   _____

▶ CROSSWORD PUZZLE

Check your answers by going back through the frames or checking the solution in Appendix C.

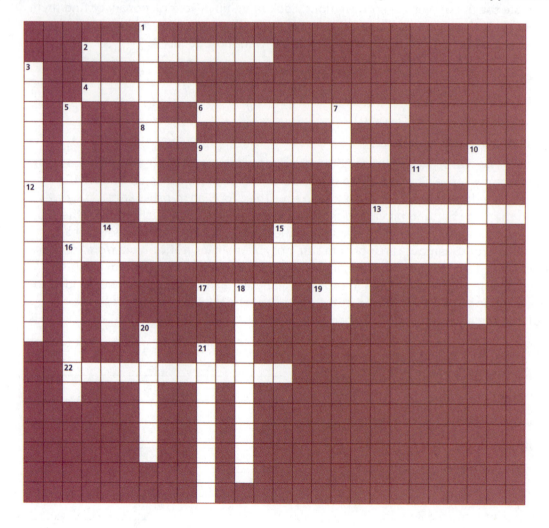

Across

2. remove a gland
4. usually benign fat tumor
6. hernia of the meninges
8. suffix for tumor
9. loss in structure size
11. suffix for instrument used to measure
12. hardening of a vessel caused by fat
13. tumor of melanocyte
16. process of producing EEG
17. watery substance produced by mucosa
19. carcinoma in situ (abbreviation)
22. high blood pressure

Down

1. tumor physician
3. glandular cancer
5. disease of lymph glands
7. synonym: cephalodynia
10. muscle tissue tumor (fibroid)
14. membrane covering closed cavities
15. blood pressure
18. incision into the skull
20. connective tissue cancer
21. inside the head, brain (word root)

▶ GLOSSARY

adenectomy	excision of a gland
adenitis	inflammation of a gland
adenoma	tumor of a gland or glandular tissue
adenopathy	disease condition of a gland or glandular tissue
atheroma	fatty (porridgelike) tissue tumor found in blood vessels
atherosclerosis	hardening of blood vessels caused by fatty growths
carcinoma	cancer of epithelial-type tissue
cephalalgia	head pain (synonym: cephalodynia)
cephalic	pertaining to the head
cephalodynic	pertaining to head pain (adjective)
cerebral	pertaining to the cerebrum (adjective)
cerebritis	inflammation of the cerebrum
cerebroma	tumor of the cerebrum
cerebrospinal	pertaining to the cerebrum and spine
cerebrovascular	pertaining to the cerebrum and blood vessels
cerebrum	largest part of the brain made of the frontal, temporal, and occipital lobes
craniectomy	excision of part of the skull
craniomalacia	softening of the skull
craniometer	instrument used to measure the size of the skull
cranioplasty	surgical repair of the skull
craniotomy	incision into the skull
cranium	skull
electroencephalogram	tracing (picture) showing brain wave activity
electroencephalograph	instrument used to turn brain waves into electrical patterns showing a picture of changes in activity
encephalitis	inflammation of the brain
encephalomalacia	softening of brain tissue
encephalomeningitis	inflammation of the brain and meninges
encephalomyelopathy	disease condition of the brain and spinal cord
glandular	pertaining to a gland
hypertension	high blood pressure
hypertrophy	overdevelopment, increase in size
hypotension	low blood pressure
hypotrophy	underdevelopment, decrease in size
lipoid	resembling fat
lipoma	fatty tissue tumor
lymphadenopathy	disease condition of the lymph glands

► **GLOSSARY**

lymphoma	lymph tissue tumor
melanocarcinoma	malignant (cancerous) melanoma
melanoma	tumor involving growth of melanocytes
meninges	three-layered membrane surrounding the brain and spinal cord
meningitis	inflammation of the meninges
meningocele	herniation of the meninges
metastasis	tumor that spreads beyond its origin (noun)
metastasize	spread beyond its origin (verb)
metastatic	pertaining to a metastasis
mucosa	mucous membrane (noun)
mucus	watery substance secreted by mucous membranes
oncologist	physician specialist in diseases involving tumors
oncology	the science that studies tumors
sarcoma	cancer of connective-type tissue
serosa	serous membrane

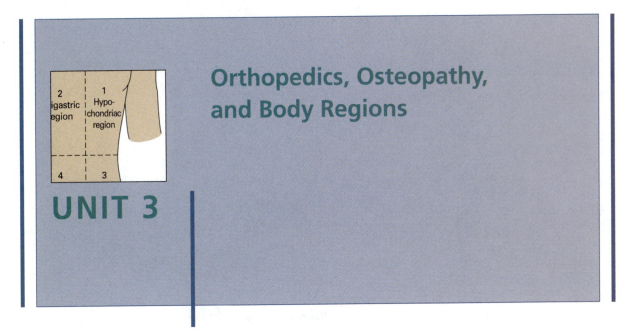

Orthopedics, Osteopathy, and Body Regions

UNIT 3

Now that you are learning more complex terms, it is time to suggest a way to remember some of the commonly mispronounced words. Begin with the suffixes -scope and -scopy. -scope is pronounced just as it looks (skōp) as in

arthroscope (**ār´** thrō skōp), endoscope (**en´** dō skōp).

But -scopy is not pronounced as it looks. The "o" from the combining form blends with the suffix and is a short "o" sound as in **os** trich or **op** tical. The accent is also placed on this vowel-suffix blend (**os´** ko pē)

arthroscopy (arthr **os´** ko pē), endoscopy (en **dos´** ko pē)

Many other suffixes follow a similar pattern; for example

o/pathy	**op´** athy	o/trophy	**ot´** rophy
o/lysis	**ol´** ysis	o/clysis	**oc´** lysis
o/stasis	**os´** tasis	o/graphy	**og´** raphy
o/meter	**om´** eter	o/metry	**om´** etry
o/stomy	**os´** tomy	o/tomy	**ot´** omy
o/logy	**ol´** ogy		

Refer back to this list as you learn these suffixes.

▶ **ANSWER COLUMN**

oste/o

3.1
Osteon is a Greek word meaning bone. Oste/o/pathy means disease of the bones. From this word, form the combining form for bone: _____ /_____.

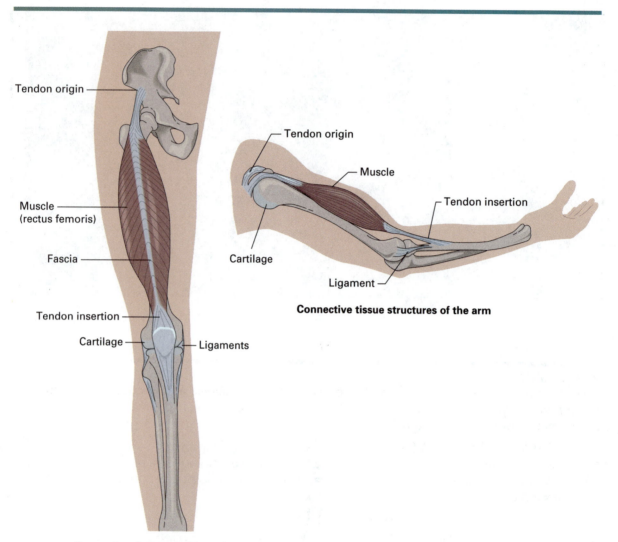

Tendon origin

Muscle
(rectus femoris)

Fascia

Tendon insertion

Cartilage

Ligaments

Tendon origin

Muscle

Tendon insertion

Cartilage

Ligament

Connective tissue structures of the arm

Connective tissue structures of the leg

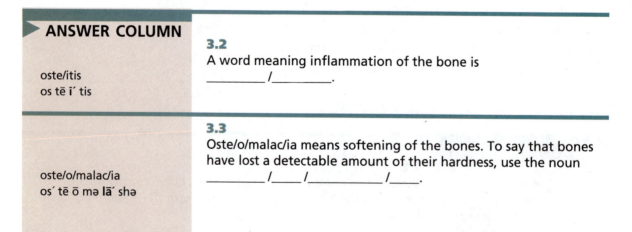

ANSWER COLUMN

oste/itis
os tē ĭ´ tis

3.2
A word meaning inflammation of the bone is
_____ /_____.

oste/o/malac/ia
os´ tē ō mə lā´ shə

3.3
Oste/o/malac/ia means softening of the bones. To say that bones have lost a detectable amount of their hardness, use the noun
_____ /_____ /_____ /_____.

► ANSWER COLUMN	
osteomalacia	**3.4** One cause of oste/o/malac/ia is the removal of calcium from the bones. When calcium is removed from the bones and they lose some of their hardness, a disorder called _____ may result.
osteomalacia	**3.5** A disorder of the parathyroid glands can cause calcium to be withdrawn from the bones. When this occurs, _____ results.
oste/o/pathy os′ tē **op**′ ə thē	**3.6** Recall **-pathy** means any disease. Form a word that means disease of bone: _____ /_____ /_____.
oste/o/path/ic os tē ō **path**′ ik	**3.7** A doctor of osteopathy (DO) receives special training about the skeleton and its relationship to disease. Using the adjectival form, we call this special type of physician an _____ /_____ /_____ /_____ doctor.
oste/oma os tē **ō**′ mə oste/o/mata os′ tē **ō**′ mə ta	**3.8** A hard outgrowth on a bone may be a bone tumor or _____ /_____. Build the plural form: _____ /__ /_____.
joint	**3.9** **-pathy** means disease. Oste/o/arthr/o/pathy is a noun that means any disease involving bones and joints. **arthr/o** is used in words to mean _____.
oste/o arthr/o pathy oste/o/arthr/o/pathy os′ tē ō är **throp**′ ə thē	**3.10** Oste/o/arthr/o/pathy is a compound noun. Analyze it: _____ /_____ bone (combining form); _____ /_____ joint (combining form); _____ disease (suffix). Now put it together: _____ /_____ /_____ /_____ /_____.

Professional Profiles ◀◀◀◀◀◀◀◀◀◀◀◀◀◀◀◀◀◀◀◀◀◀◀◀◀◀◀◀◀◀

Doctor of Osteopathy (DO): Osteopathic physicians are fully licensed to practice medicine, performing the same duties as medical doctors (MD, allopathic doctors). Because of the original philosophy of osteopathic medicine, founded by Dr. Andrew Still in 1874, they identify the musculoskeletal framework as a key element to health. They also believe that the body has a natural ability to heal itself given a favorable environment and good nutrition and so act as teachers to help patients take a responsible role for their own well-being and to change unhealthy patterns. In addition, osteopathic manipulative therapy (OMT) is incorporated in the training and practice of osteopathic physicians. Although 60 percent practice primary care, osteopathic physicians may specialize in surgery, obstetrics, anesthesiology, internal medicine, psychiatry, and other medical specialties. The American Osteopathic Association (AOA) is the national professional organization that oversees education and licensure of Doctors of Osteopathy.

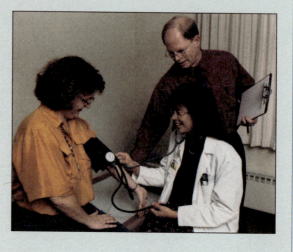

Osteopathic medical student learns proper technique for taking blood pressure (Courtesy of Osteopathic Medicine Photographic Services)

► **ANSWER COLUMN**	
	3.11 *Poros* is a Greek word meaning passageway. Oste/o/por/osis is a disease condition of the bone in which there is deterioration of the bone matrix causing pores and weakness. Calcium deficiency and hormone changes associated with menopause in women along with a hereditary predisposition can lead to _____ /____ /_____ /_____.
oste/o/por/osis os´ tē ō por ō´ sis	
	3.12 A proper diet that includes calcium and weight-bearing exercise such as walking may help to prevent porosity of the bones, called _____.
osteoporosis	
	3.13 Recall *sarcoma* is used to indicate cancer of connective tissue. Bone is connective tissue; therefore, bone cancer is called _____ /____ /_____ /_____.
oste/o/sarc/oma os´ tē ō sar cō´ mə	

ANSWER COLUMN	

	3.14
	myel/o is a combining form used to mean the bone marrow or the spinal cord. A condition characterized by increased and abnormal bone marrow development is myel/o/dys/plasia:
	    myel/o—bone marrow or spinal cord
	    dys-—prefix for difficult or poor
	    -plasia—suffix for growth and development
	When you see **myel/o**, read further to see whether it refers to

spinal cord, bone marrow	* _____ or * _____.
encephal/o/myel/o/pathy en sef´ ə lō mī el **op**´ ə thē oste/o/myel/itis os´ tē ō mī e **li**´ tis myel/o/dys/plasia mī´ el ō dis **plā**´ zha	**3.15** Any disease of the brain and spinal cord is called _____ / ____ / _____ / ____ / _____. Inflammation of the bone and marrow is called _____ / ____ / _____ / _____. Defective formation of the spinal cord is called _____ / ____ / _____ / _____.
arthr/o/scope är´ thrō skōp	**3.16** **arthr/o** is the combining form for joint. An instrument used to look at something is a **-scope**. An instrument used to look into a joint is an _____ / ____ / _____.
bone marrow germ cell myel/o	**3.17** Find the word myeloblast in your dictionary. Write the meaning here. * _____ The combining form of **myel** is _____ / ____.
myel/o/cyt/ic mī´ el ō **sit**´ ik myel/o/cele **mī**´ el ō sēl	**3.18** Find a word meaning pertaining to myelocytes _____ / ____ / _____ / ____; herniation of the spinal cord _____ / ____ / _____.
defective (poor or abnormal) formation defective formation of a joint	**3.19** **-plas/ia** means development or formation. This kind of formation occurs naturally instead of being done by a plastic surgeon. Hyper/plasia is an increase in the number of cells in a tissue (i.e., tumor). **dys-** means defective. Dys/plas/ia means * _____. Arthr/o/dys/plasia means * _____.

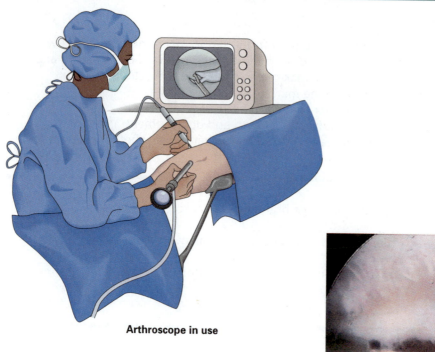

Arthroscope in use

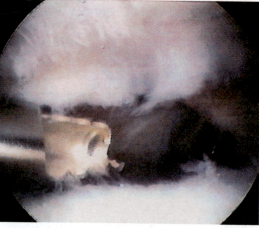

Internal view of of knee through arthroscope

ANSWER COLUMN	
myel/o/dys/plasia mī´ ə lō dis **plā**´ zhə	**3.20** Build a term that means defective (abnormal) formation of the spinal cord: _____ /_____ /_____ /_____ (body part + disorder).
hyper/plasia hī per **plā**´ zhə	**3.21** A/plasia means failure of an organ to develop properly. A word that means overgrowth or too much development is _____ /_____.
hypo/plasia hī pō **plā**´ zhə	**3.22** **Hypo-** is the opposite of **hyper-**. If excessive development is hyperplasia, deficient development is expressed as _____ /_____.

Normal size and number

Hyperplasia increased numbers

Hypertrophy increased size

Hypertrophy and hyperplasia

Dysplasia

Hyperplasia, hypertrophy, dysplasia

ANSWER COLUMN	
arthr/o/scopy är **thros´** kō pē	**3.23** Arthro is the combining form for joint. The name of the procedure for examining the joints by looking with an arthroscope is called _____ /____ /_____.
Arthr/o/plasty är´ thrō plas´ tē	**3.24** _____ /____ /_____ means surgical repair of a joint. **-plasty** means surgical repair.
surgical repair or reconstruction	**3.25** *TAKE A CLOSER LOOK* Plastic surgery has nothing to do with plastic (the material). The word root **plast** means form, mold, or rebuild. Think of a plast/ic surgeon building a new nose or molding a face. This is surgical reconstruction. The suffix **-plasty** means *_____.
arthroplasty	**3.26** Arthr/o/plasty may take many forms. When a joint has lost its ability to move, movement can sometimes be restored by an _____.
arthr/itis är **thrī´** tis arthr/itic är **thrī´** tik	**3.27** Arthr/itic means pertaining to a joint. Form a word that means inflammation of a joint: _____ /_____. A medication used to treat arthritis is an anti/_____ /_____ agent.
oste/o/arthr/itis os tē ō är **thrī´** tis	**3.28** Arthritis characterized by inflammation and destruction of bone and joint tissue is called _____ /____ /_____ /_____ (OA).

ANSWER COLUMN	
arthritis	**3.29** Rheumatoid arthritis (RA) (*rheumatoid* is Greek for resembling discharge fluid) affects the softer tissues of the joint. RA still causes inflammation of the joint or _____.
arthr/o/tomy är **throt**´ ə mē	**3.30** You're getting to be pretty good at this, aren't you? Form a word that means incision into a joint: _____ /_____ /_____.
💡 INFORMATION FRAME	**3.31** In Latin *tendo* means to stretch. Tendons are made of connective tissue and attach muscle to bone. Ligaments attach bone to bone and fascia attaches muscle to muscle.

tend/o/plasty
ten´ dō plas tē
ten/o/plasty
ten´ ō plas tē
tendin/o/plasty
ten´ din ō plas tē
	3.32 **ten/o**, **tend/o**, and **tendin/o** are all combining forms for tendon. Use your dictionary to help you. Build three terms meaning repair of the tendons:
	    _____ /_____ /_____,
	    _____ /_____ /_____, and
	    _____ /_____ /_____.

tendon/itis **ten**´ don ī´ tis tendin/itis **ten**´ din ī´ tis	**3.33** **tendon/o** and **tendin/o** are used to build words about inflammation of the tendons. Inflammation of a tendon is _____ /_____ or _____ /_____.
ten/algia ten **al**´ jē ə ten/o/dynia **ten**´ ō **din**´ ē ə	**3.34** **ten/o** is used to build the terms for pain in a tendon. Two terms for tendon pain are _____ /_____ and _____ /_____ /_____.

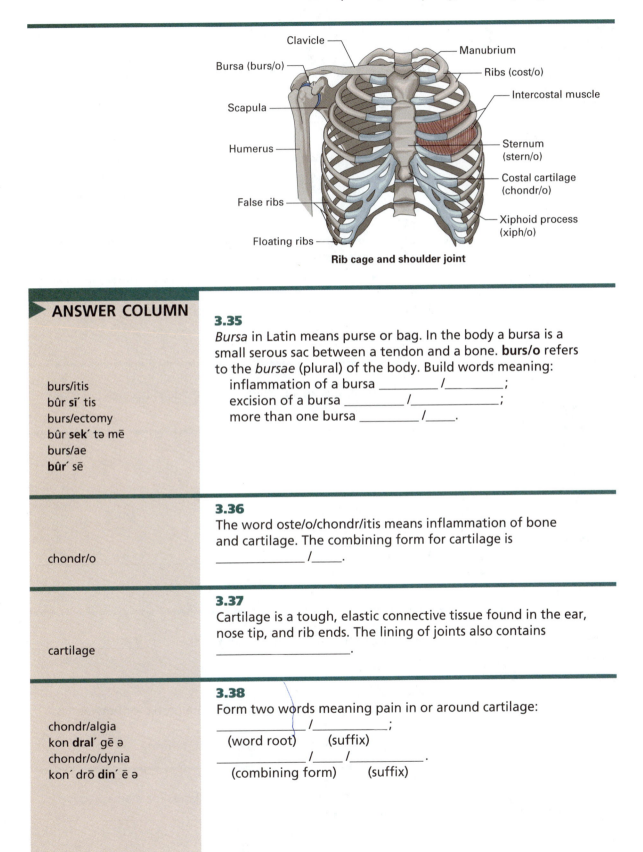

Clavicle

Bursa (burs/o)

Scapula

Humerus

False ribs

Floating ribs

Manubrium

Ribs (cost/o)

Intercostal muscle

Sternum
(stern/o)

Costal cartilage
(chondr/o)

Xiphoid process
(xiph/o)

Rib cage and shoulder joint

ANSWER COLUMN	
	3.35 *Bursa* in Latin means purse or bag. In the body a bursa is a small serous sac between a tendon and a bone. **burs/o** refers to the *bursae* (plural) of the body. Build words meaning:
burs/itis bûr **sī´** tis burs/ectomy bûr **sek´** tə mē burs/ae **bûr´** sē	inflammation of a bursa _____ /_____; excision of a bursa _____ /_____; more than one bursa _____ /____.
	3.36 The word oste/o/chondr/itis means inflammation of bone and cartilage. The combining form for cartilage is
chondr/o	_____ /____.
	3.37 Cartilage is a tough, elastic connective tissue found in the ear, nose tip, and rib ends. The lining of joints also contains
cartilage	_____.
	3.38 Form two words meaning pain in or around cartilage:
chondr/algia kon **dral´** gē ə chondr/o/dynia kon´ drō **din´** ē ə	_____ /_____; (word root) (suffix) _____ /____ /_____. (combining form) (suffix)

▶ **ANSWER COLUMN**

ten/o/plasty **ten**′ ō plast tē ten/o/dynia ten′ ō **din**′ ē ə	**3.39** Use **ten/o** to build words meaning: repair of tendons _____ /____ /_____ ; pain in tendons _____ /____ /_____ .
excision of cartilage	**3.40** Chondr/ectomy means *_____ .
ribs	**3.41** Chondr/o/cost/al means pertaining to ribs and cartilage. **cost/o** is used in words about the _____ .
cost/ectomy kos **tek**′ tə mē	**3.42** Form a word that means excision of a rib or ribs: _____ /_____ .
adjective	**3.43** Chondr/o/cost/al is an adjective. This is evident because -al is the ending for an _____ .
chondr/o cost al chondr/o/cost/al kon′ drō **kos**′ təl pertaining to cartilage and ribs	**3.44** Analyze chondr/o/cost/al: _____ /____ cartilage; _____ rib; ____ suffix. Now put them together: _____ /____ /_____ /____ . This means *_____ .
cost/al **kos**′ təl	**3.45** Form a word that means pertaining to the ribs: _____ /____ .
inter	**3.46** Inter/cost/al means between the ribs. The prefix for between is _____ . **EXAMPLE:** International means between nations.
inter/chondr/al in′ tər **kon**′ drəl	**3.47** Hypo/chondr/iac means below the cartilage. Form an adjective that means between cartilages: _____ /_____ /al.

ANSWER COLUMN	
	3.48 Inter/cost/al means between the ribs. inter- is the prefix that means _____ .
between	
	3.49 Inter/cost/al may refer to the muscles between the ribs. The muscles that move the ribs when breathing are the _____ /_____ /_____ muscles.
inter/cost/al in´ tər **kos**´ təl	
	3.50 The external intercostal muscles assist with inhalation by enlarging the rib cage. The internal intercostal muscles assist with breathing out by decreasing the size of the rib cage. Breathing is assisted by the _____ muscles.
intercostal	
	3.51 Inter/dent/al means between the teeth. The word root for tooth is _____ .
dent	

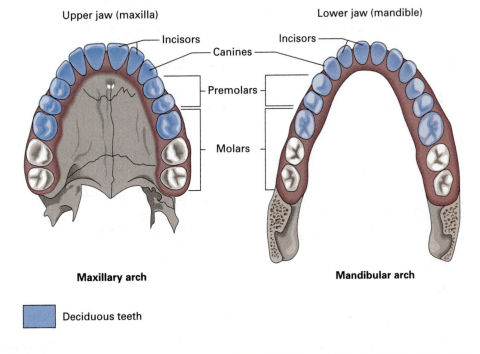

Upper jaw (maxilla)   Lower jaw (mandible)

Incisors   Incisors
Canines
Premolars
Molars

Maxillary arch   **Mandibular arch**

Deciduous teeth

	3.52 Form an adjective that means pertaining to the teeth: _____ /_____ .
dent/al **den**´ təl	

ANSWER COLUMN	
dent/algia den **tal**´ jē ə	**3.53** Pain in the teeth, or a toothache, is called _____ /_____.
dent/oid **den**´ toid	**3.54** Great! Try this: **-oid** is the suffix that means like or resembling. Form a word that means tooth shaped or resembling a tooth: _____ /_____.
teeth teeth	**3.55** A dent/ist (DDS) takes care of _____. A dent/ifrice is used for cleaning _____.
orth/odont/ist ôr´ thō **don**´ tist	**3.56** **orth/o** is a combining form taken from the Greek word *orthos,* meaning straight. **odont/o** means shaped like a tooth. A dentist who specializes in straightening abnormally positioned teeth is called an _____ /_____ /_____.
around or near	**3.57** **peri-** is a prefix meaning around or near. Peri/odont/al disease is diseased tissue *_____ the teeth.
peri/odont/al pair´ ē ō **don**´ tal	**3.58** A periodontist may perform surgery of the gums or tissues around the teeth. This is _____ /_____ /_____ surgery.

peri/oste/um
pair´ ē **os**´ tē əm
peri/chondr/ium
pair´ ē **kon**´ drē əm
peri/cardi/um
pair´ ē **kar**´ dē əm
	3.59
	Build terms meaning
	   the membrane around the bone:
	   _____ /_____ /um;
	   the membrane around the cartilage:
	   _____ /_____ /ium;
	   the membrane around the heart:
	   _____ /_____ /um.

orth/o	**3.60** An orth/o/ped/ist (ōr thō **pēd**´ ist) is a physician who specializes in the prevention and treatment of musculoskeletal disorders. The combining form indicating that "straightening" may be done is _____ /____.

ANSWER COLUMN

orth/o/ped/ist
ôr´ thō **pēd**´ ist

3.61
A person with a fractured (broken, Fx) bone or a joint injury would be treated by an _____ /_____ /_____ /_____.

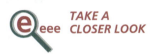

TAKE A CLOSER LOOK

orth/o/sis, orth/o/tic
ôr **thō**´ sis, ôr **tho**´ tik
prosthet/ist
pros´ the tist
prosthet/ic
pros **the**´ tik

3.62
Orth/o/tics is the science in which one studies and develops mechanical appliances used as supportive devices. The specialist who designs and fits these devices is called an orth/o/tist. This practice is closely related to the prosthet/ists who work with patients in need of replacing an amputated limb. The appliance the prosthet/ist produces is called a prosthesis. Look in the "ortho" and "prosth" sections of your dictionary to find the word that means devices used to stabilize or prevent deformity:
_____ /_____ /_____;
specialist in making artificial body parts:
_____ /_____;
pertaining to (adjective) a prosthesis:
_____ /_____.

Direction	Prefix	Word root/ Suffix
below	hypo	chondr/iac
upon	epi	gastr/ic
above	supra	lumb/ar
below	hypo	gastr/ic

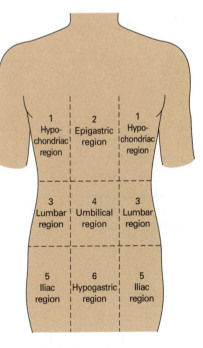

Thorax and regions of the abdomen

ANSWER COLUMN	
	3.63 **lumb/o** builds words about the lower back. Lumb/ar is the adjectival form. An adjective meaning pertaining to the lower back is _____ /_____.
lumb/ar **lum**´ bər, **lum**´ bär	
lumbar	**3.64** There are five lumbar vertebrae. Low back pain is called _____ pain.
lumbar	**3.65** There is also a reflex called the _____ reflex.
adjective pertaining to the chest and lower back or something near this	**3.66** **thorac/o** is the combining form for chest or thorax. Thorac/o/lumb/ar is a(n) (choose one) _____ (noun/adjective) meaning **_____.
INFORMATION FRAME	**3.67** supra- is a prefix that means on, higher in position, over, or above.
supra	**3.68** Supra/lumb/ar means above the lumbar region. A prefix that means above is _____.
above the lumbar region or above the lower back	**3.69** Supra/lumb/ar means *_____.
above the ribs	**3.70** Supra/cost/al means *_____.
on top of	**3.71** Supra/crani/al refers to the surface of the head *_____ the skull.
noun	**3.72** The pubis is a bone of the pelvis. Pub/is is a (choose one) _____ (noun/adjective).
pubis pubic	**3.73** From **pub/o** form a noun _____; an adjective _____. (See the illustration in Unit 14.)

ANSWER COLUMN	
pub/is py$\overline{oo}$′ bis	**3.74** The pub/ic bone is also called the _____ /____.
pubis	**3.75** Supra/pub/ic means above the pubis. **pub/o** is used in words about the _____.
supra/pub/ic s$\overline{oo}$′ prə **py$\overline{oo}$**′ bik	**3.76** The suprapubic region is above the arch of the pub/is. When the bladder is incised above the pubis, an incision is made in the _____ /_____ /_____ region.
suprapubic incision region	**3.77** "The incision is made in the suprapubic region." From this sentence pick out the adjective _____; two nouns _____ , _____.

anything close to incision
  of bladder from the
  suprapubic region
	3.78
	Try to figure out what surgery is done in a supra/pub/ic cyst/o/tomy *_____
	_____.

pelv/is pel′ vis pelves pel′ vēs	**3.79** The pelv/is is formed by the pelv/ic bones. **pelv/i** refers to the _____ /____ (noun). The plural of pelvis is _____.
pelv/i/metry pel **vim**′ ə trē	**3.80** Pelv/i/metry is done during pregnancy to find the measurements of the pelvis. To find a woman's pelvic size, the physician does _____ /____ /_____.
pelvimetry	**3.81** Look up pelvimetry or pelvis in your dictionary. Taking pelvic measurements is called _____.

ANSWER COLUMN	
	3.82 Cephal/o/pelvic disproportion (CPD) may lead to serious complications during delivery. A physician may determine whether or not a woman will have trouble during labor by doing
pelvimetry	_____.
pelv/i/meter pel **vim**´ ə tər	**3.83** Look in the dictionary for a word that names the device used for pelvimetry. It is a _____ /____ /_____.
cephal/o/pelv/ic cef´ əl ō **pel**´ vik	**3.84** A pelvimeter measures the diameter of the pelvis. When the head (**cephal/o**) of the fetus is larger than the diameter of the mother's pelvis (**pelv/o**), this is called _____ /____ /_____ /____ disproportion (CPD).
supra/pelv/ic soo´ prə **pel**´ vik	**3.85** The adjective meaning *above* the pelvis is _____ /_____ /____.
instrument instrument	**3.86** -meter is a suffix meaning an instrument used to measure. A speed/o/meter is an _____ to measure speed. A pelv/i/meter is an _____ to measure the pelvis.
measures (counts) measures thorac/o/meter thôr´ ə **kom**´ ə tər cardi/o/meter kär´ dē **om**´ ə tər	**3.87** A cyt/o/meter _____ cells. A cephal/o/meter _____ the head. A thorac/o/_____ measures the chest. A cardi/o/_____ measures the heart.
pre	**3.88** Ab/norm/al is a word that means deviating (turning away) from what is normal. ab- is a _____ /fix that means from or away from.
away from	**3.89** Abnormal is used as an ordinary English word. Abnormal means *_____ normal.
from or away from	**3.90** ab- is a prefix that means *_____.

► **ANSWER COLUMN**

wandering from (the normal course of events)	**3.91** Ab/errant uses the prefix ab- before the English word (errant) for wandering. Ab/errant means *_____. **NOTE:** Think of an error.
ab/errant ab **air**′ ənt	**3.92** Ab/errant is used in medicine to describe a structure that wanders from the normal. When some nerve fibers follow an unusual route, they form an _____ /_____ nerve.
aberrant	**3.93** Aberrant nerves wander from the normal nerve track. Blood vessels that follow a path of their own are _____ vessels.
aberrant	**3.94** Lymph vessels may be found in unexpected areas of the body. They follow an _____ course.
ab/duct/ion ab **duk**′ shun	**3.95** In Latin *ducere* (word root: **duct**) means to lead or move. Ab/duct/ion means movement away from a midline. When the arm is raised away from the side of the body, _____ /_____ /_____ has occurred.
abduction	**3.96** Abduction can occur from any midline. When the fingers of the hand are spread apart, _____ has occurred in four fingers.
abducted	**3.97** A child who has been kidnapped and taken away from home has been _____ (past tense verb).
ad/duct/ion ə **duk**′ shən ad/duct a **dukt**′	**3.98** ad- is a prefix meaning toward. Movement toward a midline is _____ /_____ /_____ (noun). When a patient is asked to move his arm toward his body, he is asked to _____ /_____ (verb) his arm.
ad/dict/ion ə **dik**′ shən	**3.99** Ad/diction means being drawn toward some habit. The person who takes drugs habitually suffers from drug _____ /_____ /_____.

ANSWER COLUMN	
addiction	**3.100** Addiction implies habit. Alcoholism is an _____ to alcohol.
addict	**3.101** A person addicted to drugs is a drug addict. A person addicted to cocaine is a cocaine _____.
ad/hes/ion ad **hē´** zhən	**3.102** An ad/hes/ion is formed when two normally separate tissues join together. They adhere to each other. Adhering to another part forms an ____ /_____ /_____.
adhesions	**3.103** Patients are usually encouraged to ambulate soon after surgery to help prevent postoperative _____.
adhesions	**3.104** Pain or intestinal obstruction may be caused by abdominal _____.
ab/domen **ab´** də mən	**3.105** **abdomin/o** is used to form words about the abdomen. When you see **abdomin/o** any place in a word, you think about the _____ /_____.
✔ **SPELL CHECK**	**3.106** In the spelling of the combining form for abdomen, the "e" changes to "i"—**abdomin/o**. **EXAMPLE:** The abdominal incision was made in the RLQ of the abdomen.
pertaining to the abdomen	**3.107** Abdomin/al is an adjective that means *_____. **NOTE:** For descriptive reference the abdomen may be divided into four quadrants including the right upper quadrant (RUQ), the left upper quadrant (LUQ), the right lower quadrant (RLQ), and the left lower quadrant (LLQ)

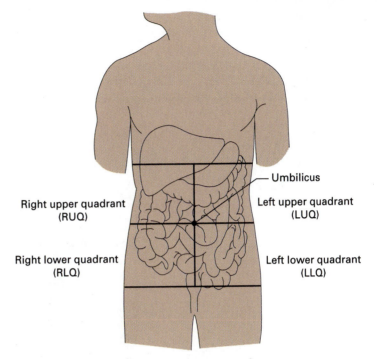

Right upper quadrant
(RUQ)

Umbilicus

Left upper quadrant
(LUQ)

Right lower quadrant
(RLQ)

Left lower quadrant
(LLQ)

Abdomen divided into quadrants

ANSWER COLUMN	
the insertion of a needle into a body cavity for the purpose of aspirating fluid	**3.108** Look up the words paracentesis and centesis in your dictionary. Write the definition here: ** _____ _____. NOTE: p. abdominal is paracentesis of the abdomen or abdominocentesis.
abdomin/o/centesis ab dom´ i nō sen tē´ sis	**3.109** Abdomin/o/centesis means tapping or puncture of the abdomen. This is a surgical puncture for the removal of fluid. The word for surgical puncture of the abdomen is _____ /_____ /_____.
abdominocentesis	**3.110** Centesis (surgical puncture) is a word in itself used as a suffix. Build a word meaning surgical puncture, or tapping of the abdomen: _____.

▶ **ANSWER COLUMN**

3.111
amni/o refers to the amnion, the protective sac that surrounds the fetus. Tapping or puncturing this sac to remove cells for genetic testing is called _____ /_____ /_____.

amni/o/centesis
am′ nē ō sen **tē**′ sis

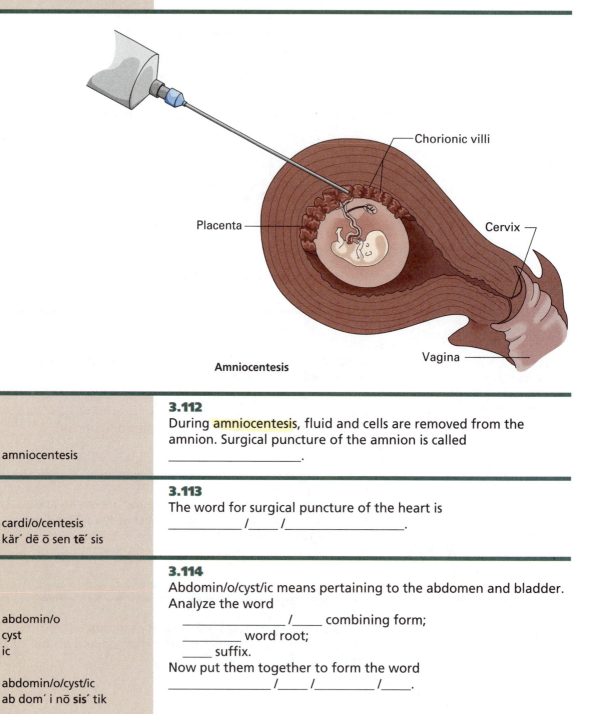

—Chorionic villi

Placenta—

Cervix ⌐

Vagina —

Amniocentesis

3.112
During <mark>amniocentesis</mark>, fluid and cells are removed from the amnion. Surgical puncture of the amnion is called _____.

amniocentesis

3.113
The word for surgical puncture of the heart is _____ /_____ /_____.

cardi/o/centesis
kär′ dē ō sen **tē**′ sis

3.114
Abdomin/o/cyst/ic means pertaining to the abdomen and bladder. Analyze the word
_____ /_____ combining form;
_____ word root;
_____ suffix.
Now put them together to form the word
_____ /_____ /_____ /_____.

abdomin/o
cyst
ic

abdomin/o/cyst/ic
ab dom′ i nō **sis**′ tik

▶ **ANSWER COLUMN**	
cyst	**3.115** From abdomin/o/cyst/ic you see that the word root for bladder is _____ .
urinary bladder	**3.116** **cyst/o** is used to form words that refer to the urinary _____ .
cyst/o/tomy sis **tot´** ə mē	**3.117** The word for incision into the urinary bladder is _____ /_____ /_____ .
cyst/ectomy sis **tek´** tə mē	**3.118** The word for excision of the urinary bladder is _____ /_____ .
cyst/o/scopy sis **tos´** cō pē	**3.119** Recall that **-scopy** is a suffix for the procedure used to look into an organ or body cavity. The process of examining by looking with an instrument into the urinary bladder is _____ /_____ /_____ .
urinary bladder	**3.120** A cyst/o/scop/ic (Cysto) exam is used to look inside the *_____ .
cyst/o/plasty **sis´** tō plas´ tē	**3.121** Surgical repair of the bladder is _____ /_____ /_____ .
cystocele	**3.122** When the bladder herniates into the vagina, a _____ is formed.
thorac/ic thô **ras´** ik	**3.123** **thorac/o** is used to form words about the thorax or chest. A word that means pertaining to the chest is _____ /_____ . See the illustration of body cavities on the next page.
thoraces **thôr´** ə sēs	**3.124** The plural form of thorax is _____ .

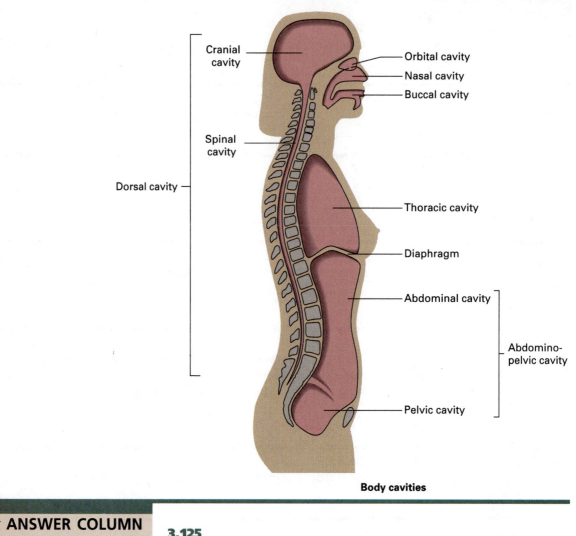

Cranial cavity

Orbital cavity

Nasal cavity

Buccal cavity

Spinal cavity

Dorsal cavity

Thoracic cavity

Diaphragm

Abdominal cavity

Abdomino-pelvic cavity

Pelvic cavity

Body cavities

▶ **ANSWER COLUMN**

3.125

Abdomin/o/thorac/ic means pertaining to the abdomen and thorax. The thorax is the chest. Supply the word parts for

abdomin/o
thorac
ic

_____ /_____ abdomen;
_____ thorax;
____ suffix—pertaining to.
Now put them together to form

abdomin/o/thorac/ic
ab dom´ i nō thô **ras´** ik

_____ /_____ /_____ /_____.

3.126

Abdomin/o/thorac/ic pain means, literally, pain in the abdomen and chest. A physician who wants to say that there were lesions in

abdominothoracic

these areas could call them _____ lesions.

► ANSWER COLUMN	**3.127** An incision may be made in the chest to insert a chest tube for the purpose of draining blood and fluid from the lung. A word that means incision of the chest is _____ /_____ /_____.
thorac/o/tomy thôr´ ə **kot´** ə mē	
thorac/o/centesis thôr´ ə kō sen **tē´** sis	**3.128** A word that means surgical tapping (puncture) of the chest to remove fluids is _____ /_____ /_____.
☑ SPELL CHECK	**3.129** Usually, thoracocentesis is shortened to thoracentesis (thôr´ ə sen **tē´** sis). Find out which form is used by your local hospital.
thorac/o/pathy thôr´ ə **kop´** ə thē	**3.130** A word that means any chest disease is _____ /_____ /_____.
thorac/o/lumbar thôr´ ak ō **lum´** bar	**3.131** Build a term meaning pertaining to the thoracic and lumbar vertebrae: _____ /_____ /_____.
head bladder	**3.132** Recall the meaning of the following word parts: **cephal/o** _____; **cyst/o** _____.
water or fluid or watery fluid	**3.133** A hydro/cyst is a sac (or bladder) filled with watery fluid. **hydro-** is used as a prefix in words to mean *_____. **NOTE:** Think of a fire hydrant.
hydro/cele **hi´** drō sēl	**3.134** An accumulation of fluid in a saclike cavity, especially in the scrotum, is called a hydro/cele. Two- to five-year-old boys are the most likely ones to develop this fluid-filled saclike swelling in the scrotum called a _____ /_____.
hydrocele	**3.135** A hydrocyst and a hydrocele are both fluid-filled sacs. The more specific term used to name the common condition found in infant and young boys is _____.

ANSWER COLUMN	
	3.136 Hydro/cephalus is characterized by an enlarged head due to increased amount of fluid in the skull. A collection of fluid in the head is called _____ /_____.
hydro/cephalus hī´ drō **sef´** ə ləs	
Hydrocephalus	**3.137** Hydrocephalus, unless arrested, results in deformity. The face seems small. The eyes are abnormal. The head is large. _____ also causes brain damage.
hydrocephalus	**3.138** Because of the damage to the brain, children with _____ are usually mentally retarded.
Hydro/cephal/ic hī´ dro se **fal´** ik	**3.139** Hydrocephalus is the noun. The adjectival suffix is **-ic**. _____ /_____ /_____ children can be seen in schools for the mentally impaired.
abnormal fear hydrophobia	**3.140** **-phobia**, from the Greek word for fear, is used as a suffix meaning any *_____. Build a word meaning abnormal fear of water: _____.
between three and twelve hydro/phobia hī´ drō **fō´** bē ə	**3.141** In a dictionary find the word phobia. It may list more than 100. How many phobias do you recognize already? **_____. An abnormal fear of water is _____ /_____.
hydrophobia	**3.142** If a person is bitten by a dog with rabies, he or she may contract rabies, which is also called _____ (so named because rabid animals are afraid of choking while drinking and will not drink water).
hydro/therapy hī´ drō **ther´** ə pē	**3.143** Therapy means treatment. Treatment by water (H_2O) is _____ /_____.
hydrotherapy	**3.144** Physical therapists (PTs) use swirling water baths to increase ease of movement. This is called _____.

Abbreviation	Meaning
AOA	American Osteopathic Association
CPD	cephalopelvic disproportion
CXR	chest x-ray
Cysto	cystoscopy
DDS	doctor of dental surgery (dentist)
DO	doctor of osteopathy
DTs	delirium tremens
FAS	fetal alcohol syndrome
Fx	fracture
H_2O	water
LLQ	left lower quadrant (abdomen)
LUQ	left upper quadrant (abdomen)
OMT	osteopathic manipulative therapy
ORTHO (ORTH)	orthopedics (orthopedist)
PT	physical therapy (therapist)
RA	rheumatoid arthritis
RLQ	right lower quadrant (abdomen)
RUQ	right upper quadrant (abdomen)

To complete your study of this unit, work the review activities on the next pages. Also, listen to the audiotapes that accompany *Medical Terminology: A Programmed Text,* 8th edition, and practice your pronunciation.

Additional practice exercises for this unit are available on the Student Practice disk found in the back of the textbook.

▶ REVIEW ACTIVITIES

Circle and Correct

Circle the correct answer for each question. Then, check your answers in Appendix A.

1. Word root for bone:
   a. calci   b. ortho
   c. oste   d. osteo

2. Combining form for joint:
   a. arther   b. artero
   c. arthero   d. arthro

3. Suffix for instrument used to look:
   a. -scope   b. -scopy
   c. -graph   d. -scopic

4. Combining form for tendon:
   a. chondro   b. teno
   c. tendonitis   d. tendon

5. Word root for rib:
   a. costal   b. chondr
   c. cost   d. ribo

6. Prefix for between:
   a. inter-   b. intra-
   c. peri-   d. endo-

7. Combining form for tooth:
   a. toid   b. dentin
   c. dontia   d. dento

8. Combining form for straight:
   a. oto   b. ortho
   c. donto   d. oligo

9. Prefix for above:
   a. inter-   b. hypo-
   c. supra-   d. infra-

10. Suffix for the process of measuring:
    a. -metro   b. -meter
    c. -metr   d. -metry

11. Prefix meaning toward:
    a. ab-   b. hyper-
    c. in-   d. ad-

12. Adjective for bladder or sac:
    a. cystosis   b. cystic
    c. cytic   d. cystal

13. Word root for move or lead:
    a. mor   b. domin
    c. duct   d. go

14. Adjective suffix:
    a. -ous   b. -ia
    c. -us   d. -sis

15. Combining form for abdomen:
    a. abdomen/o   b. stomat/o
    c. stomach/o   d. abdomin/o

▶ REVIEW ACTIVITIES

Select and Construct
Select the correct word parts from the list below and construct medical terms that represent the given meaning.

ab	abdomin(o)	ad	al	amni/o
arthr(o)	cele	centesis	cephal(ic)(o)	chondr(o)
cost	cyst	dent(o)	dont(o)	duct
errant	hydro	inter	ist	itis
lumb(o)(ar)	malacia	metr/o(y)(ic)(er)	oma	orth(o)
oste(o)	osteopathy	pelv/i(o)	phobia	plasty
pubo(is)(ic)	sarc(o)	scope(y)(ic)	supra	tendin(o)
tendon	tendon(o)	ten/o	therapy	thorac(o)(ic)
(t)ion				

1. softening of the bone _____
2. movement away from the body _____
3. water-filled sac _____
4. water on the brain (adjective) _____
5. above the pubic bone _____
6. between the ribs _____
7. surgical puncture of the abdomen _____
8. process of looking into a joint _____
9. wandering in an abnormal path _____
10. specialist in straightening teeth _____
11. inflammation of the cord that connects muscle to bone _____
12. instrument to measure the pelvis _____
13. pertaining to the head and pelvis _____
14. bone and joint specialist _____
15. bone cancer _____

Now, on your own, use the word parts list above to construct other medical terms.

16. _____ word   _____ meaning
17. _____ word   _____ meaning
18. _____ word   _____ meaning
19. _____ word   _____ meaning
20. _____ word   _____ meaning

► REVIEW ACTIVITIES

Define and Dissect
Give a brief definition and dissect each term listed into its word parts in the space provided on the right. Check your answers by referring to the frame listed in parentheses and your medical dictionary. Then, listen to the audiotapes to practice pronunciation.

1. osteomalacia (3.3)

   _____ / ____ / _____ / _____
       rt   v   rt   suffix

   _____
                definition

2. osteoarthropathy (3.10)

   _____ / ___ / _____ / ___ / _____
      rt   v   rt   v   suffix

3. arthroscopy (3.23)

   _____ / ____ / _____
         rt   v   suffix

4. tendoplasty (3.32)

   _____ / ____ / _____
         rt   v   suffix

5. chondralgia (3.38)

   _____ / _____
           rt   suffix

6. intercostal (3.49)

   _____ / _____ / _____
         rt   rt   suffix

7. orthodontist (3.54)

   _____ / _____ / _____
       rt   rt   suffix

8. suprapubic (3.76)

   _____ / _____ / _____
         pre   rt   suffix

9. thoracolumbar (3.131)

   _____ / ___ / _____ / _____
       rt   v   rt   suffix

10. pelvimetry (3.80)

    _____ / ____ / _____
          rt   v   suffix

11. aberrant (3.92)

    _____ / _____
        pre   rt

12. adduction (3.98)

    _____ / _____ / _____
        pre   rt   suffix

13. amniocentesis (3.111)

    _____ / ____ / _____
         rt   v   rt/suffix

▶ REVIEW ACTIVITIES

14. abdominocystic (3.114)

_____ / ____ / _____ / _____
rt   v   rt   suffix

15. thoracotomy (3.127)

_____ / ____ / _____
rt   v   suffix

16. hydrocephalus (3.136)

_____ / _____
pre   rt/suffix

17. hydrophobia (3.141)

_____ / _____
pre   rt/suffix

18. orthopedist (3.61)

_____ / ____ / _____ / _____
rt   v   rt   suffix

19. hypochondriac (3.47)

_____ / _____ / _____
pre   rt   suffix

20. cephalopelvic (3.84)

_____ / ____ / _____ / _____
rt   v   rt   suffix

21. cystoscopy (3.119)

_____ / ____ / _____
rt   v   suffix

22. adhesion (3.102)

____ / _____ / _____
pre   rt   suffix

23. bursectomy (3.35)

_____ / _____
rt   suffix

24. tendinitis (3.33)

_____ / _____
rt   suffix

25. osteosarcoma (3.13)

_____ / ____ / _____ / _____
rt   v   rt   suffix

26. orthotic (3.62)

_____ / ____ / _____
rt   v   suffix

27. prosthetist (3.62)

_____ / _____
rt   suffix

28. hydrocele (3.134)

_____ / _____
pre   suffix

► **REVIEW ACTIVITIES**

Abbreviation Matching
Match the following abbreviations with their definition.

_____ 1. CPD	a. cerebropulmonary disease
_____ 2. LLQ	b. fracture
_____ 3. OA	c. fetal alcohol syndrome
_____ 4. H₂O	d. cephalopelvic disproportion
_____ 5. DO	e. left upper quadrant
_____ 6. Fx	f. hydrogen
_____ 7. Cysto	g. orthopedist
_____ 8. RA	h. osteoarthritis
_____ 9. PT	i. right abdomen
_____ 10. FAS	j. bladder
	k. rheumatoid arthritis
	l. physician therapist
	m. cystoscopy
	n. left lower quadrant
	o. physical therapist
	p. water
	q. doctor of dental surgery
	r. doctor of osteopathy

Abbreviation Fill-ins
Fill in the blanks with the correct abbreviations.

11. An alcoholic experiencing withdrawal symptoms may get the _____.

12. The liver is located in the _____ of the abdomen.

13. DOs may use _____ as treatment to relieve back pain.

14. A dentist is indicated by the abbreviation _____.

15. The department that cares for patients with bone fractures is _____.

▶ CASE STUDIES

Write the term next to its meaning given below. Then, draw slashes to analyze the word parts. Note the use of medical abbreviations. Look these up in your dictionary or find them in Appendix B. If you have any questions about the answers, refer to your medical dictionary or check with your instructor for the answers in Appendix A.

CASE STUDY 3-1
REPORT SUMMARY

Preoperative diagnosis: Septic arthritis of the left knee

Orthopedic procedure: Arthroscopic examination, culture, arthroplasty left knee

A large bore cannula was introduced from the upper and medial quadrant of the knee joint through a stab incision (arthrotomy). The trocar was removed and pyorrhea was observed. A swab was sent for culture. All pus was aspirated and the knee joint irrigated then inflated with 3 L of saline. The arthroscope was introduced through the inferior lateral quadrant of the knee through a similar stab incision. The knee was inspected and everything looked inflamed. The patella showed grade II chondromalacia and the patella was tilted only in contact with the lateral condyle at about 30 degrees suggesting chronic patellar malalignment. The medial meniscus showed evidence of much more inflammation than the condyle, the margins thick, and fraying. … The scope was moved to the mediolateral side and inspected. … A motorized synovial cutter was introduced and a partial synovectomy was performed, the soft cartilage of the patellar facets were shaved off. The end of the meniscus was trimmed (meniscectomy). The wound was irrigated with saline, Maracaine instilled, and a hemovac drain inserted through one of the cannulas before the instruments were removed. A padded dressing and knee immobilizer was applied and hemovac attached to its bag. The patient was transferred to the recovery room in excellent condition.

1. reddened and swollen   _____

2. instrument used to look into a joint   _____

3. pertaining to the middle and side   _____

4. excision of the meniscus   _____

5. softening of the cartilage   _____

6. inflammation of a joint   _____

7. pertaining to the use of an arthroscope _____

8. kneecap   _____

9. pertaining to bone specialty   _____

10. middle   _____

11. discharge of pus   _____

12. cut into   _____

13. incision into a joint   _____

14. surgical repair of a joint   _____

▶ CROSSWORD PUZZLE

Check your answers by going back through the frames or checking the solution in Appendix C.

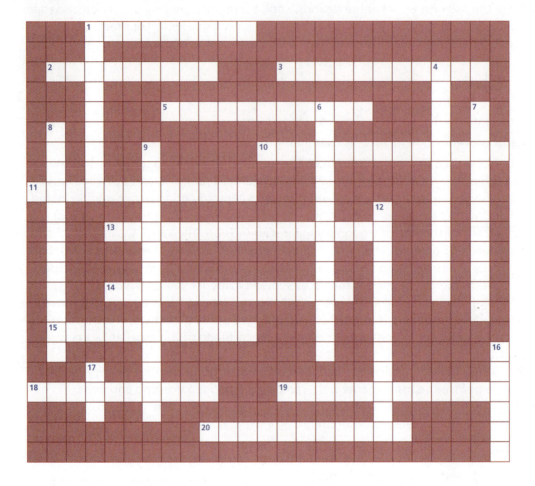

Across

1. tissues growing together that normally do not
2. pertaining to the abdomen
3. tissue around the teeth
5. physician (DO)
10. synonym for tenoplasty
11. excision of cartilage
13. surgical puncture to remove fluid from chest
14. pertaining to ribs and cartilage
15. area above the lower back or waist
18. inflamed tendon
19. bone cancer
20. person who develops artificial limbs

Down

1. raising arm to the side away from the middle
4. used to measure chest circumference
6. enlarged head due to fluid (congenital)
7. process of examining a joint with a scope
8. specialist in straightening teeth
9. defective development of bone marrow
12. condition of porous bones
16. suffix for development
17. dentist (abbreviation)

▶ GLOSSARY

abdomen	belly area, cavity below the thorax
abdominocentesis	surgical puncture of the abdomen to remove fluid
abduct	move away from the midline (verb)
abduction	movement away from the midline, e.g., arm abducted from side
aberrant	wandering from normal location, process, or behavior
abnormal	deviating from the average or expected
addiction	habitual attraction, may include physical dependence
adhesions	tissues grown together that are normally separate
amniocentesis	surgical puncture of the amnion to obtain cells for testing
arthritis	inflammation of a joint
arthroplasty	surgical repair or reconstruction of a joint
arthroscope	instrument used to look into a joint
arthoscopy	process of using an arthroscope to examine a joint
arthrotomy	incision into a joint
bursa	serous sac between a tendon and bone (bursae: plural)
bursectomy	excision of a bursa
bursitis	inflammation of a bursa
cardiocentesis	surgical puncture of the heart to remove fluid
chondralgia, chondrodynia	cartilage pain
chondrectomy	excision of cartilage
chondrocostal, costochondral	pertaining to cartilage and rib
costectomy	excision of a rib
cystocele	herniation of the urinary bladder (into the vagina)
cystoplasty	surgical repair of urinary bladder
cystoscopy	process of examining the bladder using a scope
cystotomy	incision into the urinary bladder
dentalgia	tooth pain
dentist	specialist in care of teeth
dentoid	resembling a tooth
dysplasia	poor or defective development
fascia	tissue that connects muscle to muscle
hydrocele	serous fluid accumulation in a saclike cavity
hydrocephalus	fluid in the skull causing deformity and brain damage
hydrocyst	fluid-filled sac
hydrophobia	abnormal fear of water, rabies
hydrotherapy	therapy using water
hyperplasia	abnormally increased development referring to quantity of cells
interchondral	pertaining to between the cartilage (intercartilaginous)
intercostal	pertaining to between the ribs
interdental	pertaining to between the teeth
ligament	tissue that connects bone to bone and supports visceral organs
lumbar	pertaining to the lower back, between the thorax and sacrum
meniscectomy	excision of the meniscus of the knee

► GLOSSARY

myelocytes	bone marrow cells
myelodysplasia	defective development of the bone marrow
orthodontics	dental practice of straightening teeth
orthodontist	dentist specializing in straightening teeth
orthopedist	physician specialist in treatment of skeletal and joint disorders
orthotics	pertaining to appliances used to support musculoskeletal system
orthotist	specialist that develops and assists patients with orthotics
osteitis	inflammation of the bone
osteoarthritis	inflammation of the joint and bone
osteoarthropathy	disease of bone and joint
osteochondritis	inflammation of the bone and cartilage
osteoma	bone tumor
osteomalacia	softening of the bone
osteomyelitis	inflammation of the bone and bone marrow
osteopathic	pertaining to the practice of osteopathic physicians or bone disease
osteopathy	disease of the bones
osteoporosis	porous condition of the bone due to deterioration of bone matrix
osteosarcoma	cancer of the bone
pelvis	the bony structure including the ilium, ischium, pubis, sacrum, and coccyx
pericardium	around the heart (membrane)
perichondrium	around the cartilage (membrane)
periodontal	around the tooth
periodontist	dentist specializing in treatment of diseased tissue around the teeth
periosteum	around the bone (membrane)
prosthesis	artificial limb or other body part replacement
prosthetics	pertaining to prostheses
prosthetist	specialist that develops and assists patients with prostheses
pubic	pertaining to the pubis, bone in the lower anterior pelvis
supracostal	above the ribs
supracranial	above or on top of the skull
supralumbar	above the lumbar spine
suprapubic	above the pubis
tenalgia, tenodynia	tendon pain
tendon	tissue that connects muscle to bone
tendonitis	inflammation of a tendon
tendonoplasty, tendinoplasty, tenoplasty	surgical repair of a tendon
thoracocentesis, thoracentesis	surgical pucture of the thorax to remove fluid
thoracolumbar	pertaining the chest and lower spine
thoracometer	instrument used to measure the chest
thoracopathy	disease of the chest
thoracotomy	incision into the thorax
thorax	chest, area of the back posterior to the chest (thoraces: plural)

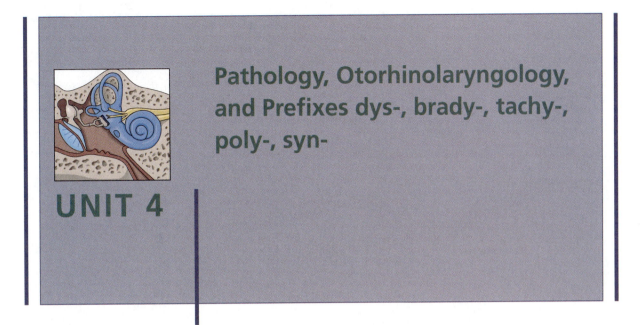

UNIT 4

Pathology, Otorhinolaryngology, and Prefixes dys-, brady-, tachy-, poly-, syn-

TAKE A CLOSER LOOK

4.1

In words such as carcinoma and coccus, the first "c" is pronounced as a hard "c" or "k" sound. When followed by o, u, a, or a consonant, "c" is pronounced like a "k" sound, e.g., coat, cut, cake, cluck.

---

hard "c" or "k"
(pronounce them aloud)

4.2

In the words colon and cardiac, the "c" is pronounced with a
*_____ sound.

NOTE: Listen to the audiotapes that accompany this text for coaching on pronunciation.

TAKE A CLOSER LOOK

4.3

In the words cerebrum and incision the "c" is pronounced as a soft "c" or "s" sound. When c is followed by i, e, or y, it is pronounced with a soft "c" or "s" sound, e.g., city, cereal, cycle.

---

soft "c" or "s"

4.4

According to the "c" rule, in the words cystocele and encephalitis each "c" is pronounced with a *_____ sound.

INFORMATION FRAME

4.5

Remember the "c" rule for those terms that follow with all of their "c's".

123

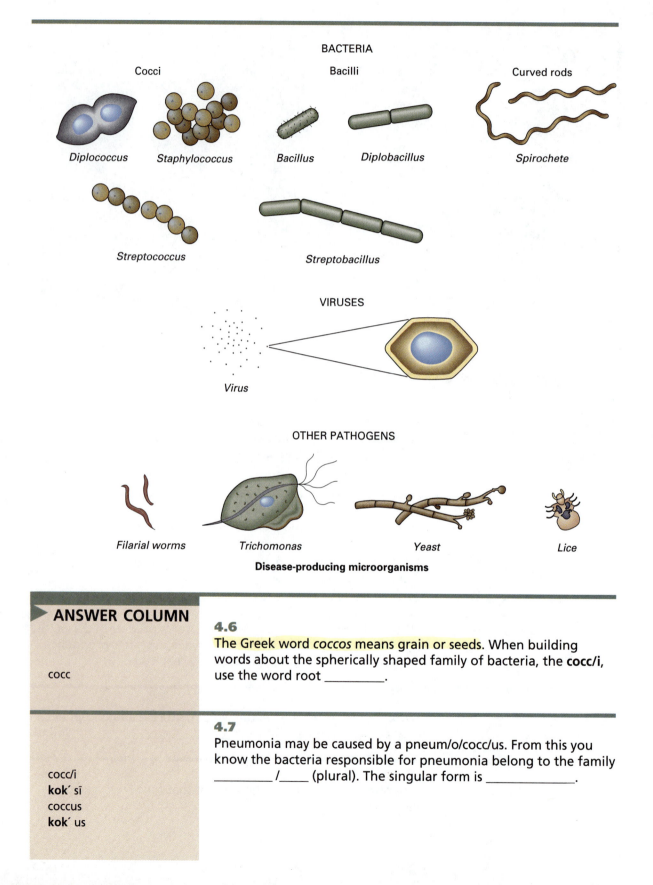

BACTERIA

Cocci

Diplococcus   *Staphylococcus*

Streptococcus

Bacilli

Bacillus   *Diplobacillus*

Streptobacillus

Curved rods

Spirochete

VIRUSES

Virus

OTHER PATHOGENS

Filarial worms   *Trichomonas*   *Yeast*   *Lice*

Disease-producing microorganisms

ANSWER COLUMN	
cocc	**4.6** The Greek word *coccos* means grain or seeds. When building words about the spherically shaped family of bacteria, the **cocc/i**, use the word root _____.
cocc/i **kok´** sī coccus **kok´** us	**4.7** Pneumonia may be caused by a pneum/o/cocc/us. From this you know the bacteria responsible for pneumonia belong to the family _____ /____ (plural). The singular form is _____.

▶ **ANSWER COLUMN**

cocci	**4.8** One form of meningitis is caused by the mening/o/cocc/us. It, too, is a member of the family _____ (plural).
cocci **kok´** sī	**4.9** There are three main types of cocci. Cocci growing in pairs are dipl/o/_____.
dipl/o/cocc/us dip´ lō **kok´** us	**4.10** Gon/o/rrhea is a venereal disease caused by *Neisseria gonorrhoeae*. This gon/o/coccus grows in pairs, so it is a _____ /_____ /_____ /_____.
cocci cocci	**4.11** Cocci growing in twisted chains are strept/o/_____. Cocci growing in clusters are staphyl/o/_____.
strept/o/cocc/i strep´ tō **kok´** sī	**4.12** **strept/o** means twisted chains or strips. Streptococci (strep) grow in twisted chains as shown here. If you should see a chain of cocci when examining a slide under the microscope, you would say they were 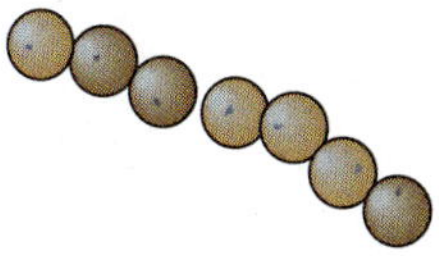 _____ /_____ /_____ /_____. **Streptococcus**
strept/o/cocc/us *Strept/o/cocc/us*	**4.13** Name the type of coccus in the following statements. Sore throat may be caused by B-hemolytic _____ /_____ /_____ /_____. Some pus formation is due to _____ /_____ /_____ /_____ *pyogenes*.
grapes	**4.14** *Staphyle* is the Greek word for bunch of grapes. **staphyl/o** is used to build words that suggest a bunch of grapes. Staphylococci (staph) grow in clusters like a bunch of _____.
staphyl/o/cocc/i staf i lō **kok´** sī	**4.15** Staphylococci grow in clusters like grapes. If you should see a cluster of cocci when using the microscope, you would say they were 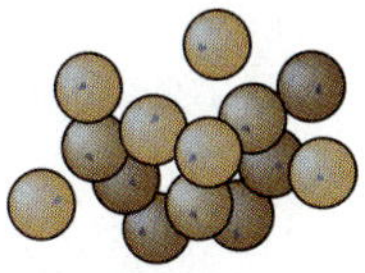 _____ /_____ /_____ /_____. **Staphylococcus**

▶ **ANSWER COLUMN**

☑ *SPELL CHECK*

4.16
Proper genus and species names are usually found italicized with genus capitalized. When using the genus initial it should also be capitalized. EXAMPLES: *Staphylococcus aureus* or *S. aureus*.

---

dipl/o/bacill/us
dip´ lō ba **sil**´ us
strept/o/bacill/us
strep´ tō ba **sil**´ us

4.17
In Latin *baculus* means staff or rod. A *bacillus* (plural bacilli) is a rod-shaped bacterium (plural bacteria). Use bacillus to form a term that means
    a rod-shaped double bacillus
    _____ /_____ /_____ /_____;
    a rod-shaped bacillus growing in twisted chains
    _____ /_____ /_____ /_____ .
Now, you've got it!

---

bacterium
bak **ter**´ ē um
bacilli
bə **sil**´ ī

4.18
We usually use the plural term bacteria because we rarely find one bacterium. Remember the plural rule: um is singular, a is plural. The singular of bacteria is _____. Now try this one: If the plural of coccus is cocci, the plural of bacillus is _____. Good.

---

staphylococci

4.19
The bacteria that cause carbuncles grow in a cluster like a bunch of grapes. Carbuncles are caused by _____.

---

staphylococci

4.20
Most bacteria that form pus grow in a cluster. They are _____.

---

staphyl/o/cocc/i

4.21
A common form of food poisoning is also caused by _____ /_____ /_____ /_____ .

---

staphyl/o

4.22
At the back of the mouth, hanging like a bunch of grapes, is the uvula. To build words about the uvula, you also use the combining form that means like a bunch of grapes. This is _____ /_____ .

---

staphyl/o/plasty
staf´ i lō plas´ tē

4.23
Surgical repair of the uvula is _____ /_____ /_____ .

► **ANSWER COLUMN**

SEXUALLY TRANSMITTED DISEASES (STDS)

Causative Agent	Disease
Bacteria	
Chlamydia trachomatis	urogenital infection
Neisseria gonorrhoeae	gonorrhea
Treponema pallidum	syphilis
Viruses	
hepatitis B virus (HBV)	hepatitis
human immunodeficiency virus (HIV)	HIV infection
	AIDS (acquired immunodeficiency syndrome)
human papilloma virus (HPV)	condylomata acuminata (venereal warts)
herpes simplex II	genital herpes, lesions
Parasites	
Trichomonas vaginalis	trichomoniasis
Phthirus pubis	pediculosis pubis, "crabs"
Sarcoptes scabiei	scabies
Fungi	
Candida albicans	candidiasis (yeast infection)

---

inflammation of the uvula

4.24
Staphyl/itis (uvul/itis) means *_____.

---

excision of the uvula
yōō′ vyōō lə

4.25
Staphyl/ectomy (uvul/ectomy) means
*_____.

---

staphyl/itis
staf′ i lī′ tis
uvul/itis
yōō vyōō lī′ tis
staphyl/ectomy
staf′ i **lek**′ tō mē
uvul/ectomy
yōō vyōō **lek**′ tō mē

4.26
uvul/o, from the Latin word meaning cluster of grapes, is also used when referring to the palatine uvula. Build words meaning
inflammation of the uvula
_____ /_____ or _____ /_____;
removal of the uvula
_____ /_____ or _____ /_____.

ANSWER COLUMN	
pus	**4.27** **py/o** is the combining form used for words involving pus. A py/o/cele is a hernia containing _____.
py/o/gen/ic pī′ ō **jen**′ ik	**4.28** **-genic** means producing or forming. Many staphylococci are pyogenic. Bacteria that produce pus are _____ /_____ /_____ /_____.
onc/o/gen/ic on′ kō **jen**′ ik path/o/gen/ic pa′ thō **jen**′ ik	**4.29** Try this one: Remember that **onc/o** refers to tumors. If a condition or substance promotes tumor production, it is said to be _____ /_____ /_____ /_____. If organisms produce disease, they are _____ /_____ /_____ /_____.
py/o/thorax pī′ ō **thôr**′ aks	**4.30** Py/o/thorax means an accumulation of pus in the thoracic cavity. When pus-forming bacteria invade the thoracic lining, _____ /_____ /_____ results.
pyothorax	**4.31** Pneumonia (fluid and infection) and lung abscess are two other diseases causing _____.
py/o/gen/ic pī′ ō **jen**′ ik	**4.32** A py/o/gen/ic bacterium is one that forms pus. You may know the noun genesis, meaning creation or beginning, as in the words generate and generation. The adjective that means something that produces or forms pus is _____ /_____ /_____ /_____.
pyogenic	**4.33** Pyogenic bacteria are found in boils. Boils become **purulent** (contain pus). This pus is formed by _____ bacteria.
pyogenic	**4.34** Look up purulent in your medical dictionary. It means pus forming or _____.
flow or discharge of pus	**4.35** **-rrhea** is a suffix meaning flow or discharge. Think of diarrhea, which means to flow through. Py/o/rrhea means *_____.

► **ANSWER COLUMN** ✓ *SPELL CHECK*	**4.36** The "rrh" in **-rrhea** is an unusual spelling for English words. It comes from the Greek language. There will be three more suffixes with "rrh" in their spelling in future frames. To indicate flow or discharge use the suffix _____.
-rrhea	
py/o/rrhea pī′ ō rē′ ə	**4.37** Py/o/rrhea alveolaris is a disease of the teeth and gums. The part of this disease's name that tells you that pus is discharged is _____ / _____ / _____.
pyorrhea	**4.38** There is also a disease of a salivary gland for which there is a flow of pus. This is _____ salivaris.
ear ear ear	**4.39** *ot* is a Greek word root meaning ear. Ot/o/rrhea means a discharge from the ear. **ot/o** is the combining form for _____. An ot/o/scope is used to examine the _____. An **ot/ic** solution is prepared for treatment of the _____.
ot/o/scopy ō **tos′** kō pē ot/ic **ō′** tik	**4.40** The process of examining the ear using an otoscope is called _____ / _____ / _____. The term that means pertaining to the ear is _____ / _____.

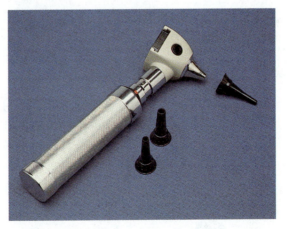

Otoscope with different sizes of reusable specula

► **ANSWER COLUMN**

ot/o/rrhea
ō tō **rē´** ə

4.41
Ot/o/rrhea is both a sign and a disease. No matter which is meant, the word _____ / _____ / _____ is used for a discharge from the ear(s).

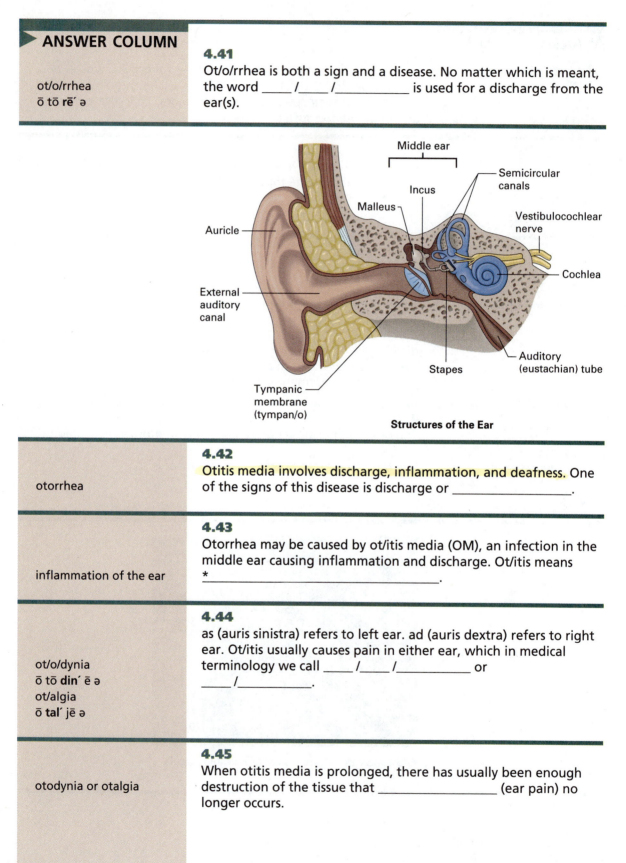

Structures of the Ear

---

otorrhea

4.42
Otitis media involves discharge, inflammation, and deafness. One of the signs of this disease is discharge or _____.

---

inflammation of the ear

4.43
Otorrhea may be caused by ot/itis media (OM), an infection in the middle ear causing inflammation and discharge. Ot/itis means
*_____.

---

ot/o/dynia
ō tō **din´** ē ə
ot/algia
ō **tal´** jē ə

4.44
as (auris sinistra) refers to left ear. ad (auris dextra) refers to right ear. Ot/itis usually causes pain in either ear, which in medical terminology we call _____ / _____ / _____ or _____ / _____.

---

otodynia or otalgia

4.45
When otitis media is prolonged, there has usually been enough destruction of the tissue that _____ (ear pain) no longer occurs.

ANSWER COLUMN	
	4.46 Small children often complain of **earache**. Medically, this could be
otodynia or otalgia	called _____.
	4.47 Recall that *as* refers to the left ear and *ad* refers to the right ear. Membrana tympani dextra (MTD) refers to the right eardrum.
eardrum	Membrana tympani sinistra (MTS) refers to the left _____.
	4.48 Look up *tympanum* in your dictionary. The tympanum is the
eardrum tympan/o	_____. One combining form for tympanum is _____ /_____.
	4.49 Build a word meaning:
tympan/ic tim **pan**´ ik tympan/o/tomy tim´ pən **ot**´ ə mē tympan/ectomy tim´ pə **nek**´ tə mē	pertaining to the eardrum _____ /_____; incision into the eardrum _____ /_____ /_____; excision of the eardrum _____ /_____. NOTE: A common synonym for tympan/o/tomy is myring/o/tomy (mī ring **ot**´ ə mē). Both are incisions for the purpose of inserting tubes in the eadrum.

Professional Profiles ◀◀◀◀◀◀◀◀◀◀◀◀◀◀◀◀◀◀◀◀◀◀◀◀◀◀◀

Audiologists, Certificate of Clinical Competency in Audiology, **(CCC-As)**, perform diagnostic hearing tests, fit hearing aids, work with patients in rehabilitation of hearing loss, and make appropriate medical referrals to physicians. In hospitals audiologists work with a variety of patients including high-risk infants and perform intraoperative monitoring during surgery. Audiologists receive a Master of Arts degree from a school accredited by the American Speech and Hearing Association (ASHA). ASHA also administers the certification process for audiologists and speech pathologists.

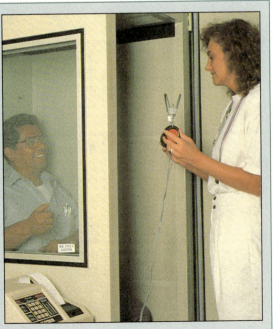

Audiologist performing audiometry

ANSWER COLUMN	

4.50
Recall that **metr** is the word root for measure. **-metry** indicates the process of measuring. The process of measuring the function of the eardrum is called _____ /____ /_____.

tympan/o/metry
tim´ pən **om**´ ə trē

4.51
audi/o is a combining form for *hearing*. The study of hearing is audi/o/logy. Build terms that mean
an instrument used to measure hearing
_____ /____ /_____ ;
the process of measuring hearing
_____ /____ /_____ ;
a record made by the instrument used to test hearing
_____ /____ /_____.
NOTE: An audience listens in an auditorium.

audi/o/meter
aw´ dē **om**´ ət ər
audi/o/metry
aw´ dē **om**´ ə trē
audi/o/gram
aw´ dē ō gram

4.52
A hearing specialist is called an: _____ /____ /_____ /_____.

audi/o/log/ist
aw´ dē **ol**´ ō jist

4.53
In your dictionary, using the word root **tympan**, find a word that means distended with gas—as tight as a drum. The word is _____ /_____.

tympan/ites
tim´ pə **ni**´ tēz

4.54
If a patient complains of a very bloated gassy feeling and has a distended abdomen, we may write _____ on the chart.

tympanites

4.55
-rrhea is a suffix meaning flow or discharge. Rhinorrhea means discharge from the nose. **rhin/o** is used in words about the _____. **-rrhea** is used to indicate
*_____.

nose
flow or discharge

4.56
The rhinoceros is from the Greek words meaning nose-horn. Using what is necessary from **rhin/o**, form a word that means inflammation of the nose: _____ /_____.

rhin/itis
rī **ni**´ tis

ANSWER COLUMN	
rhin/o/rrhea rī nō **rē´** ə	**4.57** Rhin/o/rrhea is a symptom. Drainage from the nose due to a head cold is a symptom called _____ /_____ /_____.
rhinorrhea	**4.58** A discharge from the sinuses through the nose is a form of _____.
rhinorrhea	**4.59** Nasal catarrh (ka **tär´**) is another source of _____.
rhin/o/plasty rī´ nō plas´ tē	**4.60** Build a word that means surgical repair of the nose: _____ /_____ /_____.
rhin/otomy rī **not´** ə mē	**4.61** Form a word that means incision of the nose: _____ /_____.
calculus or stone	**4.62** A rhin/o/lith is a calculus or stone in the nose. **lith/o** is the combining form for *_____.
calculi (calculus) or stones lith/o/gen/ic lith ō **jen´** ik	**4.63** -genesis is used as a noun suffix meaning generating, producing, or forming. Lith/o/genesis means producing or forming *_____. The adjectival form of lithogenesis is _____ /_____ /_____ /____.
calculi or stones	**4.64** Lith/o/logy is the science of dealing with or studying *_____.
lith/o/tomy li **thot´** ə mē lith/o/meter (You pronounce)	**4.65** Using what is necessary from **lith/o**, build a word meaning an incision for the removal of a stone _____ /_____ /_____. Name an instrument for measuring size of calculi: _____ /_____ /_____.

ANSWER COLUMN	

4.66

Calculi or stones can be formed in many places in the body. A chol/e/lith means a gallstone. **chol/e** is the combining form for

gall or bile

* _____.

4.67

Chol/e/lith means gallstone. One result of gallbladder disease is the presence of a gallstone or _____ /_____ /_____.

chol/e/lith
kō´ lə lith

INFORMATION FRAME

4.68

-iasis is a suffix used to indicate a pathological condition. -iasis may also be used when an infestation has occurred.

4.69

Lith/iasis is a disease condition characterized by the presence of stones (calculi). The presence of gallstones in the gallbladder is called _____ /_____ /_____ /_____.

chol/e/lith/iasis
ko´ lē lith ī´ ə sis

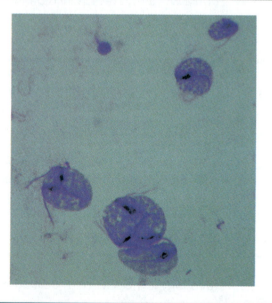

Trichomonas vaginalis

4.70

Look up the following terms in your medical dictionary. What is the "organism" that causes each infestation?

trichomonas
yeast (monilia)
filarial worm or local inflammation of lymph nodes
giardia lamblia

    trichomoniasis _____
    moniliasis   _____
    elephantiasis * _____
    giardiasis   * _____

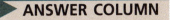

ANSWER COLUMN

gallbladder

4.71
Bile (gall) is secreted by the gallbladder (GB). Chol/e/cyst is a medical name for the _____.

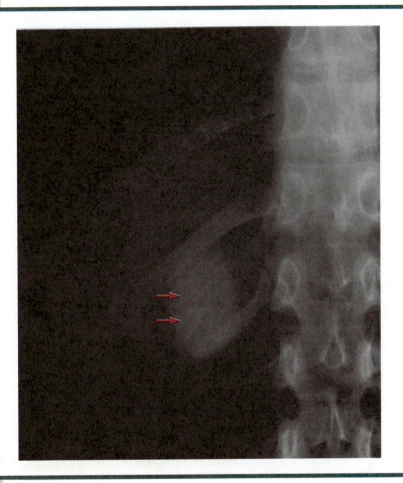

**Cholecystography:
Presence of many gallstones**

4.72
Recall that **-gram** refers to a picture and **-graphy** refers to the process of taking the picture or recording. Build terms from the following meanings:

an x-ray of the gallbladder

_____ /____ /_____ /____ /_____;

chol/e/cyst/o/gram
kō´ lē **sist´** ō gram

the process of taking a gallbladder x-ray

_____ /____ /_____ /____ /_____.

chol/e/cyst/o/graphy
kō´ lē sist **og´** raf ē

4.73
Gallstones can result in inflammation of the gallbladder (chol/e/cyst). Medically, this is called

_____ /____ /_____ /_____.

chol/e/cyst/itis
kō´ lə sist ī´ tis

NOTE: Ultrasound of the gallbladder is becoming a more common procedure for diagnosing cholecystitis.

ANSWER COLUMN	
	4.74 Cholecystitis is accompanied by pain and hyperemesis. Fatty foods aggravate these symptoms and should be avoided in cases of _____.
cholecystitis	
	4.75 Butter, cream, and even whole milk contain fat and may have to be avoided by patients with _____.
cholecystitis	
	4.76 When a cholelith causes cholecystitis, surgery may be needed. One surgical procedure is an incision into the gallbladder, called a _____ /_____ /_____ /_____.
chol/e/cyst/otomy kō′ lə sist **ot**′ ə mē	
	4.77 Usually the presence of a gallstone calls for the excision of the gallbladder. This is a _____ /_____ /_____ /_____.
chol/e/cyst/ectomy kō′ lə sist **ek**′ tə mē	
	4.78 A calculus or stone in the nose is a _____ /_____ /_____.
rhin/o/lith **rī**′ nō lith	
	4.79 brady- is used in words to mean slow. Brady/cardia means _____ heart action.
slow	
	4.80 Brady/phag/ia means slowness in eating. Abnormally slow swallowing is also called _____ /_____ /____.
brady/phag/ia brad ē **fā**′ jē ə	
	4.81 From brady/phagia you find the word root **phag** for eat. (More of **phag/o** later.) Slow eating is _____.
bradyphagia	
	4.82 Elderly people who chew and swallow very slowly are exhibiting _____.
bradyphagia	
	4.83 Abnormally slow heart action is _____ /_____ /____.
brady/cardi/a brad ē **kär**′ dē ə	

ANSWER COLUMN	
	4.84 tachy- is used in words to show the opposite of slow. tachy- means * _____ .
fast or rapid	
rapid heart action	**4.85** Tachy/cardia means * _____ .
tachy/phag/ia tak ē **fā**′ jē ə	**4.86** The word for fast eating is _____ / _____ / ____ .
tach/o/gram **tak**′ ō gram	**4.87** *Tachos* is a Greek word that means swiftness, as in tachometer. A record of the velocity of the blood flow is a _____ / ____ / _____ .
tachy/cardi/a tak ē **kär**′ dē ə	**4.88** An abnormally rapid heartbeat is called _____ / _____ / ____ .
respiration or breathing	**4.89** pne/o comes from the Greek word *pneia*, meaning breath. pne/o any place in a word means * _____ .
silent	**4.90** When pne/o begins a word, the "p" is silent. When pne/o occurs later in a word, the p is pronounced. In pne/o/pne/ic, the first "p" is _____ ; the second is pronounced (nē **op**′ nē ik).
slow breathing tachy/pnea tak ip **nē**′ ə or tak **ip**′ nē ə	**4.91** -pnea is a suffix meaning breathing. Brady/pnea (brād ip nē′ ə) means * _____ . A word for rapid breathing is _____ / _____ .
tachypnea	**4.92** The rate of respiration (R) (breathing) is controlled by the amount of carbon dioxide (CO_2) in the blood. Increased carbon dioxide speeds up breathing and causes _____ .
tachypnea	**4.93** Muscle exercise increases the amount of CO_2 in the blood. This speeds respiration (R) and produces _____ .

ANSWER COLUMN	
tachypnea	**4.94** Running a race causes _____.
without breathing	**4.95** a- and an- are prefixes meaning without or lack of. A/pnea literally means *_____.
a/pnea ap **nē**′ ə, **ap**′ nē ə	**4.96** Apnea means cessation of breathing. If the level of carbon dioxide in the blood falls very low, _____ /_____ results.
apnea brady/pnea brad ip **nē**′ ə or brad **ip**′ nē ə	**4.97** When breathing ceases for a bit, _____ results. If breathing is merely very slow, it is called _____ /_____.
a- and an-	**4.98** The prefixes meaning without are *_____. **NOTE:** a- and an- are prefixes meaning without or lack of. a- is used preceding a consonant. an- is used preceding a vowel.
without generation (origin)	**4.99** Genesis is both a Greek and an English word. It means generation (origin or beginning). A/gen/esis means *_____.
a/gen/esis ə **jen**′ ə sis	**4.100** By extension, agenesis means failure to develop or lack of development. When an organ does not develop, physicians use the word _____ /_____ /_____.
agenesis	**4.101** Agenesis can refer to any part of the body. If a hand does not develop, the condition is called _____ of the hand.
agenesis	**4.102** When the stomach is not formed, _____ of the stomach results.
carcin/o/gen/esis kär′ si nō **jen**′ ə sis	**4.103** The development of cancer is called _____ /_____ /_____ /_____.

► **ANSWER COLUMN**

4.104
A term that means pertaining to the development of cancer is
_____ /_____ /_____ /_____.

carcin/o/gen/ic
kär´ si nō **jen**´ ic

💡 *INFORMATION FRAME*

4.105
dys- is the prefix for painful, faulty, diseased, bad, or difficult.
men is the word root for menstruation. **-rrhea** means flow or discharge.

4.106
Build words that mean
  painful or difficult menstruation
  _____ /_____ /_____ /_____;
  absence of menstruation
  _____ /_____ /_____ /_____.

dys/men/o/rrhea
dis´ men ō **rē**´ ə
a/men/o/rrhea
ā´ men ō **rē**´ ə

4.107
Dysphagia means difficult swallowing. Analyze dysphagia:
_____ /_____ /_____. **dys-** in dysphagia means
_____.

dys/phag/ia
dis **fā**´ jē ə
difficult

4.108
Dys/trophy literally means poor development. The word for difficult breathing is _____ /_____.

dys/pnea
disp **nē**´ ə, **disp**´ nē ə

4.109
Pepsis is the Greek word for digestion. From this you get the combining form **peps/o** and the adjective pep/tic to use in words about _____.

digestion

4.110
Dys/peps/ia means poor _____. The result of food eaten too rapidly may be _____ /_____ /_____.

digestion
dys/peps/ia
dis **pep**´ shə

4.111
Dyspeps/ia is a noun. Eating under tension also may cause
_____.

dyspepsia

ANSWER COLUMN

a/peps/ia
a **pep´** shə
brady/peps/ia
brad i **pep´** shə
pep/tic
pep´ tik

4.112
Cessation of digestion (without digestion) is
_____ /_____ /_____ , while slow digestion is
_____ /_____ /_____ , and stomach ulcers are
_____ /_____ ulcers.

therm/o/meter
thûr **mom´** ə tər

4.113
Normal average body temperature is 37°C or 98.6°F. **therm/o**,
from the Greek word *thermos*, is the combining form that
means heat. An instrument to measure heat is a
_____ /_____ /_____ , which may be calibrated in
Celsius or Fahrenheit

therm/al or therm/ic
thûr´ məl or **thur´** mik
therm/o/esthesi/a or
thûr´ mō es **thēs´** ē ə
thûr´ mō al **jēs´** ē ə
therm/o/gen/esis
thûr´ mō **jen´** ə sis

4.114
Build words meaning
  pertaining to heat
  _____ /_____ ;
  oversensitivity to heat
  _____ /_____ /esthes/ia;
  formation of (body) heat
  _____ /_____ /gen/esis.

therm/o/phobia
thûr´ mō **fō´** bē ə
therm/o/plegia
thûr´ mō **plē´** jē ə
dia/therm/y
dī´ ə thûr mē

4.115
Build a word meaning
  abnormal fear of heat
  _____ /_____ /_____ ;
  heatstroke (paralysis)
  _____ /_____ /plegia;
  heating through tissue (treatment)
  dia/_____ /_____ .

through
heat
suffix

4.116
Diarrhea literally means to flow through and refers to a watery
bowel movement (BM). Dia/therm/y means generating heat
through (tissues).
  dia- means _____ ;
  therm means _____ ;
  -y is a noun _____ .

► **ANSWER COLUMN**

ⓔeee *TAKE A*
      CLOSER LOOK

therm or therm/o
(Try it!)

4.117
Body temperature above 101°F can indicate fever.
If you ever want information about temperature scales or
variations of body temperature, look in the dictionary for words
beginning with *_____.

hyper/therm/ia
hī′ per **thûr**′ mē ə
hypo/therm/ia
hī′ pō **thûr**′ mē ə

4.118
Using **hyper-** and **hypo-**, build a word that means
high body temperature (fever)
_____ /_____ /_____;
low body temperature
_____ /_____ /_____.

VITAL SIGNS NORMAL VALUES*

	Infant	6 Year Old	14 Year Old	Adult
Blood pressure (BP)	65–115 / 42–80	85–115 / 48–64	99–137 / 50–70	107–140 / 60–90
Respirations (R)	30–50	16–22	14–20	15–20
Pulse (P)	100–170	70–115	60–110	60–100

All Ages

Temperature (T)	
Oral	98.6°F, 37°C
Rectal	99°F, 37.7°C
Axillary	97.6°F, 36.4°C

*Values taken from *Health Assessment and Physical Examination*, by M. E. Z. Estes, 1997,
Albany, NY: Delmar.

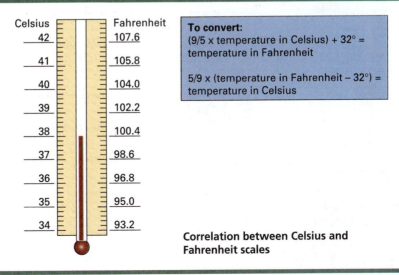

To convert:
(9/5 x temperature in Celsius) + 32° =
temperature in Fahrenheit

5/9 x (temperature in Fahrenheit – 32°) =
temperature in Celsius

**Correlation between Celsius and
Fahrenheit scales**

ANSWER COLUMN	
	4.119
	micro- means small. Hydr/o/cephalus is a condition involving fluid in the head. A condition of an abnormally small head is called
micro/cephal/us mī´ krō **sef´** ə ləs	_____ /_____ /_____.
	4.120
	Microcephalus limits the size of the brain. Most microcephalic people are mentally retarded. Occasionally a baby is born with an
microcephalus	unusually small head, or _____.
	4.121
	A cyst is a sac containing fluid.
	A very small cyst is a
micro/cyst	_____ /_____.
mī´ krō sist	A very small cell is a
micro/cyte	_____ /_____.
mī´ krō sīt	A condition of having a small heart is
micro/cardi/a	_____ /_____ /____.
mī´ krō **kär´** dē ə	One thousandth of a milligram is a
micro/gram **mī´** krō gram	_____ /_____.
	4.122
micro/surgery	Surgery performed on minute structures using a microscope and
mī´ krō **sûr´** jər ē	small instruments is _____ /_____.
	4.123
large	macro- is the opposite of micro-. macro- is used in words to mean _____.
	NOTE: micro- and macro- are combining forms used as prefixes.
	4.124
macro/cyte(s)	Things that are macro/scop/ic can be seen with the naked eye.
mak´ rō sīt(s)	Very large cells are called _____ /_____.
	4.125
macro/cephal/us	An abnormally large head is a
	_____ /_____ /____.
macro/blast	A large embryonic (germ) cell is a
	_____ /_____.
macro/cocc/us	A very large coccus is a
(You pronounce)	_____ /_____ /____.

ANSWER COLUMN	
abnormally: large tongue large ear(s) large nose large lips	**4.126** Use your dictionary to help you define the following conditions: macro/gloss/ia *_____ macrot/ia *_____ macro/rhin/ia *_____ macro/cheil/ia *_____
dactyl	**4.127** *Dactylos* is a Greek word meaning finger. Macro/dactyl/ia is a condition of abnormally large fingers or toes. The word root for fingers or toes is _____.
dactyl/o	**4.128** Another way of saying large fingers or toes is dactyl/o/megal/y. The combining form for finger or toe is _____ /_____.
dactyl/itis dak ti lī′ tis **dak′** ti lō spaz əm dactyl/o/gram dak **til′** ə gram	**4.129** A finger or toe is also called a digit. (When you see digit, finger, or toe, use **dactyl/o**.) Build a word meaning inflammation of a digit _____ /_____; cramp or spasm of a digit _____ /_____ /spasm; a fingerprint _____ /_____ /gram. (picture)

condition of having
  abnormally large
  fingers or toes (digits)
fingers or toes (digits)
	4.130
	Macro/dactyl/ia means *_____
	_____.
	Poly/dactyl/ism means too many *_____.

syn	**4.131** syn- is a prefix meaning with or together. Syn/dactyl/ism means a joining together of two or more digits. The prefix that means together or with is _____.
syn/dactyl/ism sin **dak′** til izm	**4.132** A person with two or more fingers joined together has a condition called _____ /_____ /_____.

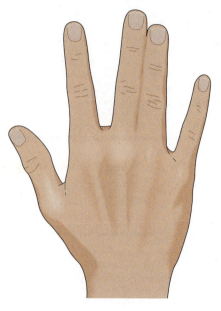

Syndactylism

ANSWER COLUMN	
syn/erg/istic sin er **jis´** tik	**4.133** Syn/erg/ism occurs when two or more drugs or organs working together produce an increased effect (**syn-**, join; **erg**, work; **-ism**, condition or state). Drugs that work together to increase each other's effects are called _____ /_____ /_____ (adjective) drugs.
syn/erg/etic sin er **jet´** ik	**4.134** Syn/ergetic also means working (**erg**) together (**syn**), but usually it refers to muscles that work together. The three muscles in the forearm that work together are _____ /_____ /_____ muscles.
synergistic	**4.135** Tylenol with codeine tablets are frequently more effective for killing pain than Tylenol alone. This is because Tylenol and codeine are _____ drugs.
synergistic	**4.136** Alcohol intake is contraindicated (recommended against) when taking analgesics because the effects can multiply central nervous system depression. This is a dangerous _____ effect.

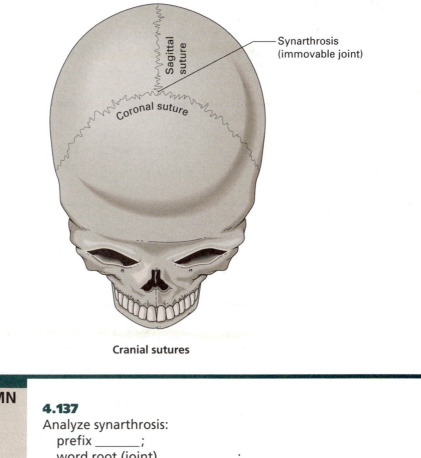

Cranial sutures

▶ **ANSWER COLUMN**	**4.137**
	Analyze synarthrosis:
	    prefix _____;
	    word root (joint) _____;
	    condition _____.

syn arthr osis	
	4.138 Syn/arthr/osis indicates an immovable joint. The joined bones are fused together. When bones are fused at a joint so that there is no movement, _____ /_____ /_____ occurs. **EXAMPLE:** sacrum, pelvis, skull.
syn/arthr/osis sin är **thrō´** sis	
🏛 *WORD ORIGINS*	**4.139** **drom/o** comes from the Greek word for *run*. Drom/o/mania is an insane impulse to wander or roam. You usually use **drom** with the prefixes **syn-** and **pro-**.
	4.140 A syn/drome is a variety of symptoms occurring (running along) together. The complete picture of a disease is its _____.
syndrome **sin´** drōm	

ANSWER COLUMN	
Korsakoff's syndrome	**4.141** Look up syndrome in your dictionary. Read about Korsakoff's syndrome or sudden infant death syndrome (SIDS). A syndrome due to alcoholism is * _____.
syndrome	**4.142** Expectant mothers are warned not to drink alcohol during pregnancy to prevent deformities in the newborn, known as fetal alcohol _____ (FAS).
syndrome	**4.143** Behavior changes and hyperemesis following a viral infection are symptoms occurring together that may indicate Reye's _____.
pro/drome **prō´** drōm	**4.144** Pro/drome means running before (a disease). A symptom indicating an approaching disease is a _____ /_____.
prodromes	**4.145** The sneezes that come before a common cold are the _____ (plural) of the cold.
pro/dromal prō **drō´** məl	**4.146** Chicken pox has a macular rash that precedes the papules. This is known as a _____ /_____ (adjective) rash.
dips	**4.147** *Dipsia* is Greek for thirst. Poly/dipsia means excessive thirst (desire for much fluid). The root word for thirst is _____.
poly/dipsia pol ē **dip´** sē ə	**4.148** **poly-** is a prefix meaning too much or too many. Poly/dipsia can be caused by something as simple as eating too much salt. A highly salted meal may cause _____ /_____.

ANSWER COLUMN	
polydipsia	**4.149** Polydipsia can be caused by something as complex as an upset in pituitary secretion. If the pituitary gland secretes too much of one hormone, salt is retained in the body, and _____ results.
polydipsia	**4.150** High blood sugar levels and lack of insulin in diabetes also cause _____ (excessive thirst).
dips/o/mania dip sō **mā′** nē ə	**4.151** Dips/o/mania is an old term for alcoholism. A person who drinks alcohol excessively and becomes physically and psychologically addicted suffers from _____ /____ /_____ or alcoholism.
alcohol/ism **al′** kō hol izm	**4.152** Korsakoff's syndrome characterized by nerve inflammation, insomnia, hallucinations, disorientation, and nerve pain is a sequel to chronic _____ /_____.
TAKE A CLOSER LOOK	**4.153** Alcoholism, a chronic physical and psychological disease, has grave consequences for the individuals who are afflicted as well as for the family members surrounding them. Read more about this disease in your dictionary or encyclopedia. Treatment of alcoholism includes carefully planned withdrawal from alcohol, nutrition, rest, and psychotherapy. Alcoholics Anonymous (AA) offers many support group programs for the alcoholic, spouses (Al-anon), and children (Ala-Teen). There are even groups for adults whose parents were alcoholic (ACOA) and who still suffer the effects of being raised in an alcoholic or dysfuntional home.

Abbreviation	Meaning	Abbreviation	Meaning
AA	Alcoholics Anonymous	HPV	human papilloma virus
ACOA	Adult Children of Alcoholics	LMP	last menstrual period
ad	right ear, *auris dextra* (Latin)	mcg	microgram
		mg	milligram
AFB	acid fast bacillus (i.e., TB)	MTD	right eardrum (*membrana tympani dextra*)
Al-Anon	AA support group for spouses of alcoholics	MTS	left eardrum (*membrana tympani sinistra*)
Ala-Teen	AA support group for children of alcoholics		
as	left ear, *auris sinistra* (Latin)	NVS	neurological vital signs
C°	Celsius degrees (metric temperature)	OM	otitis media
		O&P	ova and parasites
C&S	culture and sensitivity (antibiotic susceptibility)	P	pulse
		PAR	perennial allergic rhinitis
CO_2	carbon dioxide	R	respiration (rate)
DM	diabetes mellitus	SIDS	sudden infant death syndrome
F°	Fahrenheit degrees		
FAS	fetal alcohol syndrome	SOB	short of breath
GB	gallbladder	staph	staphylococcus
GNID	gram negative intra-cellular diplococcus	strep	streptococcus
		T, temp	temperature
HBV	hepatitis B virus	TB	tuberculosis
HIV	human immuno-deficiency virus	VS	vital signs (T, P, R, BP)
		°	degree symbol

To complete your study of this unit, work the review activities on the next pages. Also, listen to the audiotapes that accompany *Medical Terminology: A Programmed Text,* 8th edition, and practice your pronunciation.

Additional practice exercises for this unit are available on the Student Practice disk found in the back of the textbook.

► **REVIEW ACTIVITIES**

Circle and Correct
Circle the correct answer for each question. Then, check your answers in Appendix A.

1. Sound made by c followed by an o, as in costal:
   a. s   b. k   c. j   d. x

2. Sound made by c followed by an i, as in cervicitis:
   a. s   b. k   c. j   d. x

3. Plural for round-shaped bacteria:
   a. bacilli   b. bacillus
   c. coccus   d. cocci

4. Prefix for double:
   a. tri-   b. diplo-
   c. daplo-   d. ex-

5. Combining form for twisted chains:
   a. strep   b. strepto
   c. stretp   d. strept

6. Combining form for uvula:
   a. staphylo   b. strepto
   c. vulvo   d. uvul

7. Suffix for flow or discharge:
   a. -itis   b. -rrhagia
   c. -pnea   d. -rrhea

8. Combining form for ear:
   a. audio   b. tympano
   c. oto   d. oculo

9. Suffix for surgical repair:
   a. -acopy   b. -tomy
   c. -ectomy   d. -plasty

10. Combining form for bile (gall):
    a. chole   b. calcul
    c. lith   d. bil

11. Singular for rod-shaped bacteria:
    a. bacilla   b. bacillus
    c. coccus   d. bacterium

12. Combining form for pus:
    a. genic   b. gen/o
    c. staphyl/o   d. py/o

13. Word root for nose:
    a. ot   b. rhin
    c. nas/o   d. lith

14. Suffix meaning infestation (condition):
    a. -iasis   b. -pathy
    c. -lith   d. -oid

15. Suffix for breathing:
    a. -pne   b. -pneo
    c. -pnea   d. -pepsia

16. Combining form for heat:
    a. tempero   b. thermal
    c. thermo   d. Fahrenheit

17. Prefix for small:
    a. incro-   b. macro-
    c. micro-   d. hypo-

18. Prefix for large:
    a. macro-   b. megaly-
    c. micro-   d. poly-

19. Prefix for join together:
    a. inter-   b. intra-
    c. osis-   d. syn-

20. Suffix for thirst:
    a. -hydro   b. -dipsia
    c. -mania   d. -poly

21. Word root for finger or toe (digits):
    a. acro   b. dactyl
    c. digit   d. phalang

22. Prefix for many or much:
    a. poly-   b. olig-
    c. hyper-   d. sub-

▶ **REVIEW ACTIVITIES**

Select and Construct
Select the correct word parts from the list below and construct medical terms that represent the given meaning.

a	algia	audio	blast	brady	cardio(a)	cephalus
chole	cysto	cyte	dactylo(ia)	dia	dipso(ia)	drome(al)
dynia	dys	ectomy	ergetic(ergy)	geno(ic) esis	graphy(gram)	hemat
hyper	hypo	ia	iasis	ic	ism	ites
itis	lith(o)	macro	metry	micro	neur	osis
ot(o)(ia)	pepsia	phago(ia)	pnea	poly	pro	pyo
rhino	rrhea	spasm	staphyl	syn	tachy	therapy
therm(o)(al)(y)	tomy	tympan(o)	uvul(o)			

1. slow heart rate   _____
2. fast eating (swallowing)   _____
3. inflammation of the uvula   _____
4. stones in the gallbladder   _____
5. earache   _____
6. process of measuring hearing ·   _____
7. difficulty with digestion   _____
8. pus-forming (adjective)   _____
9. discharge from the nose   _____
10. record of eardrum function   _____
11. distended with gas   _____
12. x-ray picture of gallbladder   _____
13. absence of breathing   _____
14. heat therapy (heating through)   _____
15. excessive thirst   _____
16. working together   _____
17. abnormally small head   _____
18. very large cell   _____
19. before the onset of illness   _____
20. low body temperature   _____

Mix and Match
Match the organism on the left with its description or disease name on the right.

_____ 1. streptococcus   a.   double dot-shaped bacteria

_____ 2. staphylococci   b.   HIV is a _____.

_____ 3. diplococcus   c.   parasite protozoan with flagella

_____ 4. trichomonas   d.   skin bacteria growing in bunches

_____ 5. virus   e.   moniliasis

_____ 6. yeast   f.   B hemolytic _____ causes throat infection.

_____ 7. filarial worm   g.   elephantiasis

_____ 8. giardia   h.   giardiasis

▶ **REVIEW ACTIVITIES**

Define and Dissect
Give a brief definition and dissect each term listed into its word parts in the space provided on the right. Check your answers by referring to the frame listed in parentheses and your medical dictionary. Then, listen to the audiotapes to practice pronunciation.

1. diplococci (4.9)

   _____ / ____ / _____ / ____
   rt   v   rt   suffix

   _____
   definition

2. staphylococcus (4.15)

   _____ / ____ / _____ / ____
   rt   v   rt   suffix

3. uvulectomy (4.26)

   _____ / _____
   rt   suffix

4. pyocele (4.27)

   ____ / ____ / _____
   rt   v   suffix

5. otorrhea (4.41)

   ____ / ____ / _____
   rt   v   suffix

6. tympanotomy (4.49)

   _____ / ____ / _____
   rt   v   suffix

7. audiogram (4.51)

   _____ / ____ / _____
   rt   v   suffix

8. rhinolith (4.78)

   _____ / ____ / _____
   rt   v   rt

9. cholecystitis (4.73)

   _____ / ____ / _____ / ____
   rt   v   rt   suffix

10. trichomoniasis (4.70)

    _____ / ____ / ____ / _____
    rt   v   rt   suffix

11. bradyphagia (4.80)

    _____ / _____ / ____
    pre   rt   suffix

12. tachypnea (4.91)

    _____ / _____
    pre   suffix

13. dyspepsia (4.110)

    _____ / _____ / ____
    pre   rt   suffix

▶ REVIEW ACTIVITIES

14. cholecystography (4.72)

_____ / ___ / _____ / ___ / _____
   rt   v   rt   v   suffix

15. staphyloplasty (4.23)

_____ / ____ / _____
      rt   v   suffix

16. gonorrhea (4.10)

_____ / ____ / _____
    rt   v   suffix

17. diplobacillus (4.17)

_____ / ____ / _____ / _____
    rt   v   rt   suffix

18. tympanometry (4.50)

_____ / ____ / _____
     rt   v   suffix

19. audiologist (4.52)

_____ / ____ / _____
    rt   v   suffix

20. pyogenic (4.32)

_____ / ____ / _____ / _____
  rt   v   rt   suffix

21. lithotomy (4.65)

_____ / ____ / _____
     rt   v   suffix

22. cholelithiasis (4.69)

_____ / ___ / _____ / _____
    rt   v   rt   suffix

23. carcinogenesis (4.103)

_____ / ___ / _____
     rt   v   rt/suffix

24. dyspnea (4.108)

_____ / _____
    pre   suffix

25. tympanites (4.53)

_____ / _____
     rt   suffix

26. thermometer (4.113)

_____ / ____ / _____
     rt   v   suffix

27. microsurgery (4.122)

_____ / _____
    pre   rt/suffix

28. macrocephalus (4.125)

_____ / _____
    pre   rt/suffix

29. polydactylism (4.130)

_____/_____/_____
pre   rt   suffix

30. synergistic (4.133)

_____/_____/_____
pre   rt   suffix

31. synarthrosis (4.138)

_____/_____/_____
pre   rt   suffix

32. syndrome (4.140)

_____/_____
pre   rt/suffix

33. prodromal (4.146)

_____/_____/_____
pre   rt   suffix

34. polydipsia (4.148)

_____/_____/_____
pre   rt   suffix

35. dipsomaniac (4.151)

_____/__/_____/_____
rt   v   rt   suffix

36. dipsomania (4.151)

_____/__/_____
rt   rt   suffix

37. microgram (4.121)

_____/_____
pre   suffix

38. hyperthermia (4.118)

_____/_____/_____
pre   rt   suffix

39. syndactylism (4.132)

_____/_____/_____
pre   rt   suffix

40. dactylospasm (4.129)

_____/__/_____
rt   v   suffix

41. diathermy (4.115)

_____/_____/_____
pre   rt   suffix

42. microcyst (4.121)

_____/_____
pre   rt

43. thermoalgesia (4.114)

_____/__/_____/_____
rt   v   rt   suffix

▶ REVIEW ACTIVITIES

Matching Abbreviations
Match the following abbreviations with their definition.

_____ 1. AA
_____ 2. T
_____ 3. °F
_____ 4. mcg
_____ 5. SIDS
_____ 6. VS
_____ 7. FAS
_____ 8. GB
_____ 9. MTD
_____ 10. HPV
_____ 11. as
_____ 12. OM

a. microgram
b. milligram
c. degrees Celsius
d. fetal alcohol syndrome
e. oculomotor
f. degrees Fahrenheit
g. acid fast bacillus
h. gonorrhea
i. left ear
j. Al-Anon
k. microscopic
l. temperature
m. otitis media
n. right eardrum
o. human papilloma virus
p. vital signs
q. sudden infant death syndrome
r. Alcoholics Anonymous
s. gallbladder

▶ CASE STUDIES

Write the term next to its meaning given below. Then, draw slashes to analyze the word parts. Note the use of medical abbreviations. Look these up in your dictionary or find them in Appendix B. If you have any questions about the answers, refer to your medical dictionary or check with your instructor for the answers in Appendix A.

CASE STUDY 4-1

OPERATIVE REPORT—**CHOLECYSTECTOMY**

Pt: female, age 39, Ht: 5'3", Wt: 192 lbs., BP: 130/84, T: 99.6°F, P: 80, R: 18

Summary: Ms. Colette Stone is a 39-year-old female who was seen in the office with complaints of repeated pain in the **epigastric** region and **RUQ** of the abdomen. The pain radiates to her shoulder and back. Ms. Stone states that the pain becomes aggravated with consumption of any kind of food, particularly greasy, fatty, or fried food. A complete workup was done, including **ultrasound** of the **gallbladder**. This revealed the presence of a **cholelith**.

Surgery Report Findings: The gallbladder was **edematous** and somewhat thick-walled. There was a stone impacted in the outlet of the gallbladder, measuring about 1.0 **cm** in diameter. Operative **cholangiograms** showed a small **ductal** system, but there were no filling defects and there was good emptying of the contrast medium into the duodenum.

1. pertaining to a duct   _____

2. swollen   _____

3. cholecyst   _____

4. gallstone   _____

5. x-ray of bile ducts   _____

6. centimeter   _____

7. upon the stomach   _____

8. right upper quadrant   _____

9. excision of the gallbladder   _____

10. use of high frequency sound waves _____

11. temperature, degrees   _____

► CROSSWORD PUZZLE

Check your answers by going back through the frames or checking the solution in Appendix C.

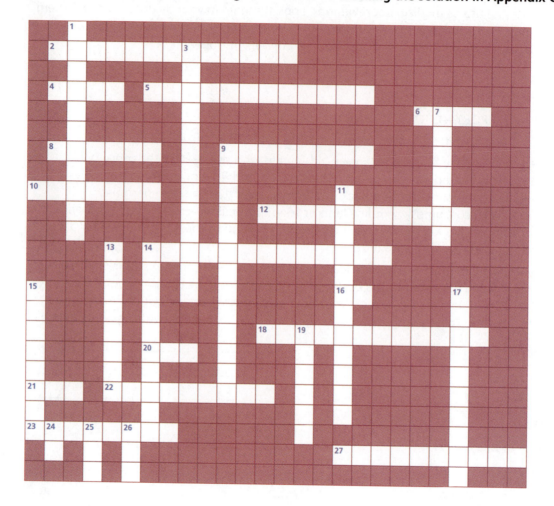

Across

2. inflamed gallbladder
4. suffix for breathing
5. promoting cancer growth
6. prefix for many
8. suffix for paralysis
9. Korsakoff's _____
10. having trouble breathing
12. slow heart rate
14. enlarged fingers
16. tuberculosis (abbreviation)
18. fever
20. culture and sensitivity (abbreviation)
21. human immuno-deficiency virus (abbreviation)
22. large cell
23. failure to develop
27. organism that produces disease

Down

1. surgical repair of the nose
3. round bacteria in twisted chains
7. ear pain
9. excision of the uvula
11. joined joint with no movement
13. eardrum
14. Gram neg intracellular _____
15. purulent discharge
17. runny nose
19. suffix for eating (swallowing)
24. gallbaldder (abbreviation)
25. neurological vital signs (abbreviation)
26. prefix for joined

▶ GLOSSARY

agenesis	lack of development
alcoholism	chronic physical and psychological addiction to alcohol
amenorrhea	absence of menstruation
apepsia	cessation of digestion
apnea	absence of breathing
audiogram	graphic record of hearing function
audiologist	hearing specialist
audiometer	instrument to test hearing
audiometry	process of testing hearing
bacillus	rod-shaped bacterium
bradycardia	slow heart rate
bradypepsia	slow digestion
bradyphagia	slow eating (swallowing)
bradypnea	slow breathing
calculi	small stones
carcinogenesis	formation of cancer
cholangiogram	x-ray of the bile ducts
cholecyst	gallbladder
cholecystitis	inflammation of the gallbladder
cholecystogram	x-ray of the gallbladder
cholecystography	process of obtaining x-ray of the gallbladder
cholecystotomy	incision into the gallbladder
cholelith	gallstone
cholelithiasis	infestation with gallstones
coccus	sphere-shaped bacterium

dactylitis	inflammation of the fingers and/or toes
dactylogram	fingerprint
dactylospasm	spasm of a digit
diplobacillus	double bacillus
diplococci	cocci growing in pairs
dipsomania	abnormal compulsion to drink (alcohol)
dysmenorrhea	painful menstruation
dyspepsia	poor digestion
dysphagia	difficulty swallowing
dyspnea	difficulty breathing
hydrocephalus	enlarged head due to fluid accumulation (congenital)
hyperthermia	abnormally high body temperature (synonym: fever)
hypothermia	abnormally low body temperature
lithometer	instrument to measure stones
lithotomy	incision for the removal of stones
macroblast	abnormally large immature
macrocephalus	large head size
macrocheilia	enlarged lips
macrococcus	large coccus
macrocyte	large cell
macrodactylia	abnormally large digits
macroglossia	enlarged tongue
macrorhinia	enlarged nose
microcardia	abnormally small-sized heart
microcephalus	abnormally small head

► GLOSSARY

microcyst	a small cyst
microcyte	a small cell
microgram	one millionth of a milligram
microsurgery	surgery performed using a microscope or other magnifying device
moniliasis	yeast infection
oncogenic	tumor-forming
otic	pertaining to the ear
otodynia	earache (synonym: otalgia)
otorrhea	discharge from the ear
otoscope	instrument used to look into the ear
pathogenic	disease-producing
peptic	pertaining to digestion
polydactylism	condition of having more than five digits on hands or feet
polydipsia	condition of excessive thirst
prodrome	the time before the onset of a disease
pyogenic	pus-forming
pyorrhea	flow or discharge of pus
pyothorax	pus in the chest cavity
rhinitis	inflammation of the nose
rhinolith	calculus in the nasal passages
rhinoplasty	surgical repair of the nose
rhinorrhea	runny nose
staphylectomy	excision of the uvula (synonym: uvulectomy)
staphylitis	inflammation of the uvula (synonym: uvulitis)
staphylococci	bacteria growing in bunches (like grapes)
staphyloplasty	surgical repair of the uvula
streptobacillus	bacillus growing in twisted chains
streptococci	round bacteria growing in twisted chains
synarthrosis	joints that are fused and immovable
syndactylism	fingers or toes that are fused together (can be congenital)
syndrome	symptoms that occur together to characterize a disease
synergistic	works together
tachycardia	fast heart rate
tachyphagia	fast eating
tachypnea	fast breathing
thermal	pertaining to heat (synonym: thermic)
thermoesthesia	oversensitivity to heat (synonym: thermoalgesia)
thermogenesis	generation of heat
thermophobia	abnormal fear of heat
thermoplegia	paralysis caused by a person being exposed to too high of a temperature (synonym: heat stroke)
trichomonas	infestation with thricomonas
tympanectomy	excision of the eardrum
tympanic	pertaining to the eardrum
tympanites	distended with gas
tympanometry	process of measuring eardrum function
tympanotomy	incision into the eardrum (synonym: myringotomy)

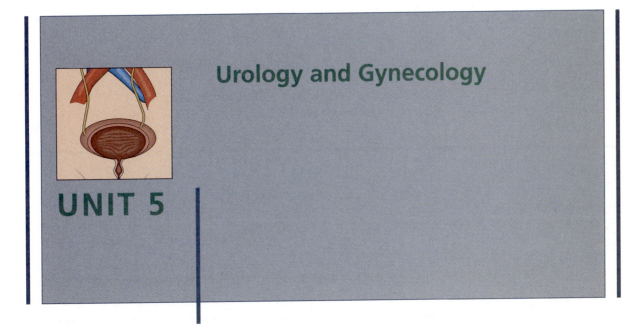

Urology and Gynecology

UNIT 5

Information for Frames 5.1–5.32.

Word	Combining Form	New Suffix to Use When Needed
urine	ur/o	-lith (stone)
kidney	nephr/o	-lysis (destruction)
	ren/o	-pexy (surgical fixation)
renal pelvis	pyel/o	-ptosis (prolapse)
ureter	ureter/o	-rrhagia (hemorrhage or "bursting forth" of blood)
bladder	cyst/o	
urethra	urethr/o	-rrhaphy (suturing or stitching)
		-uria (urine, urination)

5.1

Urology is the study of the urinary tract. The urinary tract is responsible for forming urine from waste materials in the blood and eliminating urine from the body. What would you guess to be the combining form for urine? ____.

(See the illustration of a kidney on page 161.)

ur/o

> **ANSWER COLUMN**

5.2

A ur/o/logist is a physician specialist with expertise in treating disorders of the male and female urinary system and male reproductive system. Men with concerns about infertility or impotence may consult a _____ /_____ /_____.

ur/o/logist
yōō **rol′** ō jist

5.3

Build words meaning
    pertaining to urinary tract and genitals
    _____ /_____ /_____ (genitourinary);
    any disease of the urinary tract
    _____ /_____ /_____.

When nephroptosis occurs, one treament option could be to put the kidney back in place using surgery. Nephr/o/pexy is fixation of a prolapsed kidney. The suffix for fixation is _____.

ur/o/genital
yōō rō **jen′** i tal
ur/o/pathy
yōō **rop′** ə thē

-pexy

5.4

Nephr/o/plasty is also a repair of the kidney. The specific type of repair to treat nephroptosis is _____ /_____ /_____.

nephr/o/pexy
nef′ rō peks ē

5.5

poly- is a prefix that means many or much. **-uria** is a suffix meaning condition of the urine. Poly/uria means excessive amount of urine. When a person drinks too much water, _____ /_____ results.

poly/uria
pol ē **yōōr′** ē ə

CONDITIONS INVOLVING URINATION	
Condition	**Description**
poly/uria	too much (frequent) urination
noct/uria	excessive urination at night
an/uria	suppressed (lack of) urination
olig/uria	abnormally low amount of urine
hemat/uria	blood in the urine
albumin/uria	protein (albumin) in the urine
glycos/uria	sugar in the urine
keton/uria	ketones in the urine
nocturn/al en/ur/esis	bed wetting

▶ **ANSWER COLUMN**

noct/uria
nok **tyoor′** ē ə
poly/uria
pol ē **yoor′** ē ə
hemat/uria
hem at **yoor′** ē ə
olig/uria
ō lig **yoor′** ē ə

5.6
Now, cover the table listing conditions of urination. Build words meaning
    urinating at night
    _____ /_____;
    frequent urination
    _____ /_____;
    blood in the urine
    _____ /_____;
    low (scant) amount of urine
    _____ /_____.

poly/neur/itis
pol ē noo **rī′** tis

5.7
Poly/neur/o/pathy means disease of many nerves. The word for inflammation of many nerves is _____ /_____ /_____.

poly/arthr/itis
pol ē är **thrī′** tis
poly/neur/algia
pol ē noo **ral′** jē ə
poly/ot/ia
pol ē **ō′** shē ə

5.8
Build words meaning
    inflammation of many joints
    _____ /_____ /_____;
    pain in many nerves
    _____ /_____ /_____;
    state of having too many or more than two ears
    _____ /_____ /_____.

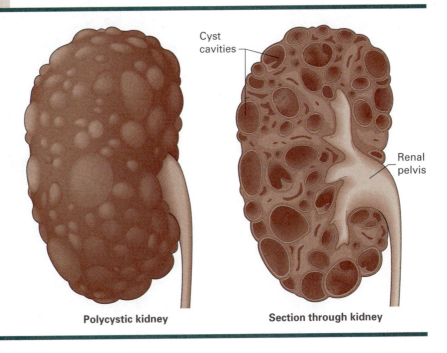

Polycystic kidney   **Section through kidney**

Cyst cavities

Renal pelvis

▶ **ANSWER COLUMN**

having many cysts eating too much excessive fear of things (many phobias)	**5.9** Define the following terms: poly/cyst/ic * _____ ; poly/phagia * _____ ; poly/phobia * _____ .
ren/o	**5.10** **ren** is one word root for *kidney*. The combining form for kidney is _____ /____.

ren/al
rē´ nəl
ren/o/pathy
re **nop´** ə thē
ren/o/gram
rē´ nō gram
	5.11
	Build words meaning
	  pertaining to the kidney
	  _____ /____;
	  any kidney disease
	  _____ /____/_____;
	  record from an x-ray of the kidney
	  _____ /____ /_____.
	NOTE: A KUB is an x-ray of the kidneys, ureters, and bladder.

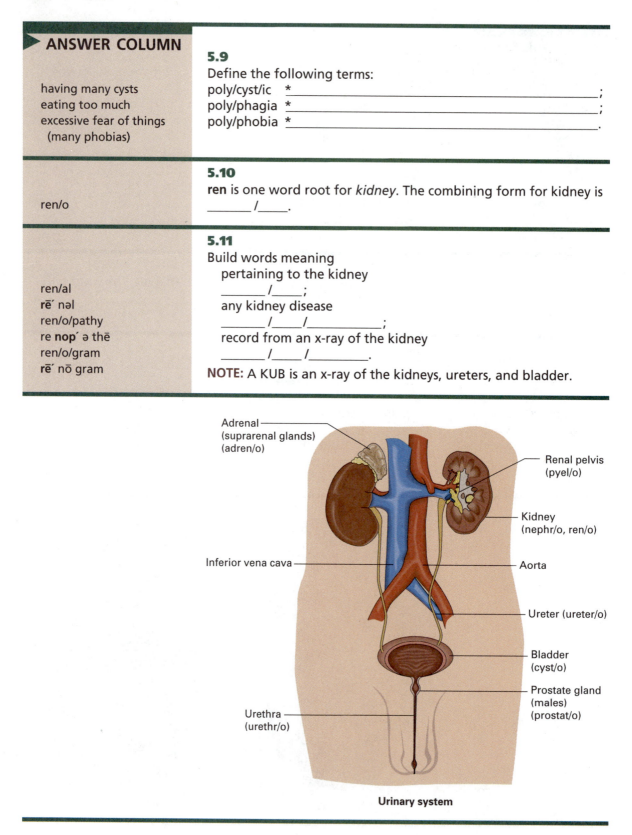

Urinary system

ANSWER COLUMN	
	5.12 Renointestinal means * _____. Renogastric means * _____.
pertaining to the kidney and intestine pertaining to the kidney and stomach	
	5.13 **nephr/o** is also used in words to refer to the kidney. A word that means inflammation of the kidney is _____ /_____.
nephr/itis nef **rī´** tis	
⊖eee *TAKE A CLOSER LOOK*	**5.14** **nephr/o** comes from Greek, **ren/o** from Latin. Nephrons, the functional units of the kidney, are tiny structures in the renal cortex. They filter blood to remove waste and excess water and form urine. Look up **nephr/o** and **ren/o** in your dictionary. Make a list of terms beginning with each and then compare them.
	5.15 -**ptosis** is a suffix meaning prolapsed. Nephr/o/ptosis can occur from a hard blow or jolt to the kidney. People who ride motorcycles often wear special clothing or a kidney belt to protect against _____ /_____ /_____ .
nephr/o/ptosis nef´ rop **tō´** sis	

	5.16
	Recall the suffixes for stone, softening, enlargement, and
	destruction. Build words meaning
	    stone in the kidney
	    _____ /_____ /_____;
	    softening of kidney tissue
	    _____ /_____ /_____ /____;
	    enlargement of the kidney
	    _____ /_____ /_____ /____;
	    destruction of kidney tissue
	    _____ /_____ /_____ .

nephr/o/lith **nef´** rō lith nephr/o/malac/ia nef rō mə **lā´** shə nephr/o/megal/y nef rō **meg´** ə lē nephr/o/lysis nef **rol´** ə sis	

	5.17
	For review try this: Build terms that mean
	    gallstone
	    _____ /_____ /_____;
	    condition (infestation) of gallstones
	    _____ /_____ /_____ /_____;
	    nasal stones
	    _____ /_____ /_____ .
	Good.

chol/e/lith chol/e/lith/iasis rhin/o/lith	

5.18
Locate the renal pelvis in the illustration of the kidney. The renal pelvis is formed at the juncture of the calyces. **pyel/o** refers to the

renal pelvis

*_____.

5.19
Using what you need from the combining form for renal pelvis, form words meaning
   inflammation of the renal pelvis

pyel/itis
pī ə lī′ tis
pyel/o/plasty
pī′ e lō plas′ tē

   _____ /_____;
   surgical repair of the renal pelvis
   _____ /_____ /_____.

5.20
Pyel/o/nephr/osis means *_____.
Form words that means
   inflammation of the renal pelvis and kidney

condition of renal pelvis
  and kidney

pyel/o/nephr/itis
pī′ e lō nef rī′ tis
pyel/o/gram
pī′ ə lō gram

   _____ /_____ /_____ /_____;
   x-ray of the renal pelvis
   _____ /_____ /_____.

NOTE: An IVP is an intravenous pyelogram as shown in the x-ray below.

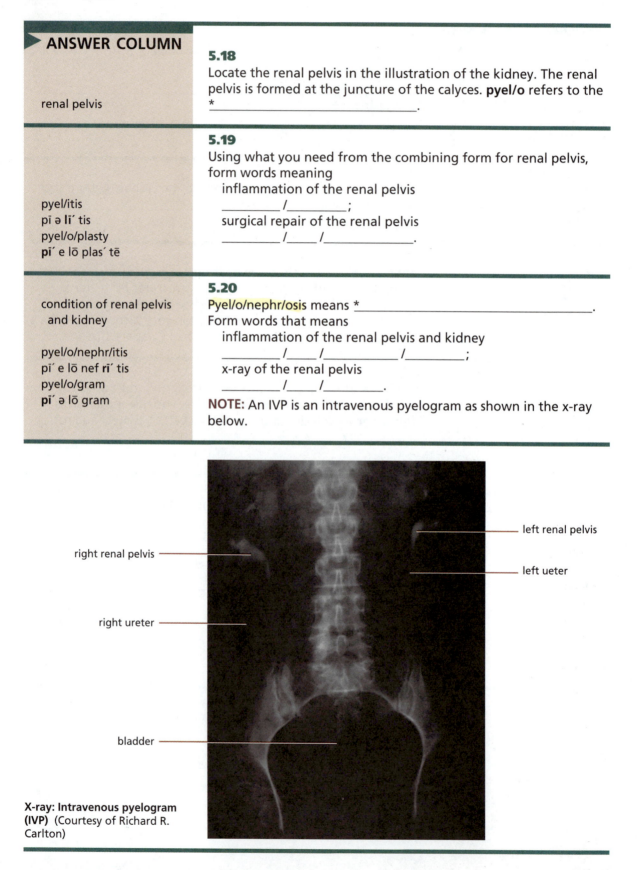

right renal pelvis

right ureter

bladder

left renal pelvis

left ueter

X-ray: Intravenous pyelogram (IVP) (Courtesy of Richard R. Carlton)

ANSWER COLUMN

stone or calculus in the ureter	**5.21**
	Ureter/o/lith means *_____.
	Form words that mean
	   herniation of the ureter
	   _____ /____ /_____;
	   any disease of the ureter
	   _____ /____ /_____.

ureter/o/cele
yōō rē′ tər ō sēl
ureter/o/pathy
yōō rē′ tər **op**′ ə thē

---

plastic surgery of the
  ureter and renal pelvis
ureter/o/pyel/itis
yōō rē′ tər ō pī ə **lī**′ tis

5.22
Ureter/o/pyel/o/plasty means *_____
_____.
Form a word meaning inflammation of the ureter and renal pelvis:
_____ /____ /_____ /_____.

---

ureter/o/cyst/o/stomy
yōō rē′ tə rō sis **tos**′ tə mē
ureter/o/py/osis
yōō rē′ tər ō pī **ō**′ sis

5.23
Form words meaning
   making a new opening between the ureter and bladder
   _____ /____ /_____ /____ /_____;
   a condition of the ureter involving pus
   _____ /____ /____ /_____.

---

suturing or stitching of
  the ureters

5.24
Ureter/o/rrhaphy introduces a new word part: -rrhaphy.
-rrhaphy means suturing or stitching. Ureterorrhaphy means
*_____.

NOTE: The "rrh" is pronounced as a plain "r". The "h" in "rrh" is silent.

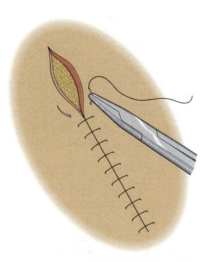

Interrupted (individual) sutures

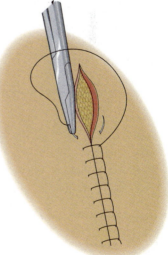

Continuous sutures

▶ **ANSWER COLUMN**

ureter/o/rrhaphy
yo͞o rē′ tər ôr′ ə fē

5.25
Form the word that means suturing of the ureter:
_____ /_____ /_____.

nephr/o/rrhaphy
nef rôr′ ə fē
cyst/o/rrhaphy
sis tôr′ ə fē

5.26
Form words meaning
   suturing of a kidney
   _____ /_____ /_____;
   suturing of the bladder
   _____ /_____ /_____.

neur/o/rrhaphy
noo rôr′ ə fē
colp/o/rrhaphy
kol pôr′ ə fē

5.27
Use **neur/o** and **colp/o** to form words meaning
   suturing of a nerve
   _____ /_____ /_____;
   suturing of the vagina
   _____ /_____ /_____.

☑ *SPELL CHECK*

5.28
The combining form for urethra is **urethr/o**. Take care not to confuse the spelling with **uter/o** or **ureter/o**.

suturing of the urethra

urethr/o/tomy
yo͞o rē throt′ ə mē
urethr/o/spasm
yo͞o rē′ thrō spaz əm

5.29
Urethr/o/rrhaphy means *_____.
Form words meaning
   incision into the urethra
   _____ /_____ /_____;
   spasm of the urethra
   _____ /_____ /_____.

urethra
yo͞o rē′ thrə
urethr/o/cyst/itis
yo͞o rē′ thrō sis tī′ tis

5.30
Urethr/o/rect/al means pertaining to the urethra and rectum. Urethr/o/vagin/al means pertaining to the _____ and vagina. Form a word that means inflammation of urethra and bladder: _____ /_____ /_____ /_____.

💡 *INFORMATION FRAME*

5.31
-rrhagia is another complex word part that can be used as a suffix because it follows a word root and ends a word. -rrhagia means hemorrhage, or bursting forth of blood.

ANSWER COLUMN	

ANSWER COLUMN

hem/o/rrhage
hem´ ôr əg
urethr/o/rrhagia
yōō rē´ thrō **rā´** jē ə
men/o/rrhagia
men´ ō **rā´** jē ə
cyst/o/rrhagia
sis tə **rā´** jē ə
ureter/o/rrhagia
yōō rē´ tər ō **rā´** jē ə

5.32
Gastr/o/rrhagia means stomach hemorrhage. Encephal/o/rrhagia means brain _____ /_____ /_____.
A word that means hemorrhage of the urethra is
_____ /_____ /_____.
Excessive bleeding during menstruation is
_____ /_____ /_____.
hemorrhage of the bladder
_____ /_____ /_____;
hemorrhage of the ureter
_____ /_____ /_____.

---

formation of spermatozoa
or formation of sperm or
formation of male germ
cells

5.33
Now turn your studies to a new body system. Look at the diagram of the male reproductive system on page 168. *Sperma* is the Greek word meaning seed. **spermat/o** and **sperm/o(i)** are two combining forms for *spermatozoa* or male germ cells (sperm).
Spermat/o/genesis means *_____
_____.

---

sperm/o/lysis or
spûr **mol´** ə sis
spermat/o/lysis
spûr mə **tol´** ə sis
spermat/o/blast or
spûr **mat´** ō blast
sperm/o/blast
spûr´ mō blast

5.34
Build words meaning
the destruction of spermatozoa
_____ /_____ /_____;
an immature sperm cell
_____ /_____ /_____.

---

spermat/o/cyst
spûr **mat´** ō sist
spermat/oid
spûr´ mə toid
spermat/o/pathy
spûr´ mə **top´** ə thē

5.35
A bladder or sac containing sperm is a
_____ /_____ /_____.
A word for resembling sperm is
_____ /_____.
A word for disease of the sperm is
_____ /_____ /_____.

---

sperm/i/cide
spûr´ mə sīd

5.36
-cide is a Latin suffix meaning to kill or destroy. Think of suicide or genocide. An agent used to kill sperm is a
_____ /_____ /_____.

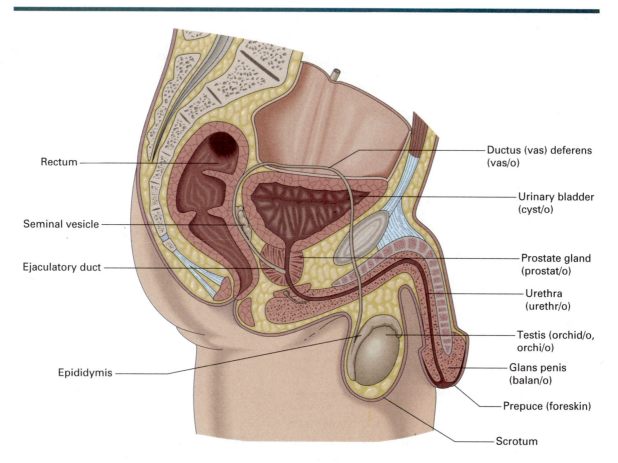

Rectum

Seminal vesicle

Ejaculatory duct

Epididymis

Ductus (vas) deferens (vas/o)

Urinary bladder (cyst/o)

Prostate gland (prostat/o)

Urethra (urethr/o)

Testis (orchid/o, orchi/o)

Glans penis (balan/o)

Prepuce (foreskin)

Scrotum

Male reproductive system

ANSWER COLUMN	
spermicide	**5.37** A condom (flexible sheath) placed over the erect penis provides a barrier to sperm. For contraceptive purposes condoms are used with creams and foams that contain a _____.
excision of the testicle	**5.38** **orchid/o, orchi/o,** and **orch/o** are all Greek combining forms for *testicle*. Orchid/ectomy, orchi/ectomy, and orch/ectomy all mean * _____. **NOTE:** Look up **orchid/o, orchi/o,** and **orch/o** to discover how each is used.
orchid/algia ôr´ kid **al´** gē ə orchid/o/dynia ôr´ kid ō **din´** ē ə	**5.39** For this study use only **orchid/o** to build two terms that mean pain in the testes: _____ / _____; _____ / ____ / _____.

► **ANSWER COLUMN**

testicul/ar
tes **ti**´ kōō lar

5.40
The Latin adjectival form for testicle is testicular. A person with orchidalgia is experiencing _____ /_____ pain.

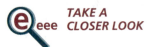
TAKE A CLOSER LOOK

5.41
Look at the terms listed below. They all refer to the testicles.

test/is	singular noun
test/es	plural noun
test/icle	singular noun
test/icles	plural noun
test/icular	adjectival form

testicular

5.42
Cancer of the testes is a very serious condition occurring more frequently in males between the ages of 18 and 35. Testicular self-exam (TSE) is recommended for early detection of _____ cancer.

orchid/o/plasty
or´ kid ō plas tē

5.43
Around the time of birth the testicles normally descend from the abdominal cavity into the scrotum. Sometimes this fails to happen (crypt/orchid/ism). Surgical repair may be indicated. The operation is called an _____ /_____ /_____. This operation is also called orchiopexy.

orchid/o/cele
ôr´ kid ō sēl
orchid/o/tomy
ôr´ kid **ot**´ ə mē

5.44
Build words meaning
   herniation of a testicle
   _____ /_____ /_____;
   incision into a testicle
   _____ /_____ /_____.

crypt/orchid/ism
krip **tôr**´ kid iz əm

5.45
Crypt/orchid/ism means undescended testicle. **crypt** means hidden. When a testicle is hidden in the abdominal cavity, the condition is known as _____ /_____ /_____.

▶ **ANSWER COLUMN**	**5.46** A crypt/ic remark is one with a hidden meaning. A crypt/ic belief is one whose meaning is _____. Cryptorchidism refers to a _____ testicle.
hidden hidden (undescended)	

5.47

prostat/o is used for words relating to the prostate gland. Prostat/ic is the adjectival form, as in the condition benign prostatic hyperplasia (BPH, enlargement of the prostate due to increase in number of cells and aging). Build a term meaning inflammation of the prostate gland: _____ /_____.
See the case study on Transurethral Resection (TUR) at the end of this unit.

prostat/itis
pros tā **ti**´ tis

5.48

The normal functioning prostate secretes a fluid that is added to sperm to create semen (**semin/o**). The combination of fluids and sperm is called _____ /_____ (adjective) fluid. The _____ /_____ vesical secretes fluid to lubricate and nurture sperm.

semin/al
sem´ i nal
semin/al

Single nodule   Multiple nodules

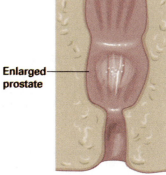

Enlarged prostate

Hard, irregular mass

Hard, irregular, fixed mass

Benign prostatic hyperplasia (BPH)   **Cancer of the prostate**

5.49

The seminal vesicles also secrete a fluid that combined with the prostatic fluid and sperm is called _____.

semen
sē´ men

5.50

An abnormal flow or discharge from the prostate gland is called _____ /_____ /_____.

prostat/o/rrhea
pros´ tā to **rē**´ ə

ANSWER COLUMN	
prostat/algia pros´ tā **tal**´ jē ə prostat/ectomy pros´ tāt **ek**´ tō mē	**5.51** Prostatic pain is called _____ /_____. Excision of the prostate is _____ /_____.
balan/o/plasty **bal**´ an ō plas tē	**5.52** **balan/o** is the combining form for glans penis. Balan/itis is inflammation of the glans penis. Surgical repair of the glans penis is called _____ /_____ /_____.
balan/o/rrhea bal an ō **rē**´ ə	**5.53** An infection may cause a flow or discharge from the glans penis. This is called _____ /_____ /_____.
pen/itis pē **ni**´ tis	**5.54** The male external genitalia includes the scrotum and penis. **pen/o** is used to build words about the penis. Pen/ile is the adjectival form. Inflammation of the penis is _____ /_____.
pen/ile **pē**´ nil	**5.55** Trauma, prostatectomy, or diabetes may cause impotence (the inability to have an erection). A device can be implanted into the penis that is filled with fluid to produce an erection. This is called a _____ /_____ prosthesis (implant).
scrot/um **skrō**´ təm	**5.56** The saclike structure that contains the testes is the _____ /_____. Build a term that means pertaining to the penis and scrotum.

an embryonic egg cell
  (a cell that will become
  an ovum)
	5.57
	The Greek word for egg is *oon.* In scientific words, **o/o** (pronounce both o's) means egg or ovum. An o/o/blast is
	* _____.

o/o/gen/esis ō ə **jen**´ ə sis	**5.58** O/o/gen/esis is the formation and development of an ovum. The changes that occur in the cell from ooblast to mature ovum are called _____ /_____ /_____ /_____.

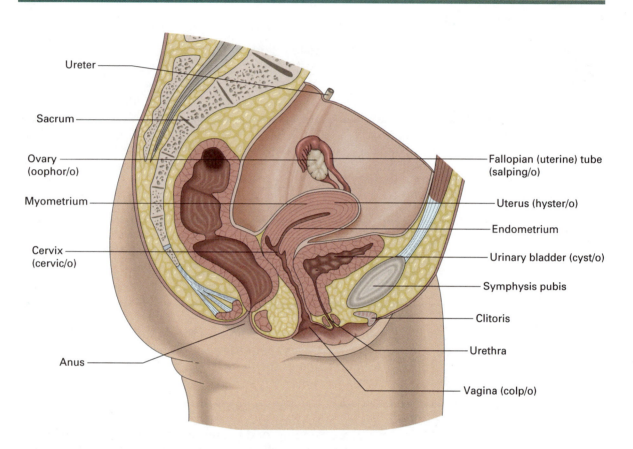

Female reproductive system

ANSWER COLUMN	
	5.59 O/o/gen/esis must be complete for the ovum to be mature. It is impossible for a spermatozoon to fertilize an ovum until _____ is complete.
oogenesis	
ovary	**5.60** The combining form used in words that refer to the ovary is **oophor/o**. (This literally means egg bearing.) When you see **oophor** in a word, you think of the _____.
ovary	**5.61** The ovary is the organ that is responsible for maturing and discharging the ovum (ovulation). About every 28 days an ovum (plural ova) is discharged from the _____.

ANSWER COLUMN

🏛 **WORD ORIGINS**

5.62
This frame shows the development of the word oophorectomy:

o/o	egg	from Greek, *oon*
phor/o	bear	from Greek, *phoros*
ect/o	out	from Greek, *ektos*
-tomy	cut	from Greek, *tomos*

Ovary comes from Latin. An ovarium is a place that holds eggs. Think of aquarium amd solarium. Ovarian is the adjective derived from ovarium.

---

excision of the ovary

5.63
oophor/o is used in words to refer to the ovary. Oophorectomy means *_____.

---

oophor/itis
ō ə fôr ĭ´ tis
oophor/ectomy
ō ə fôr ek´ tə mē
oophor/oma
ō ə fôr ō´ mə

5.64
Using what you need from **oophor/o**, build words that mean
inflammation of an ovary
_____ /_____;
excision of an ovary
_____ /_____;
tumor of an ovary (ovarian tumor)
_____ /_____.

---

fixation
orchi/o/pexy or
ōr´ kē ō peks´ ē
orchid/o/pexy
or´ kid ō peks´ ē

5.65
Recall that **-pexy** is a suffix meaning *fixation*. Oophor/o/pexy means fixation of a displaced ovary. **-pexy** is a suffix that means _____. Fixation of a displaced testicle is _____ /_____ /_____.

---

oophor/o/pexy
ō of´ ə rō peks´ ē

5.66
An oophor/o/pexy is a surgical procedure. When an ovary is displaced, an _____ /_____ /_____ may be performed.

PRONUNCIATION NOTE

5.67
An alternative pronunciation of terms containing **oophor** is "o͞o´ fer" as in oophoropexy (o͞o´ fer ō pek sē) or oophorectomy (o͞o fer ek´ tō mē).

---

oophoropexy

5.68
The surgical procedure to fixate a prolapsed (dropped or sagged) ovary is called an _____.

ANSWER COLUMN	
-pexy	**5.69** In the male, fixation of a prolapsed or undescended testicle is called orchid/o/pexy (orchiopexy). The suffix that means fixation is _____.
fallopian tube(s)	**5.70** **salping/o**, from the Greek word *salpinx*, meaning trumpet (describing the shape), is used to build words about the fallopian tube(s). A salping/o/scope is an instrument used to examine the *_____.
salping/o/stomy sal pin **gos´** tō mē	**5.71** A new surgical opening made in a fallopian tube is called a _____ /_____ /_____.
salping/itis sal pin **ji´** tis salping/ectomy sal pin **jek´** tə mē	**5.72** Using what you need of **salping/o**, build words meaning inflammation of a fallopian tube (or eustachian tubes) _____ /_____; excision of a fallopian tube (uterine tube) _____ /_____. **NOTE: salping/o** is also used to refer to the eustachian tubes in the ears. The context of the medical report should tell you if it refers to ears or uterine tubes.
salping/o-/oophor/itis sal ping´ gō ō ə fôr ī´ tis	**5.73** When you are building compound medical words and use two like vowels between word roots or combining forms, separate them with a hyphen. For a model use salpingo-oophorectomy, and build a word that means inflammation of the fallopian tube and ovary. _____ /_____-/_____ /_____
☑ SPELL CHECK	**5.74** Do not drop the o in **salping/o** when joining it to **oophor/o** because oo means egg. Remember to use a hyphen: salpingo-oophoritis.
salping/o-/oophor/o/cele sal ping´ gō ō **of´** ə rō sēl	**5.75** A hernia that encloses the fallopian tube and ovary is a _____ /_____-/_____ /_____ /_____.
inflammation of the vagina	**5.76** **colp/o** is used in words about the vagina. Colp/itis means *_____.

ANSWER COLUMN	
vaginal pain colp/o/pathy kol **pop**′ ə thē	**5.77** Colp/o/dynia means *_____. Any disease of the vagina is called _____ /_____ /_____ (vaginopathy).
vaginal spasm colp/ectomy kol **pek**′ tə mē	**5.78** Colp/o/spasm is a *_____. Excision of a part of the vagina is a _____ /_____ (vaginectomy).

colp/o/pexy
kol′ pō peks ē
colp/o/plasty
kol′ pō plast′ ē
	5.79
	Build words meaning
	   fixation of the vagina
	   _____ /_____ /_____;
	   surgical repair of the vagina (vaginoplasty)
	   _____ /_____ /_____.

colp/o/scope
kol′ pō skōp
colp/o/tomy
kol **po**′ tōm ē
	5.80
	Build words meaning
	   instrument for examining the vagina
	   _____ /_____ /_____;
	   incision into the vaginal wall
	   _____ /_____ /_____.

Explanation for next frame	**5.81** In words built from **laryng/o**, **pharyng/o**, **salping/o**, and **mening/o**, the g is pronounced as a hard g when followed by o, u, a, or a consonant. The g in good, gut, gate, and glad is a hard g. **NOTE:** Listen to the audiotapes that accompany *Medical Terminology: A Programmed Text*, 8th edition, for assistance with these rules.
hard (Pronounce them)	**5.82** In laryng/oscope and salpingocele, the "g" of the word root is pronounced hard, as in "goat." In pharyngalgia and meningocele, the word root "g" also is given a _____ pronunciation.
hard (Pronounce them)	**5.83** In laryngostomy, pharyngotomy, salpingopexy, and meningomalacia, the "g" is given a _____ sound.

ANSWER COLUMN	
o u a consonant	**5.84** A hard g precedes the vowels _____, _____, and _____ or a _____.
Explanation for next frame	**5.85** In words built from **laryng/o**, **pharyng/o**, **salping/o**, and **mening/o**, the "g" is soft when followed by e, i, or y. The "g" in germ, giant, and gymnast is soft.
soft (Pronounce them)	**5.86** In laryngectomy and salpingitis, the "g" is a soft "g", as in germ. In meningeal and pharyngitis, the "g" also is given a _____ pronunciation.
soft (Pronounce them)	**5.87** In meningitis, salpingectomy, laryngitis, and pharyngectomy, the "g" is given a _____ sound.
e i y	**5.88** A soft "g" precedes the vowels _____, _____, and _____.
a o u e i y	**5.89** "g" is given a hard sound when followed by the vowels _____, _____, and _____. "g" is given the soft "j" sound when followed by the vowels _____, _____, and _____.
two like vowels join word roots or combining forms	**5.90** In compound words a hyphen (-) is often used when *_____ _____. **EXAMPLE:** salpingo-oophoritis.
INFORMATION FRAME	**5.91** The spermatozoon is the male germ cell; the ovum, the female egg cell. When they unite in the fallopian tube, fertilization occurs. The fertilized ovum moves to the uterus, implants itself into the endometrium, and grows until birth.

ANSWER COLUMN	
uterus yōō′ ter əs	**5.92** **hyster/o** is of Greek origin and is used to build words about the uterus as an organ. A hyster/ectomy is an excision of the _____.
uterus uterus	**5.93** A hyster/o/tomy is an incision into the _____, and a hysterospasm is a spasm of the _____.
hyster/o/salping/o/gram his′ tər ō sal **ping**′ ō gram	**5.94** A hyster/o/gram is an x-ray (picture) of the uterus. There is a special x-ray (HSG) procedure performed to determine patency (openness) of the fallopian tubes by injecting a contrast medium. This "picture," an x-ray of the uterus and fallopian tubes, is called a _____ /_____ /_____ /_____ /_____.
hyster/o/pathy his′ tər **op**′ ə thē	**5.95** A general term for any disease of the uterus is _____ /_____ /_____.
hyster/o salping/o oophor -ectomy	**5.96** A hyster/o/salping/o-/oophor/ectomy is the excision of the uterus, fallopian tubes, and ovaries. Analyze this word: _____ /_____ combining form for uterus _____ /_____ combining form for fallopian tubes _____ word root for ovary _____ suffix—excision

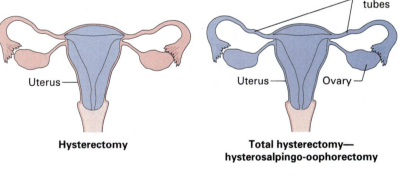

Uterine tubes

Uterus

Uterus — Ovary

Hysterectomy

Total hysterectomy— hysterosalpingo-oophorectomy

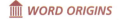

WORD ORIGINS

5.97

hyster/o is used in words pertaining to the uterus as an organ. **metr/o** refers to the tissues of the same organ. **metr/o** comes from the Greek word *metra*, meaning womb.

ANSWER COLUMN	
	5.98 In order to view the uterus more closely, an instrument (**-scope**) with a light source is used to see into the uterus. This instrument is called a _____ /_____ /_____. The procedure is called _____ /_____ /_____.
hyster/o/scope **his**´ ter ō skōp hyster/o/scopy his´ ter **os**´ kō pē	
	5.99 Uterus (word root **uter**) comes from a Latin word meaning womb. The adjectival form is uterine. The tubes that attach to the uterus leading to the ovaries are the _____ /_____ (fallopian) tubes.
uter/ine **yoo**´ ter in	
	5.100 There are exceptions to the rule, but in general **hyster/o** means the uterus as an _____. **metr/o** refers to the uterine _____.
organ tissues	
	5.101 Metr/itis means an inflammation of the uterine musculature. Metr/o/paralysis and metr/o/plegia mean paralysis of the *_____.
uterus or uterine musculature	
	5.102 Using **metr/o** (**mē**´ trō) and **-rrhea**, build a word meaning abnormal flow or discharge from the uterine tissues: _____ /_____ /_____. **NOTE: -metry** and **-meter** are suffixes meaning measure and instrument used to measure. They are pronounced **me**´ trē and **me**´ ter, as in audiometry (aw dē **om**´ et rē) and cytometer (sī **tom**´ et er).
metr/o/rrhea mē trō **rē**´ ə, or met rō **rē**´ ə	

	5.103
	Build words meaning
	  any uterine disease
	  _____ /_____ /_____;
	  herniation of the uterus
	  _____ /_____ /_____.

metr/o/pathy or mē **trop**´ ə thē hyster/o/pathy his´ ter **op**´ ə thē metr/o/cele or **mēt**´ rō sēl hyster/o/cele **his**´ ter ō sēl	

▶ **ANSWER COLUMN**

5.104
The endo/metr/ium is the lining of the uterus.
Build words meaning
   inflammation of the uterine lining
   _____ /_____ /_____;
   disease of the uterine tissue
   _____ /_____ /_____.

endo/metr/itis
en dō mē **trī**′ tis
metr/o/pathy
mē **trop**′ ə thē

5.105
Endo/metr/iosis is a condition in which tissue that looks and acts like endometrial tissue is found in places other than the lining of the uterus. When endometriallike tissue is found on the outside of the uterus, the ovaries, or bowel, this condition is called
_____ /_____ /_____.

endo/metr/iosis
en′ dō mē trē **ō**′ sis

5.106
Build the word that means excision of the uterus, fallopian tubes, and ovaries: _____ /_____ /_____ /_____-/
_____ /_____.

hyster/o/salping/o-/
oophor/ectomy
his′ te rō sal ping′ gō-
ō′ ə fôr **ek**′ tə mē

💡 *INFORMATION FRAME*

5.107
-ptosis is a suffix meaning prolapse or downward displacement.

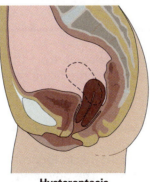
Hysteroptosis

5.108
Hyster/o/ptosis means prolapse of the uterus. *Ptosis* is a Greek word that means *_____.

prolapse, falling, or to fall

ANSWER COLUMN	
	5.109 Hyster/o/ptosis (his ter op **tō´** sis) is a compound word constructed from
hyster/o ptosis	_____ /_____ the combining form for uterus; _____ a word meaning prolapse.
	5.110 When prolapse occurs, a fixation is usually done. A hyster/o/pexy would be done to correct or fixate
hyster/o/ptosis his´ tər op **tō´** sis	_____ /_____ /_____.
	5.111 Many organs can prolapse or sag. When the uterus prolapses, it is called _____.
hysteroptosis	
	5.112 Build a word meaning prolapse of the vagina: _____ /_____ /_____.
colp/o/ptosis kol´ pop **tō´** sis	
	5.113 A word meaning surgical fixation of the uterus is _____ /_____ /_____. A word meaning uterine hernia is _____ /_____ /_____.
hyster/o/pexy **his´** tə rō pek sē hyster/o/cele **his´** tə rō sēl	
	5.114 **gynec/o** and **gyn/e** come from the Greek word *gyne*, which means woman. The field of medicine called gynec/o/logy deals with diseases of _____.
women	
	5.115 Gynec/o/log/ic or gynec/o/log/ical are adjectival forms of gynecology (GYN). The physician who specializes in female disorders is called a _____ /_____ /_____.
gynec/o/logist gī nə **kol´** ə jist, or jin ə **kol´** ə jist	

ANSWER COLUMN	
	5.116 Build words meaning resembling woman _____ /_____; any disease peculiar to women _____ /_____ /_____; abnormal fear of women _____ /_____ /_____.

gynec/oid
gī´ nə koid, or **jin´** ə koid
gynec/o/pathy
gī´ nə **kop´** ə thē, or
jin ə **kop´** ə thē
gyn/e/phobia
gī nə **fō´** bē ə, or
jin ə **fō´** bē ə

5.117
Vas is a Latin word meaning vessel. **vas/o** is another combining form for blood vessel. Vas/o/dilatation means enlarging the diameter of a _____.
NOTE: Dilatation and dilation are synonyms.

vessel

5.118
Vas/o/constriction is the opposite of vas/o/dilatation. Vas/o/constriction means *_____
_____.

decreasing the size of the diameter of a vessel

5.119
Nitroglycerine is a vas/o/dilator. People with angina pectoris experience chest pain due to vas/o/constriction of the blood vessels to the heart. After taking a _____ /_____ /_____, the vessels allow more blood to flow to the heart and the pain stops.

vas/o/dilator
vas´ ō **dī´** lā ter

5.120
Vas/o/motor is an adjective that refers to nerves that control the tone of the blood _____ walls.

vessel

5.121
Using **vas/o**, build words meaning
pertaining to a vessel
_____ /____;
spasm of a vessel
_____ /____ /_____;
crushing of a vessel (with forceps to stop hemorrhage)
_____ /____ /_____.

vas/al
vā´ səl, or **vā´** zəl
vas/o/spasm
vas´ ō spaz əm, or
vā´ zō spaz əm
vas/o/tripsy
vas´ ō trip sē, or
vā´ zō trip sē

► **ANSWER COLUMN**

💡 *INFORMATION FRAME*

5.122

vas/o can be used to mean many types of vessels. Look at the words used in your dictionary beginning with **vas** or **vas/o**. Only six of them use the common medical forms and could be confused with **angi/o**. The four words in Frame 5.123 refer to the vas deferens only—no other vessel. The vas deferens is shown in the illustration on page 168.

5.123

Build words meaning
    incision into the vas deferens

vas/o/tomy	_____ /_____ /_____;
vas **ot**´ ə mē	

    suture of the vas deferens

vas/o/rrhaphy	_____ /_____ /_____;
vas **or**´ ə fē	

    making a new opening into the vas deferens

vas/o/stomy	_____ /_____ /_____;
vas **os**´ tə mē	

    removal of a segment of the vas deferens

vas/ectomy	_____ /_____.
vas **ek**´ tə mē	

NOTE: Tubal ligation of the fallopian tubes is the equivalent sterilization surgery in women.

5.124

The combining form that refers to tissue is **hist/o**. Hist/o/lysis is the destruction of _____.

tissue

5.125

A hist/o/genous substance is a substance that is made by _____.

tissue

5.126

Build words meaning
    the study of tissue

hist/o/logy	_____ /_____ /_____;
his **tol**´ ə jē	

    one who studies tissues

hist/o/log/ist	_____ /_____ /_____ /_____.
his **tol**´ ə jist	

5.127

Build words meaning
    an embryonic tissue (cell)

hist/o/blast	_____ /_____ /_____;

    a tissue cell

hist/o/cyte	_____ /_____ /_____;

    resembling tissue

hist/oid	_____ /_____.
(You pronounce)	

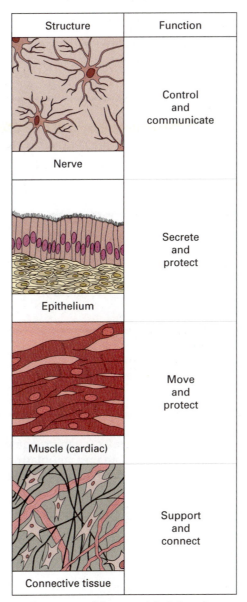

Structure	Function
Nerve	Control and communicate
Epithelium	Secrete and protect
Muscle (cardiac)	Move and protect
Connective tissue	Support and connect

Four types of tissue and their function

5.128

new   neo- from the Greek *neos* means new. Neo/genesis means generation of _____ tissue.

5.129

new
new

Neo/natal refers to the _____ born. A neo/plasm is a tumor or _____ growth (formation—**plasm/o**).

ANSWER COLUMN	
	5.130 A special unit for the newborn is the _____ /_____ intensive care unit.

ANSWER COLUMN

neo/natal
nē ō **nāt**′ əl

5.130
A special unit for the newborn is the _____ /_____ intensive care unit.

neo/plasm
nē′ ō plaz əm

5.131
Neo/plasm refers to any kind of tumor or abnormal growth of cells. A nonmalignant tumor is called a benign
_____ /_____.

neoplasm
neoplasm
neoplasms

5.132
A neoplasm can also be a malignant tumor. Carcinoma is a
_____. A melanoma can be a malignant
_____. An onc/ologist is a physician who studies
_____ (plural).

neoplasm
neoplasm

5.133
A sarcoma is also a _____ of connective tissue.
Oste/o/sarcoma is a malignant _____ of the bone.

anti/neo/plas/tic
an′ ti nē ō **plas**′ tik

5.134
Recall anti- is a prefix meaning against. A therapeutic
agent that works against neoplasms is called an
_____ /_____ /_____ /plast/ic agent.

Abbreviation	Meaning
AID	artificial insemination (donor's sperm)
AIH	artificial insemination (husband's sperm)
BPH	benign prostatic hyperplasia (hypertrophy)
Cysto	cystoscopy
ESRD	end stage renal disease
F, ♀	female
GYN	gynecology (ist)
HSG	hysterosalpingogram
IVP	intravenous pyelogram
KUB	kidney, ureter, bladder, x-ray, radiography
M, ♂	male
MD	doctor of medicine
PAP	Papanicolaou test (smear)
PID	pelvic inflammatory disease
PSA	prostate specific antigen
RPG	retrograde pyelogram
sp gr	specific gravity
TAH	total abdominal hysterectomy
TSE	testicular self-exam
TUR (P)	transurethral resection (prostate)
Ua	urinalysis
UTI	urinary tract infection

To complete your study of this unit, work the review activities on the next pages. Also, listen to the audiotapes that accompany *Medical Terminology: A Programmed Text,* 8th edition, and practice your pronunciation.

Additional practice exercises for this unit are available on the Student Practice disk found in the back of the textbook.

▶ **REVIEW ACTIVITIES**

Circle and Correct
Circle the correct answer for each question. Then, check your answers in Appendix A.

1. Sound made by "g" followed by e:
   a. "k"   b. "j"
   c. "s"   d. "g" as in gut

2. Suffix for destruction:
   a. -plasty   b. -rrhexis
   c. -lysis   d. -malacia

3. Plural form for sperm:
   a. sperms   b. spermat
   c. spermatozoon   d. spermatozoa

4. Word root for penis:
   a. penile   b. pen
   c. balan   d. orchid

5. Suffix for prolapse:
   a. -ptosis   b. -ectomy
   c. -cele   d. -pexy

6. Suffix for surgical fixation:
   a. -ptosis   b. -ectomy
   c. -plasty   d. -pexy

7. Suffix for suturing:
   a. -rrhea   b. -rrhaphy
   c. -rrhia   d. -rrhagia

8. Word root for uterus (the organ):
   a. utero   b. hyster
   c. metro   d. meter

9. Adjective for testis:
   a. testes   b. orchidic
   c. testicular   d. testicle

10. Suffix for instrument used to make a picture (x-ray):
    a. -graph   b. -scope
    c. -meter   d. -tome

11. Combining form for woman:
    a. hystero   b. andro
    c. gyneco   d. femino

12. Adjective for ovary:
    a. ovarian   b. ova
    c. oophoral   d. uterine

13. Combining form for kidney:
    a. pyelo   b. nephro
    c. oophoro   d. renal

14. Suffix for abnormal bleeding:
    a. -rrhea   b. -rrhaphy
    c. -rrhagia   d. -rrhia

15. Suffix for flow or discharge:
    a. -clysis   b. -trophy
    c. -rrhea   d. -hydro

16. Adjective for kidney:
    a. nephral   b. nephroc
    c. cystic   d. renal

17. Combining form for the tube that leads from the kidneys to the bladder:
    a. cysto   b. uretero
    c. urethro   d. pyelo

18. Correct spelling for term meaning bleeding:
    a. hemorage   b. hematorrhagia
    c. hyperemia   d. hemorrhage

▶ REVIEW ACTIVITIES

Select and Construct

Select the correct word parts from the list below and construct medical terms that represent the given meaning.

algia	ary	balano	centesis	colpo	crypt(o)
cyst(o)	dermato	dynia	ectomy	endo	fibro
genesis	gram	gyneco	hystero	ic	ism
itis	logy(ist)	lysis	metritis	metro	nephr/o
oma	oo	oophoro	orchid(o)	osis	ostomy
pathy	pexy	plasty	pneumono	prostato	ptosis
pulmon/o	pyelo	reno(al)	rrhagia	rrhaphy	rrhea
salpingo	scope	scopy	spasm	testiculo	uretero
urethro	uro				

1. inflammation of the renal pelvis and the kidney _____

2. suture of the tube that goes from the kidney to the urinary bladder _____

3. process of examining the urinary bladder by looking through an instrument _____

4. prolapsed kidney _____

5. x-ray of the kidney _____

6. fixation of the bladder _____

7. abnormal bleeding of the urethra _____

8. destruction of kidney tissue _____

9. make a new opening in the urinary bladder _____

10. inflammation of the inner lining of the uterus _____

11. prolapse of the uterus _____

12. undescended testicles _____

13. excision of the prostate gland _____

14. specialist in women's health _____

15. formation of ova _____

16. discharge from the glans penis _____

17. vaginal pain _____

18. instrument used to look into the uterus _____

19. specialist in men's health _____

20. x-ray of uterus and fallopian tubes _____

21. fixation of a prolapsed testicle _____

22. process of viewing the inside of the vagina with a scope _____

▶ **REVIEW ACTIVITIES**

Define and Dissect
Give a brief definition and dissect each term listed into its word parts in the space provided on the right. Check your answers by referring to the frame listed in parentheses and your medical dictionary. Then, listen to the audiotapes to practice pronunciation.

1. nephropexy (5.4)

    _____ /_____ /_____
         rt   v   suffix

    _____
    definition

2. ureterocele (5.21)

    _____ /_____ /_____
         rt   v   suffix

3. ureteropyelitis (5.22)

    _____ /_____ /_____ /_____
      rt   v   rt   suffix

4. cystorrhaphy (5.26)

    _____ /_____ /_____
      rt   v   suffix

5. urethrotomy (5.29)

    _____ /_____ /_____
         rt   v   suffix

6. nephroptosis (5.15)

    _____ /_____ /_____
         rt   v   suffix

7. renopathy (5.11)

    _____ /_____ /_____
         rt   v   suffix

8. nephrolith (5.16)

    _____ /_____ /_____
         rt   v   rt

9. renal (5.11)

    _____ /_____
         rt   suffix

10. ureterocystostomy (5.25)

    _____ /_____ /_____ /_____ /_____
      rt   v   rt   v   suffix

11. renogram (5.11)

    _____ /_____ /_____
         rt   v   suffix

12. spermatozoa (5.34)

    _____ /_____ /_____
         rt   v   suffix

13. orchidoplasty (5.43)

    _____ /_____ /_____
         rt   v   suffix

14. testicular (5.40)

    _____ /_____
         rt   suffix

15. prostatorrhea (5.50)

    _____ /_____ /_____
         rt   v   suffix

16. hysterosalpingogram (5.94)

_____ / __ / _____ / __ / _____
rt   v   rt   v   suffix

17. salpingo-oophorocele (5.75)

_____ / __ / _____ / __ / _____
rt   v   rt   v   suffix

18. colposcope (5.80)

_____ / __ / _____
rt   v   suffix

19. endometriosis (5.105)

_____ / _____ / _____
pre   rt   suffix

20. hysteroptosis (5.110)

_____ / __ / _____
rt   v   suffix

21. seminal (5.48)

_____ / _____
rt   suffix

22. hysteroscopy (5.98)

_____ / __ / _____
rt   v   suffix

23. hysterosalpingo-oophorectomy (5.106)

_____ / __ / _____ / __ / _____ / _____
rt   v   rt   v   rt   suffix

24. orchidalgia (5.40)

_____ / _____
rt   suffix

25. spermicide (5.36)

_____ / __ / _____
rt   v   suffix

26. gynecologist (5.115)

_____ / __ / _____
rt   v   suffix

27. vasotripsy (5.121)

_____ / __ / _____
rt   v   suffix

28. vasectomy (5.123)

_____ / _____
rt   suffix

29. histolysis (5.124)

_____ / __ / _____
rt   v   suffix

30. vasoconstriction (5.118)

_____ / __ / _____ / _____
rt   v   rt   suffix

31. neoplasm (5.133)

_____ / _____
pre   suffix

▶ REVIEW ACTIVITIES

Abbreviation Matching

Match the following abbreviations with their definition.

_____ 1. HSG

_____ 2. Cysto

_____ 3. BPH

_____ 4. F, ♀

_____ 5. TUR(P)

_____ 6. M, ♂

_____ 7. GYN

_____ 8. UTI

_____ 9. AID

_____ 10. TSE

_____ 11. RPG

_____ 12. IVP

_____ 13. Ua

_____ 14. TAH

a. urinalysis (testing)

b. testicular self-exam

c. transluminal upper restoration

d. hysterectomy (total abdominal)

e. retrograde pyelogram

f. arteriosclerosis

g. benign prostatic hyperplasia (hypertrophy)

h. female

i. transurethral resection of the prostate

j. gynecophobia

k. artificial insemination using husband's sperm

l. intravenous pyelogram

m. male

n. artificial insemination by donor's sperm

o. gynecology (ist)

p. urinary tract infection

q. hysterosalpingogram

r. upper respiratory infection

s. cystoscopy

Abbreviation Fill-ins

Fill in the blanks with the correct abbreviations.

15. doctor of medicine _____

16. prostate specific antigen _____

17. testicular self-exam _____

18. artificial insemination using donor sperm _____

19. end stage renal disease _____

20. Papanicolaou test _____

▶ **CASE STUDIES**

Write the term next to its meaning given below. Then, draw slashes to analyze the word parts. Note the use of medical abbreviations. Look these up in your dictionary or find them in Appendix B. If you have any questions about the answers, refer to your medical dictionary or check with your instructor for the answers in Appendix A.

CASE STUDY 5-1

DISCHARGE SUMMARY—**TRANSURETHRAL** RESECTION OF THE PROSTATE

Pt: male, age 72

Dx: Benign prostatic **hyperplasia** with retention and **hydronephrosis**

Mr. Travis Reese was brought to the hospital for a **TUR** for reasons itemized in the **H&P**. He underwent a TUR of the trilobar gland on 9/21. On 9/22 **cystoclysis** was clear. He had one degree of temperature and went to straight drainage. On 9/23 his temperature was normal, with slight **hematuria**. The **catheter** was removed. On 9/24 he was **afebrile**, urine: light diluted cherry Kool-aid color. A **postoperative** instruction sheet was given to Mr. Reese. He read it and had no questions. He was given a prescription for Achromycin 250 **mg qid** and discharged.

Pathology report: 40 grams of **benign** tissue with mild focal, acute, and **chronic prostatitis**.

1. milligrams four times a day   _____
2. noncancerous   _____
3. study of disease   _____
4. overdevelopment   _____
5. inflammation of the prostate   _____
6. long-term less severe   _____
7. history and physical exam   _____
8. urine (water) in the kidney   _____
9. transurethral resection   _____
10. blood in the urine   _____
11. without a fever   _____
12. irrigation of the bladder   _____
13. tube inserted in the bladder   _____
14. after surgery   _____
15. across the urethra   _____

▶ CROSSWORD PUZZLE

Check your answers by going back through the frames or checking the solution in Appendix C.

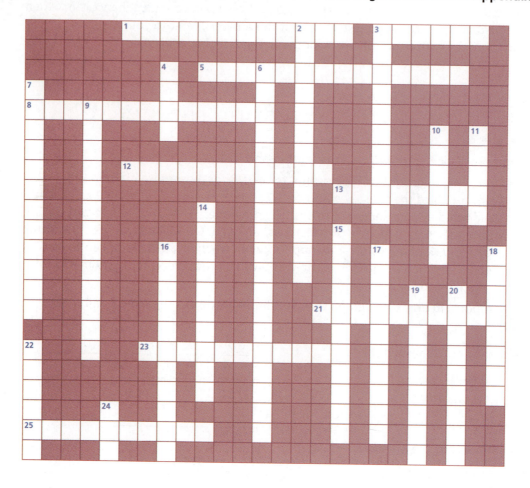

Across

1. suturing of the urinary bladder
3. pertaining to the penis
5. inflammation of the kidney and renal pelvis
8. condition of endometrial tissue on other organs
12. discharge from the glans penis
13. scant amount of urine
21. surgical fixation of orchidoptosis
23. stone in the tube from kidney to bladder
25. pertaining to the testes

Down

2. excision of the prostate gland
3. excessive hunger and eating
4. transurethral resection of the prostate
6. HSG
7. prolapsed kidney
9. surgical repair of testis
10. pertaining to the uterus
11. pertaining to the kidney
14. hysteropathy (synonym)
15. excessive bleeding with menses
16. metrocele (synonym)
17. inflamed ovaries
18. having three ears
19. colpodynia (synonym)
20. blood in the urine
22. combining form: hidden
24. pelvic inflammatory disease (abbreviation)

▶ GLOSSARY

antineoplastic	agent that works against tumor growth
anuria	unable to produce urine
balanoplasty	surgical repair of the glans penis
balanorrhea	discharge from the glans penis
colpalgia	vaginal pain
colpitis	inflammation of the vagina
colpopathy	any disease of the vagina (vaginopathy)
colpoptosis	prolapse of the vagina
colposcope	instrument used to examine the vagina and cervix closely
colposcopy	the process of using a colposcope to examine tissues of vagina and cervix
colpotomy	incision into the vaginal wall
cryptorchidism	condition of an undescended testis
cystorrhagia	hemorrhage of the bladder
cystorrhaphy	suturing of the urinary bladder
endometriosis	condition of endometrial tissue growing outside of the endometrium
endometritis	inflammation of the endometrium
glycosuria	glucose (sugar) in the urine
gynecoid	resembling a woman or female structures
gynecologist	physician specialist in women's health
gynecology	the science studying women's health
gynecopathy	any disease peculiar to women
gyneophobia	abnormal fear of women
hematuria	blood in urine
hemorrhage	bleeding
histoblast	embryonic tissue
histocyte	tissue cell
histoid	resembling tissue
histologist	specialist in tissue studies
histology	study of tissues
histolysis	destruction of tissue
hysterectomy	excision of the uterus
hysteropathy	any disease of the uterus
hysteropexy	fixation of a prolapsed uterus
hysterosalpingogram	x-ray of the uterus and fallopian tubes (uses contrast media)
hysterosalpingo-oophorectomy	total abdominal hysterectomy
hysteroscope	instrument used to examine the inside of the uterus closely
hysteroscopy	the process of using a hysteroscope
menorrhagia	abnormally excessive menstruation
metrocele	herniation of uterine tissues (hysterocele)
metropathy	any disease of the uterine tissues (hysteropathy)

▶ GLOSSARY

metrorrhea	discharge from the uterine tissues
neonatal	pertaining to newborns
neoplasm	abnormal or new growth—tumor
nephritis	inflammation of the kidney
nephrolith	kidney stone
nephromalacia	softening of kidney tissue
nephromegaly	enlargement of a kidney
nephropexy	surgical fixation of a prolapsed kidney
nephroptosis	prolapsed or displaced kidney
nephrorrhaphy	suturing of kidney tissue
neurorrhaphy	suturing of a nerve
nocturia	excessive urination at night
oliguria	abnormally low amount of urine
oogenesis	formation of ova
oophorectomy	excision of an ovary
oophoritis	inflammation of an ovary
oophoroma	tumor of an ovary
oophoropexy	surgical fixation of a prolapsed ovary
oophoroptosis	prolapsed ovary
orchidalgia	testicular pain (orchidodynia)
orchidectomy	excision of a testis (orchiectomy, orchectomy)
orchidocele	herniation of the testes
orchidoptosis	prolapsed condition of a testis
orchiopexy	fixation of a prolapsed testis (orchidopexy)
orchioplasty	surgical repair of the testes
orchiotomy	incision into a testis
penile	pertaining to the penis
penitis	inflammation of the penis
polyarthritis	inflammation of many joints
polycystic	having many cysts
polyneuralgia	pain in many nerves
polyneuritis	inflammation of many nerves
polyotia	having more than two ears
polyphagia	excessive hunger and eating
polyphobia	having many fears
polyuria	abnormally excessive urination
prostatalgia	prostate pain
prostatectomy	excision of the prostate
prostatitis	inflammation of the prostate gland
pyelitis	inflammation of the renal pelvis
pyelogram	x-ray of the renal pelvis
pyelonephritis	inflammation of the renal pelvis and the kidney
pyeloplasty	surgical repair of the renal pelvis
renal	pertaining to the kidney
renogastric	pertaining to the kidney and stomach
renogram	x-ray of the kidney (renograph)

▶ GLOSSARY

renointestinal	pertaining to the kidney and intestine
renopathy	any disease of the kidney
salpingectomy	excision of a fallopian tube
salpingitis	inflammation of the fallopian tube (or eustachian tube)
salpingo-oophoritis	inflammation of the ovary and fallopian tube
salpingo-oophorocele	herniation of the ovary and fallopian tube
salpingostomy	forming a new opening in the fallopian tube
spermatoblast	immature sperm cell (spermoblast)
spermatocyst	saclike structure containing sperm
spermatoid	resembling sperm
spermatolysis	destruction of sperm (spermolysis)
spermatopathy	any disease of the sperm
spermicide	agent that kills sperm
testicular	pertaining to the testes
ureterocele	herniation of the ureter
ureterocystostomy	procedure to form a new opening between the ureter and the urinary bladder
ureterolith	stone in the ureter
ureteropathy	any disease involving the ureter
ureteropyelitis	inflammation of the ureter and the renal pelvis

ureteropyosis	condition of pus in the ureter
ureterorrhagia	hemorrhage of the ureter
ureterorrhaphy	suturing of the ureter
urethrocystitis	inflammation of the urethra and urinary bladder
urethrorrhagia	hemorrhage of the urethra
urethrorrhaphy	suturing of the urethra
urethrospasm	spasm of the muscles of the urethra
urethrotomy	incision into the urethra
urogenital	pertaining to the urinary tract and genitals
urologist	physician specialist in disorders of the urinary and male reproductive systems
urology	the medical specialty that studies the urinary system
uropathy	any disease of the urinary system
uterine	pertaining to the uterus
vasectomy	excision of the vas deferens (for sterilization)
vasoconstriction	decrease in vessel diameter
vasodilation (vasodilatation)	increase in vessel diameter
vasorrhaphy	suturing of vessel or vas deferens
vasostomy	procedure to make a new opening in the vas deferens
vasotomy	incision into the vas deferens
vasotripsy	surgical crushing of a vessel

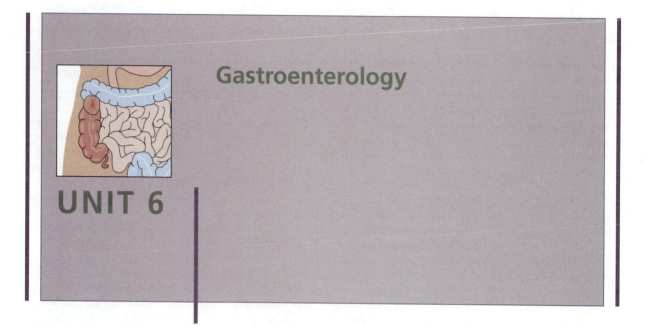

UNIT 6

Gastroenterology

Read through the digestive system information in the table below. Locate the organs named by studying the illustration on page 197. Then, work Frames 6.1–6.63.

▶▶▶▶▶◀◀◀◀◀

Organ	Combining Form	Suffixes	Examples
mouth	stomat/o	-itis	stomat/itis
teeth	dent/o, odont/o	-ist	dent/ist
tongue	gloss/o, lingu/o	-plegia*	gloss/o/plegia
lips	cheil/o	-plasty	cheil/o/plasty
gums	gingiv/o	-ectomy	gingiv/ectomy
esophagus	esophag/o	-spasm	esophag/o/spasm
stomach	gastr/o	-ectasia*	gastr/ectasia
small intestine	enter/o	-logy	enter/o/logy
duodenum	duoden/o	-ostomy	duoden/o/stomy
jejunum	jejun/o	-rrhaphy	jejun/o/rrhaphy
ileum	ile/o	-tomy	ile/o/tomy
large intestine	col/o	-clysis*	col/o/clysis
sigmoid colon	sigmoid/o	-scopy	sigmoid/o/scopy
rectum	rect/o	-cele	rect/o/cele
anus and rectum	proct/o	-scope	proct/o/scope
accessory organs			
liver	hepat/o	-megaly	hepat/o/megaly
gallbladder	cholecyst/o	-gram	chol/e/cyst/o/gram
pancreas	pancreat/o	-lith	pancreat/o/lith

*New suffix.

196

ANSWER COLUMN	
	6.1 *Stoma* is a Greek word meaning mouth. The combining form for mouth is _____ /_____.
stomat/o	
inflammation of the mouth surgical repair of the mouth	**6.2** Stomat/itis means *_____. Stomat/o/plasty means *_____.

stomat/algia
stō mə **tal´** jē ə
stomat/o/rrhagia
stō´ mə tō **rā´** jē ə
	6.3
	Using the word root for mouth, form words meaning
	    pain in the mouth
	    _____ /_____;
	    hemorrhage of the mouth
	    _____ /_____ /_____.

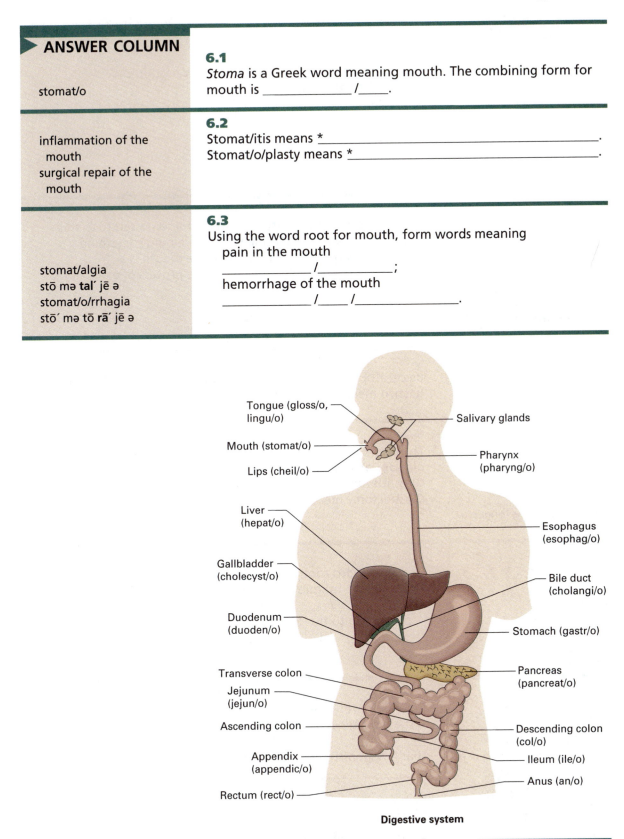

Digestive system

ANSWER COLUMN

6.4
Using the combining form (**stomat/o**) for mouth, build words meaning
  condition of mouth fungus
  _____ /_____ /myc/osis;
  any disease of the mouth
  _____ /_____ /_____.

stomat/o/myc/osis
stō´ mə tō mī **kō´** sis
stomat/o/pathy
stō´ mə **top´** ə thē

6.5
Recall that **-scope** is a suffix for an instrument used to examine. A micr/o/scope is an instrument for examining something small. An instrument for examining the mouth is a
_____ /_____ /_____. The process of examining with this instrument is _____ /_____ /_____.

stomat/o/scope
stō **mat´** ō skōp
stomat/o/scopy
stō mə **tos´** kə pē

✔ SPELL CHECK

6.6
Be careful to use **stomat/o** for mouth, not stomach. Remember, **gastr/o** means stomach.

6.7
The Greek combining form for tongue is **gloss/o** (think of a glossary of words).
Gloss/itis means *_____.
Gloss/ectomy means *_____.

inflammation of the
  tongue
excision of the tongue

6.8
Using the word root, build words meaning
  pain in the tongue
  _____ /_____;
  pertaining to the tongue
  _____ /al.

gloss/algia
glos **al´** jē ə
gloss/al
glos´ əl

6.9
hypo- is a prefix meaning below or under. Cranial nerve XII is the hypo/gloss/al nerve. It supplies nerve impulses
*_____. A medication that is administered under the tongue is a
_____ /_____ /_____ medication.

under the tongue or
  to the tongue
hypo/gloss/al or
hī pō **glos´** əl
sub/lingu/al
sub **lin´** gwal

► **ANSWER COLUMN**

🏛 *WORD ORIGINS*

6.10
sub- and lingual are Latin word parts. hypo- and glossal are Greek word parts. Generally, original languages are not mixed as they form words. So sublingual and hypoglossal are usually used.

sub/lingu/al
sub **lin**′ gwal

6.11
lingu/o is a Latin combining form for tongue (think of lingusitics or language). Lingu/al is the adjectival form. sub- is a prefix used with **lingu/o**. Build an adjective that means pertaining to under the tongue: _____ /_____ /____.

under the tongue

6.12
Nitroglycerin tablets are administered sub/lingual/ly. This means they are placed *_____.

hypo/gloss/al
sub/lingu/al

6.13
Two words that you have learned that mean under the tongue are
_____ /_____ /____;
_____ /_____ /____.

gloss/o/ptosis
glos op **tō**′ sis
gloss/o/scopy
glos **os**′ kə pē

6.14
Using the combining form for tongue, build words meaning
    prolapse of the tongue
    _____ /____ /_____;
    examination of the tongue
    _____ /____ /_____.

gloss/o/plegia
glos ō **plē**′ jē ə
gloss/o/plegic
glos ō **plē**′ jik

6.15
-plegia is a suffix meaning paralysis. Build words meaning
    paralysis of the tongue
    _____ /____ /_____ (noun);
    paralysis of the tongue
    _____ /____ /_____ (adjective).

inflammation of the lips
plastic surgery of the lips

6.16
cheil/o (note: e before i) is a combining form for lips. Cheil/itis means *_____.
Cheil/o/plasty means *_____.

cheil
cheil/o
kī′ lō

6.17
The word root for lip is _____.
The combining form for lip is _____ /____.

> **ANSWER COLUMN**

cheil/o/tomy
kī **lot**´ ə mē
cheil/osis
kī **lō**´ sis

6.18
Build words meaning
 incision of the lips
 _____ / _____ / _____ ;
 condition or disorder of the lips
 _____ / _____ .

cheil/o/stomat/o/plasty
kī´ lō stō **mat**´ ə plas tē

6.19
A word meaning plastic surgery of the lips and mouth is
_____ / _____ / _____ / _____ / _____ .
 lips   mouth   repair

pertaining to the gums
gingiv/o

6.20
gingiv/o is the combining form for gums. Gingiv/al means
* _____ .
The combining form for gums is _____ / _____ .

gingiv/itis
jin ji **vī**´ tis
gingiv/algia
jin ji **val**´ jē ə

6.21
Build words meaning
 inflammation of the gums
 _____ / _____ ;
 gum pain
 _____ / _____ .

gingiv/ectomy
jin ji **vek**´ tə mē
gingiv/o/gloss/itis
jin´ ji vō glos **ī**´ tis
lingu/o/gingiv/al
lin´ gwō **jin**´ ji vəl

6.22
Build words meaning
 excision of gum tissue
 _____ / _____ ;
 inflammation of the gums and tongue
 _____ / _____ / _____ / _____ ;
 tongue and gums (adjective)
 _____ / _____ / _____ / _____ .

esophag/eal
ē so fa **jē**´ al

6.23
eso- means in or toward and **phag/o** means swallow. **esophag/o** is used in words about the esophagus used for swallowing. The adjective is _____ /eal.
 word root   suffix

esophag/u
ē **so**´ fə gus

6.24
sten/osis is a condition of narrowing that may occur in a tube or passageway. Mitral stenosis is a narrowing of the mitral valve opening in the heart. Esophag/o/sten/osis is a narrowing of the _____ / _____ .

ANSWER COLUMN

6.25

A person experiencing dysphagia may have a narrowing of the esophagus or

_____ /_____ /_____ /_____.

esophag/o/stenosis
ē so′ fə gō sten ō′ sis

6.26

Build an adjective meaning pertaining to the esophagus and stomach: _____ /_____ /_____ /_____ or

_____ /_____ /_____ /_____.

esophag/o/gastr/ic
gastr/o/esophag/eal
(You pronounce)

6.27

Gastr/o/esophag/eal reflux disease (GERD) causes the gastric and duodenal juices to enter and irritate the esophagus. A person who has chronic heartburn and throat irritation may be suffering from

_____ /_____ /_____ /_____ reflux disease.

gastr/o/esophag/o/eal
gas′ trō ē sof ə **gē**′ əl

6.28

Not eating just before going to bed, avoiding fatty foods, losing weight, and elevating the head of the bed are all recommendations for people who have GERD or

*_____.

gastroesophageal reflux
   disease

6.29

Gastr/o/rrhagia means *_____.
Gastr/itis means *_____.
Gastr/ic means *_____.

stomach hemorrhage
inflammation of the
   stomach
pertaining to the
   stomach

TAKE A
CLOSER LOOK

6.30

An organism called *Helicobacter pylori* (HP) has been reported to be the most common cause of gastritis in children and adults in the world. It is transmitted through contamination with gastrointestinal substances like feces or vomitus. Symptoms of HP gastritis include epigastric pain, nausea, vomiting, and dyspepsia and this infection can be successfully treated with antibiotics. If you are curious about the many forms of gastritis, look up the classifications of gastritis in your dictionary or a textbook of medicine.

ANSWER COLUMN	

	6.31
	-ectasia (or ectasis) is a suffix meaning stretching or dilatation.
	Form words meaning
	    dilatation (stretching) of the stomach
	    _____ /_____;
	    prolapse of the stomach and small intestine
	    _____ /____ /_____ /____ /_____.

gastr/ectasia
gas trek **tā´** shə
gastr/o/enter/o/ptosis
gas´ trō en´ tər op **tō´** sis

6.32
enter/o is used in words about the small intestine or the intestine in general. Tablets that dissolve in the intestine may have been treated with an enter/ic coating. Inflammation of the intestine is
_____ /_____.

enter/itis
en ter **ī´** tis

6.33
The internal medicine specialty that studies diseases of the stomach and intestine is
_____ /____ /_____ /____ /_____.

gastr/o/enter/o/logy
gas´ trō en´ ter **ol´** ō gē

6.34
Recall the prefix **dys-**, meaning difficulty or pain. Dysentery is a disorder of the intestine characterized by inflammation, pain, and diarrhea. When caused by an amoeba-type parasite, it is called amoebic _____ /_____ /____.

dys/enter/y
dis´ en tair ē

Hiatal hernia

Inguinal hernia

Umbilical hernia

ANSWER COLUMN

6.35
Form words meaning
    pertaining to the stomach and small intestine

gastr/o/enter/ic
gas´ trō en **tair**´ ik
enter/o/rrhagia
en tə rō **rā**´ jē ə

    _____ /____ /_____ /____;
    hemorrhage of the small intestine
    _____ /____ /_____.

6.36
Build words meaning
    intestinal hernia

enter/o/cele
en´ tə rō sēl
enter/o/clysis
en tə **rok**´ lə sis

    _____ /____ /_____;
    washing or irrigation of the small intestine
    _____ /____ /_____.

6.37
Build words meaning
    paralysis of the small intestine

enter/o/plegia
en tə rō **plē**´ jē ə
enter/ectasia
en tə rek **tā**´ shə

    _____ /____ /_____;
    dilatation of the small intestine
    _____ /_____.

6.38

prolapse of the small
  intestine
surgical puncture of the
  small intestine

Enter/o/ptosis means *_____
_____.
Enter/o/centesis means *_____
_____.

6.39

pertaining to the colon
  or large intestine
surgical puncture of the
  colon

col/o is the combining form for colon (large intestine).
Col/ic or colonic means
*_____.
Col/o/centesis means *_____.

6.40
Build words meaning
    surgical fixation of the colon

col/o/pexy
kō´ lō pek sē, **kol**´ ō pek sē
col/ostomy
ko **los**´ tə mē
col/o/ptosis
kōl´ op **tō**´ sis

    _____ /____ /_____;
    making a new opening into the colon
    _____ /_____;
    prolapse of the colon
    _____ /____ /_____.

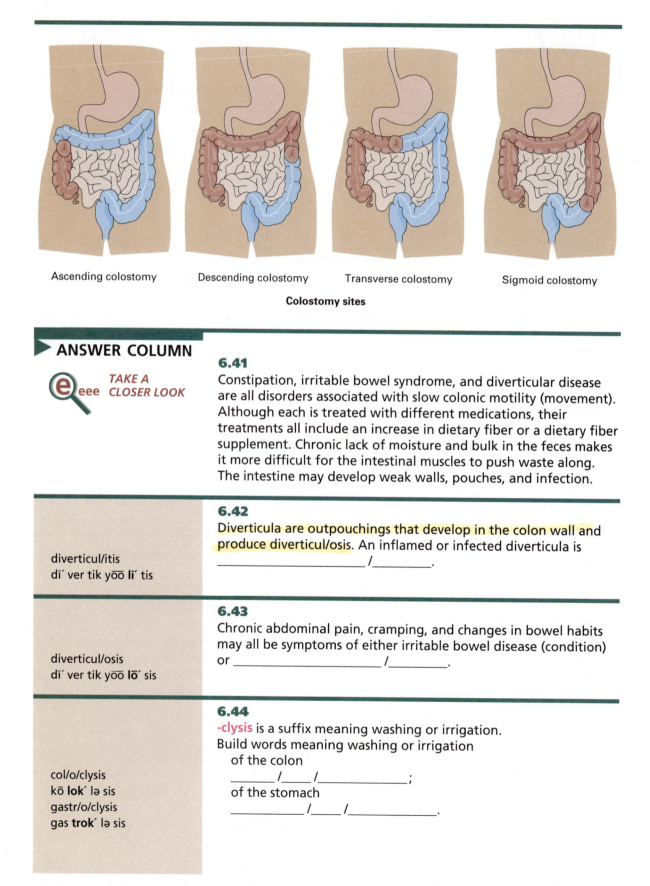

Ascending colostomy   Descending colostomy   Transverse colostomy   Sigmoid colostomy

Colostomy sites

ANSWER COLUMN

ⓔeee   *TAKE A*
         CLOSER LOOK

6.41
Constipation, irritable bowel syndrome, and diverticular disease
are all disorders associated with slow colonic motility (movement).
Although each is treated with different medications, their
treatments all include an increase in dietary fiber or a dietary fiber
supplement. Chronic lack of moisture and bulk in the feces makes
it more difficult for the intestinal muscles to push waste along.
The intestine may develop weak walls, pouches, and infection.

---

diverticul/itis
dī′ ver tik yo͞o lī′ tis

6.42
Diverticula are outpouchings that develop in the colon wall and
produce diverticul/osis. An inflamed or infected diverticula is
_____ /_____.

---

diverticul/osis
dī′ ver tik yo͞o lō′ sis

6.43
Chronic abdominal pain, cramping, and changes in bowel habits
may all be symptoms of either irritable bowel disease (condition)
or _____ /_____.

---

col/o/clysis
kō **lok**′ lə sis
gastr/o/clysis
gas **trok**′ lə sis

6.44
-clysis is a suffix meaning washing or irrigation.
Build words meaning washing or irrigation
   of the colon
   _____ /____ /_____;
   of the stomach
   _____ /____ /_____.

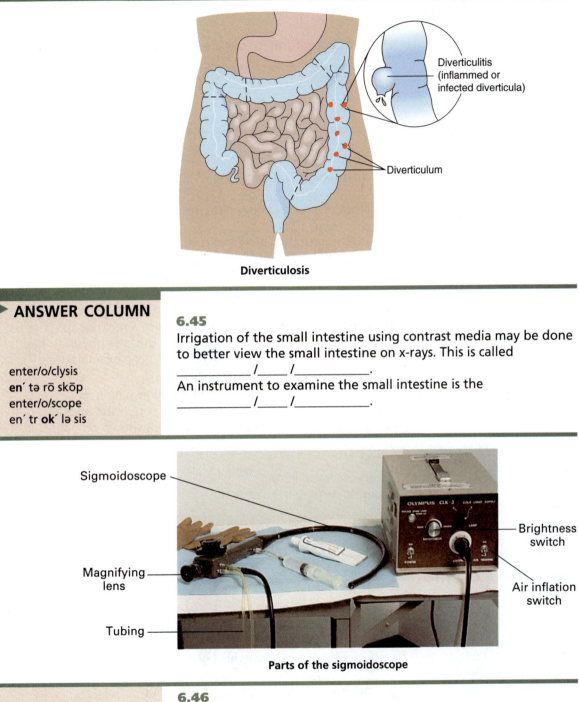

Diverticulosis

Diverticulitis (inflamed or infected diverticula)

Diverticulum

Parts of the sigmoidoscope

Sigmoidoscope

Brightness switch

Air inflation switch

Magnifying lens

Tubing

OLYMPUS CLK-3   COLD LIGHT SUPPLY

▶ **ANSWER COLUMN**

enter/o/clysis
en´ tə rō skōp
enter/o/scope
en´ tr **ok´** lə sis

6.45
Irrigation of the small intestine using contrast media may be done to better view the small intestine on x-rays. This is called
_____ /_____ /_____.
An instrument to examine the small intestine is the
_____ /_____ /_____.

sigmoid/o/scope
sig **moid´** ō skōp
sigmoid/o/scopy
sig moid **ōs´** kō pē

6.46
sigmoid/o refers to the sigmoid colon. An instrument used to examine the sigmoid colon is the
_____ /_____ /_____.
The procedure is called _____ /_____ /_____.

▶ ANSWER COLUMN

pertaining to the rectum
a rectal hernia or
   herniation of the
   rectum

6.47
The combining form for rectum is **rect/o**. Rect/al means
*_____.
A rect/o/cele is *_____.

rect/o/clysis
rek **tok´** lə sis
rect/o/scope
rek´ tə skōp
col/o/rect/al
kō lō **rek´** təl

6.48
Build words meaning
   washing or irrigation of the rectum
   _____ /_____ /_____;
   instrument for examining the rectum
   _____ /_____ /_____;
   pertaining to the colon and rectum
   _____ /_____ /_____ /_____.

rect/o/scopy
rek **tos´** kə pē
rect/o/scopic
rek tə **skop´** ik

6.49
The process of examining the rectum with a rect/o/scope is called
_____ /_____ /_____. In doing this, the physician has
performed a _____ /_____ /_____ examination.
                                    (adjective)

NOTE: A more common procedure is a sigmoid/o/scopy. This is
done using an endoscope introduced through the anus and
rectum to the sigmoid colon. This scope is shown on page 205.

rect/o/plasty
rek´ tə plas tē
rect/o/rrhaphy
rek **tôr´** ə fē

6.50
Build words meaning
   plastic surgery of the rectum
   _____ /_____ /_____;
   suturing (stitching) of the rectum
   _____ /_____ /_____.

rect/o/urethr/al
rek tō yoo **rē´** thrəl
rect/o/cyst/o/tomy
rek´ tō sis **tot´** ə mē

6.51
Build words meaning
   pertaining to the rectum and urethra
   _____ /_____ /_____ /_____;
   incision of the bladder through the rectum
   _____ /_____ /_____ /_____ /_____.
      rectum   bladder   incision

specializes in diseases of
   the anus and rectum
the study of diseases of
   the anus and rectum

6.52
proct/o is the combining form for anus and rectum.
A proct/o/logist is one who *_____
_____.
Proct/o/logy is *_____
_____.

ANSWER COLUMN	

6.53
Build words meaning
  washing or irrigation of anus and rectum
  _____ /_____ /_____;
  paralysis of the anus and rectum
  _____ /_____ /_____.

proct/o/clysis
prok **tok**´ lə sis
proct/o/plegia
prok tə **plē**´ jē ə

6.54
A proct/o/logist examines the rectum and anus with a
  _____ /_____ /_____.
This examination is called
  _____ /_____ /_____.

proct/o/scope
prok´ tə skōp
proct/o/scopy
prok **tos**´ kə pē

6.55
Build words meaning
  suturing of the rectum and anus
  _____ /_____ /_____;
  surgical fixation of the rectum and anus
  _____ /_____ /_____.

proct/o/rrhaphy
prok **tôr**´ ə fē
proct/o/pexy
prok´ tō peks ē

6.56
The liver has many functions including the production of heparin, which affects the blood-clotting mechanism. It also produces bile. **hepat/o** is the combining form for liver. It comes from the Greek word *hepar*, meaning liver. Hepat/ic means
* _____.
Hepat/o/megaly means * _____.

pertaining to the liver
enlargement of the liver

6.57
Build words meaning
  inspection (examination) of the liver
  _____ /_____ /_____;
  any disease of the liver
  _____ /_____ /_____.

hepat/o/scopy
hep ə **tos**´ kə pē
hepat/o/pathy
hep ə **top**´ ə thē

6.58
Build words meaning
 incision into the liver
  _____ /_____ /_____;
  excision of (part of) the liver
  _____ /_____.

hepat/o/tomy
hep ə **tot**´ ə mē
hepat/ectomy
hep ə **tek**´ tə mē

ANSWER COLUMN	
	6.59 Hepat/itis B is a serious condition of the liver caused by a viral infection. Hepatitis B vaccine (HBV) may be administered as an immunization protection against _____ /_____.
hepat/itis hep ə **tīt´** is	
hepat/itis (spread of infection)	**6.60** Using standard precautions to avoid contact with body fluids of others helps to prevent _____ /_____.

pertaining to the
  pancreas
destruction of pancreatic
  tissue
	6.61
	The pancreas is both a digestive and endocrine organ.
	pancreat/o is used in words about the pancreas.
	Pancreat/ic means
	* _____.
	Pancreat/o/lysis means
	* _____.

pancreat/o/lith
pan krē **at´** ō lith
pancreat/o/pathy
pan´ krē ə **top´** ə thē
	6.62
	Build words meaning
	    a stone or calculus in the pancreas
	    _____ /_____ /_____;
	    any pancreatic disease
	    _____ /_____ /_____.

pancreat/ectomy
pan´ krē ə **tek´** tə mē
pancreat/o/tomy
pan´ krē ə **tot´** ə mē
	6.63
	Build words meaning
	    excision of part or all of the pancreas
	    _____ /_____;
	    incision into the pancreas
	    _____ /_____ /_____.

chol/e/cyst/o/graph or chol/e/cyst/o/gram	**6.64** Recall that cholelithiasis is a condition in which gallstones have formed in the gallbladder. Choleliths can also lodge in the biliary duct blocking bile flow or the pancreatic ducts causing pancreatitis. An x-ray of the gallbladder is called _____ /_____ /_____ /_____ /_____. **NOTE:** -graph is supposed to mean machine, but in practice it has come to mean the x-ray picture (film) itself.

ANSWER COLUMN

pancreat/itis
pan´ krē ə **tīt**´ is
chol/e/cyst/itis
kōl´ ē sis **tīt**´ is

6.65
Build words meaning inflammation of the
pancreas
_____ /_____ ;
gallbladder
_____ /_____ /_____ /_____ .

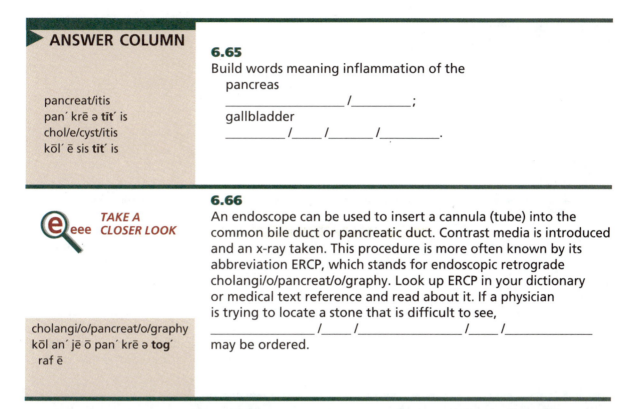

TAKE A CLOSER LOOK

cholangi/o/pancreat/o/graphy
kōl an´ jē ō pan´ krē ə **tog**´
raf ē

6.66
An endoscope can be used to insert a cannula (tube) into the common bile duct or pancreatic duct. Contrast media is introduced and an x-ray taken. This procedure is more often known by its abbreviation ERCP, which stands for endoscopic retrograde cholangi/o/pancreat/o/graphy. Look up ERCP in your dictionary or medical text reference and read about it. If a physician is trying to locate a stone that is difficult to see,
_____ /_____ /_____ /_____ /_____
may be ordered.

Normal ERCP

ERCP with stones

hepat/o/rrhagia
hep ə tō **rā**´ jē ə
hepat/o/rrhaphy
hep ə **tôr**´ ə fē

6.67
Build words meaning
hemorrhage of the liver
_____ /_____ /_____ ;
suture of a wound of the liver
_____ /_____ /_____ .

▶ **ANSWER COLUMN**	**6.68**
	Build words meaning
	    hernia of the liver
	    _____ /_____ /_____ ;
	    pain in the liver
	    _____ /_____ /_____ ;
	    stone in the liver
	    _____ /_____ /_____ .

hepat/o/cele hep **at**´ ō sēl hepat/o/dynia hep at ō **din**´ ē ə hepat/o/lith hep **at**´ ō lith	
	6.69 <mark>A/tresia literally means not perforated or not open.</mark> Biliary atresia is a condition in which the bile ducts are not open. A congenital condition in which a part of the intestine is closed is intestinal _____ /_____ .
a/tresia a **trē**´ zē ə	
closed atresia	**6.70** If a baby is born with esophageal atresia, the esophagus would be _____ . In the heart, congenital closure of the mitral valve is mitral _____ .
atresia	**6.71** Bile backs up into the liver if the ducts are closed or blocked. Biliary _____ is a serious condition.
℮eee TAKE A CLOSER LOOK	**6.72** Another debilitating liver disease is <mark>cirrh/osis</mark> of the liver. In Greek *kirrhos* means orange-yellow. This disease occurs as a result of malnutrition, alcoholism, poisoning, or a history of hepatitis. Treatment of cirrhosis depends on its cause and may include diet modifications, vitamin supplements, cessation of alcohol use and related support groups, energy conservation, and surgery.
cirrh/osis si **rō**´ sis	**6.73** Chronic alcoholism or hepatitis may lead to a dysfunctional liver disease called _____ /_____ .

splen/ectomy
spli **nek**´ tə mē
splen/o/megaly
splen ō **meg**´ ə lē
splen/o/ptosis
splen op **tō**´ sis
	6.74
	splen/o is used in words about the *spleen*. Build words meaning
	    excision of the spleen
	    _____ /_____ ;
	    enlargement of the spleen
	    _____ /_____ /_____ ;
	    prolapse of the spleen
	    _____ /_____ /_____ .

ANSWER COLUMN

✔ *SPELL CHECK*

6.75
Watch your spelling in words about the spleen. The noun spleen has two "e's", but the combining form has one "e", i.e., **splen/o**.

---

splen/o/pexy
splen´ ō peks ē
splen/o/pathy
splen **op´** ə thē
splen/o/rrhaphy
splen **ôr´** ə fē
splen/o/rrhagia
splen ō **rā´** jē ə

6.76
Build words meaning
   surgical fixation of the spleen
   _____ /____ /_____;
   any disease of the spleen
   _____ /____ /_____;
   suture of the spleen
   _____ /____ /_____;
   hemorrhage from the spleen
   _____ /____ /_____.

---

pain in the spleen

6.77
The spleen is one of the blood-forming organs.
Splen/algia means *_____.

---

pertaining to the spleen

6.78
Splen/ic means *_____.

---

esophag/o/duoden/ostomy
i **sof´** ə gō dōō ə də **nos´**-
   tə mē

6.79
Recall the suffix -ostomy. Anastomosis is a surgical connection between tubular structures. The combining form for esophagus is **esophag/o**. When an entire gastrectomy is performed, a new connection is made between the esophagus and the duodenum. This particular anastomosis can also be called an
_____ /____ /_____ /_____.

---

stomach, small intestine,
   and large intestine
esophagus, stomach

small intestine, gallbladder

6.80
All of the operations below are types of anastomoses. Using what you have learned about the digestive system, list the body parts indicated in the following procedures:
gastr/o/enter/o/col/ostomy
*_____
esophag/o/gastr/ostomy
*_____
enter/o/cholecyst/ostomy
*_____

ANSWER COLUMN

jejun/o/ile/itis
inflammation of the
  jejunum and ileum
chole/cyst/o/duoden/ostomy
new opening between the
  duodenum and gallbladder
esophag/o/gastr/o/duoden/-
  o/scopy
examination of the
  esophagus, stomach, and
  duodenum
chol/e/angi/o/pancreat/o/-
  graphy
x-ray of the biliary and
  pancreatic ducts

6.81

Some of these medical words get pretty long. Insert the slashes and define the following terms:

jejunoileitis

_____ ,

* _____ ;

cholecystoduodenostomy

_____ ,

* _____ ;

esophagogastroduodenoscopy (EGD)

_____ ,

* _____ ;

cholangiopancreatography

_____ ,

* _____ .

Good!

Abbreviation	Meaning
BM	bowel movement
PO	by mouth (Latin: *per os*)
NPO	nothing by mouth
EGD	esophagogastroduodenoscopy
ERCP	endoscopic retrograde cholangiopancreatography
GERD	gastroesophageal reflux disease
HB	hepatitis B
HBV	hepatitis B vaccine
HP	Helicobacter pylori
GI	gastrointestinal
GB	gallbladder
NG	nasogastric

To complete your study of this unit, work the review activities on the next pages. Also, listen to the audiotapes that accompany *Medical Terminology: A Programmed Text,* 8th edition, and practice your pronunciation.

Additional practice exercises for this unit are available on the Student Practice disk found in the back of the textbook.

▶ REVIEW ACTIVITIES

Circle and Correct

Circle the correct answer for each question. Then, check your answers in Appendix A.

1. Suffix for dilatation or stretching:
   a. -dilatate   b. -clysis
   c. -ectomy   d. -ectasia

2. Prefix for below:
   a. epi-   b. inter-
   c. sub-   d. supra-

3. Combining form for small intestine or intestine:
   a. colpo   b. entero
   c. duodeno   d. intestino

4. Combining form for liver:
   a. hepat   b. hepato
   c. heparin   d. livo

5. Suffix for paralysis:
   a. -plasia   b. -phagia
   c. -plegia   d.- phasia

6. Prefix for difficult or painful:
   a. sub-   b. dynia-
   c. algia-   d. dys-

7. Combining form for spleen:
   a. spleno   b. spleeno
   c. spleen   d. splenic

8. Suffix for making a new opening:
   a. -tomy   b. -ostomy
   c. -tome   d. -scopy

9. Suffix for irrigation or washing:
   a. -colo   b. -ecstasia
   c. -clysis   d. -enema

10. Word root for stomach:
    a. stomato   b. stomacho
    c. cheilo   d. gastr

11. Stenosis means:
    a. dilation   b. discharge
    c. tubelike   d. narrowing

12. The term for a congenital condition in which a tube is closed is:
    a. stenosis   b. coloclysis
    c. atresia   d. anastomosis

► REVIEW ACTIVITIES

Select and Construct
Select the correct word parts from the list below and construct medical terms that represent the given meaning.

al	algia	angi/o	cele	cheilo
chol(e)	clysis	colo	duoden(o)	dys
ectasia	ectomy	entero(ic)	esophago(eal)	gastr(o)(ic)
gingiv(o)(a)	glosso(al)	graphy	hepato(i)c	hypo
ileo	itis	jejuno	linguo(al)	lith
megaly	myc(osis)	ostomy	pancreato	pathy
plasty	pleg(ic)(ia)	procto	ptosis	rect(o)(al)
rrhagia	rrhaphy	rrhea	scope(y)(ic)	sigmoid(o)
sis	spleno	stomato	sub	tomy

1. fungus infection of the mouth _____

2. below the tongue _____

3. surgical repair of the lips _____

4. inflammation of the gums _____

5. bleeding of the small intestine _____

6. process of examining the esophagus, stomach, and duodenum by looking with an instrument _____

7. prolapse of the small intestine _____

8. irrigation of the rectum _____

9. paralysis of the anus and rectum _____

10. stone in the pancreas _____

11. enlargement of the spleen _____

12. dilatation of the stomach _____

13. instrument for looking in the sigmoid colon _____

14. inflammation of the liver _____

15. herniation of the rectum _____

16. pertaining to stomach and esophagus _____

17. x-ray process of biliary and pancreatic ducts _____

18. pertaining to colon and rectum _____

▶ **REVIEW ACTIVITIES**

Define and Dissect

Give a brief definition and dissect each term listed into its word parts in the space provided on the right. Check your answers by referring to the frame listed in parentheses and your medical dictionary. Then, listen to the audiotapes to practice pronunciation.

1. cheilostomatoplasty (6.19)

   _____ / ___ / _____ / ___ / _____
   rt   v   rt   v   suffix

   _____
              definition

2. gingivoglossitis (6.22)

   _____ / ___ / _____ / _____
   rt   v   rt   suffix

   _____

3. gastrorrhagia (6.29)

   _____ / ___ / _____
   rt   v   suffix

   _____

4. esophageal (6.23)

   _____ / _____
            rt   suffix

   _____

5. enterocentesis (6.38)

   _____ / ___ / _____
   rt   v   rt/suffix

   _____

6. dysentery (6.34)

   _____ / _____ / _____
   pre   rt   suffix

   _____

7. colopexy (6.40)

   _____ / ___ / _____
   rt   v   suffix

   _____

8. rectocele (6.47)

   _____ / ___ / _____
   rt   v   suffix

   _____

9. proctologist (6.52)

   _____ / ___ / _____
   rt   v   suffix

   _____

10. hepatomegaly (6.56)

    _____ / ___ / _____
    rt   v   suffix

    _____

11. pancreatolysis (6.61)

    _____ / ___ / _____
    rt   v   suffix

    _____

12. splenorrhagia (6.76)

    _____ / ___ / _____
    rt   v   suffix

    _____

13. esophagoduodenostomy (6.79)

    _____ / ___ / _____ / ___ / _____
    rt   v   rt   v   suffix

    _____

▶ REVIEW ACTIVITIES

14. jejunoileitis (6.81)   _____ / ____ / _____ / _____
    _{rt}   _v   _{rt}   _{suffix}

15. gastroenteric (6.35)   _____ / ____ / _____ / ____
    _{rt}   _v   _{rt}   _{suffix}

16. sigmoidoscopy (6.49)   _____ / ____ / _____
    _{rt}   _v   _{suffix}

17. coloclysis (6.44)   _____ / ____ / _____
    _{rt}   _v   _{suffix}

18. enterectasia (6.37)   _____ / _____
    _{rt}   _{suffix}

19. glossoplegia (6.15)   _____ / ____ / _____
    _{rt}   _v   _{suffix}

20. sublingual (6.11)   _____ / _____ / ____
    _{pre}   _{rt}   _{suffix}

21. gastroenterology (6.33)   _____ / ___ / _____ / ___ / _____
    _{rt}   _v   _{rt}   _v   _{suffix}

22. hepatitis (6.59)   _____ / _____
    _{rt}   _{suffix}

23. esophagospasm (table)   _____ / ____ / _____
    _{rt}   _v   _{suffix}

24. gingivectomy (6.22)   _____ / _____
    _{rt}   _{suffix}

25. stomatomycosis (6.4)   _____ / ____ / _____ / _____
    _{rt}   _v   _{rt}   _{suffix}

26. esophagostenosis (6.24)   _____ / ____ / _____ / _____
    _{rt}   _v   _{rt}   _{suffix}

27. cholangiopancreatography (6.66)   _____ / ____ / _____ / ____ / _____
    _{rt}   _v   _{rt}   _v   _{suffix}

28. cirrhosis (6.72)   _____ / _____
    _{rt}   _{suffix}

▶ REVIEW ACTIVITIES

Abbreviation Matching
Match the following abbreviations with their definition.

_____ 1. GB

_____ 2. EGD

_____ 3. GI

_____ 4. PO

_____ 5. NPO

_____ 6. HBV

_____ 7. GERD

_____ 8. ERCP

_____ 9. NG

_____ 10. BM

_____ 11. HP

a. Helicobacter pylori
b. hepatomegaly
c. gums and incisors
d. sublingually
e. bowel movement
f. gallbladder
g. nothing by mouth
h. hepatitis B vaccine
i. gastrointestinal
j. orally
k. esophagogastroduodenostomy
l. esophagogastroduodenoscopy
m. AIDS virus
n. Escherichia coli
o. gastroesophageal reflux disorder
p. after meals
q. endoscopic retrograde choleangiopancreatography
r. nasogastric (tube)

Suffix Matching
Match the suffixes on the left with their meanings on the right.

_____ 1. -plegia

_____ 2. -clysis

_____ 3. -ectasia

_____ 4. -rrhagia

_____ 5. -megaly

_____ 6. -ostomy

a. stretching, dilation
b. uncontrolled twitching
c. new permanent opening
d. suturing
e. washing, irrigation
f. hemorrhage
g. herniation
h. enlarged
i. incision into
j. paralysis

▶ CASE STUDIES

Write the term next to its meaning given below. Then, draw slashes to analyze the word parts. Note the use of medical abbreviations. Look these up in your dictionary or find them in Appendix B. If you have any questions about the answers, refer to your medical dictionary or check with your instructor for the answers in Appendix A.

CASE STUDY 6-1
ENDOSCOPY REPORT
Pt: female, age 89

Dx: **Gastrointestinal hemorrhage**, duodenal ulcer   Tx: **EGD**

Ms. Dena Jitters was admitted through the emergency room because of **vomiting** coffee ground material and passing **melenic** stools. The **nasogastric** tube introduced, showed bright red blood. The patient became **hypotensive** and two units of packed red cells were given. Then, Ms. Jitters became stable with a BP of 120/80. She was lavaged with iced **isotonic** saline and an endoscopy was performed.

REPORT: Premedication: Cetacaine locally. The **endoscope** was easily passed into the esophagus. Numerous amounts of **thrombi** were noted. The scope was introduced into the stomach, which showed increased amounts of bright red blood in the fundus. No **mucosal** lesions could be seen; however, half of the stomach was full of blood. The scope was then passed into the **duodenal** bulb, where clots were also noted. This patient could have a duodenal **ulcer**, but because of the amount of blood, it is difficult to delineate an ulcer crater.

A great clot was located on the **anterior** wall. As the scope was withdrawn, the antrum of the stomach could be seen with no lesion noted. It was difficult to clean up all the blood clots and, because of the status of the patient, the procedure was discontinued. Ms. Jitters tolerated the procedure well and did not vomit or **aspirate**.

1. front _____

2. ejecting from the stomach through the mouth _____

3. bleed _____

4. pertaining to the intestine and stomach _____

5. instrument used to look into _____

6. pertaining to mucosa _____

7. breathe in (suck in) _____

8. having the same concentration _____

9. sore _____

10. stomach and intestine _____

11. black (old blood) _____

12. low blood pressure (adjective) _____

13. first part of small intestine (adjective) _____

14. clots _____

15. esophagogastroduodenoscopy _____

▶ CROSSWORD PUZZLE

Check your answers by going back through the frames or checking the solution in Appendix C.

Across

1. specialty in the study of the stomach and the intestine
3. stretching of the stomach
4. enlarged spleen
5. gallbladder x-ray
7. surgical repair of the gums
12. x-ray of the bile ducts (vessels) and pancreatic ducts (process)
13. esophagogastro-duodenoscopy (abbreviation)
14. suffix for stone
17. inflammation of the pancreas
19. endoscopic retrograde cholangiopancreato-graphy (abbreviation)
20. condition of a closed tube or duct (often congenital)

Down

1. pertaining to the stomach and esophagus
2. inflamed gums and tongue
3. gastrointestinal (abbreviation)
6. hemorrhage of the liver
8. instrument used to look into the sigmoid colon
9. irrigation of the anus and rectum
10. suture of the rectum
11. sublingual (synonym)
15. herniation of the intestine
16. nothing by mouth (abbreviation)
18. Greek for mouth

▶ GLOSSARY

anastomosis	connecting two tubular structures
atresia	closed ducts or tubes
cheiloplasty	surgical repair of the lips
cheilosis	condition of the lips
cheilostomatoplasty	repair of the lips and mouth
cheilotomy	incision into the lip
cholangio-pancreatography	process of taking x-ray with contrast media of the biliary and pancreatic ducts
cholecystograph (cholecystogram)	x-ray picture of the gallbladder
cirrhosis	chronic liver disease causing loss of liver function and resistance to blood flow through the liver. Etiology: poor nutrition, alcoholism, previous hepatitis
colic	pertaining to the colon (synonym: colonic)
colocentesis	surgical puncture of the colon to remove fluid
coloclysis	irrigation of the colon
colopexy	surgical fixation of the colon
coloptosis	prolapsed colon
colorectal	pertaining to the colon and rectum
colostomy	making a new opening (stoma) in the colon
diverticulitis	inflammation of diverticula of the intestine
diverticulosis	condition of having diverticula
dysentery	inflammation of the intestine, pain, diarrhea
enterectasia	stretching of the intestine
enteritis	inflammation of the intestine
enterocele	intestinal hernia
enterocentesis	surgical puncture of the intestine to remove fluid
enteroclysis	irrigation of the intestine
enteroplegia	paralysis of the intestine
enteroptosis	prolapse of the intestine
enterorrhagia	hemorrhage of the intestine
enteroscope	instrument for examining the intestine
esophageal	pertaining to the esophagus
esophago-duodenostomy	anastomosis between the esophagus and duodenum
esophagogastric	pertaining to the esophagus and stomach
esophagostenosis	narrowing of the esophagus
gastrectasia	dilatation of the stomach
gastric	pertaining to the stomach
gastritis	inflammation of the stomach
gastroclysis	irrigation of the stomach
gastroenteric	pertaining to the stomach and intestine

► GLOSSARY

gastroenterology	the study of disease of the stomach and intestine
gastroenteroptosis	prolapse of stomach and intestine
gastrorrhagia	hemorrhage of the stomach
gingival	pertaining to the gums
gingivalgia	gum pain
gingivectomy	excision of the gums
gingivoglossitis	inflammation of the gums and tongue
glossal	pertaining to the tongue
glossalgia	tongue pain
glossoplegia	tongue paralysis (adjective: glossoplegic)
glossoptosis	prolapse of the tongue
glossoscopy	examination of the tongue with a scope
hepatectomy	excision of the liver
hepatitis	inflammation of the liver
hepatocele	herniation of the liver
hepatodynia	liver pain (hepatalgia)
hepatolith	liver stone
hepatopathy	any disease of the liver
hepatorrhagia	hemorrhage of the liver
hepatorrhaphy	suture of the liver
hepatoscope	instrument for examining the liver
hepatoscopy	process of using a hepatoscope
hypoglossal	pertaining to below the tongue (synonym: sublingual)
linguogingival	pertaining to the gums and tongue
pancreatectomy	excision of the pancreas
pancreatic	pertaining to the pancreas
pancreatolith	pancreas stone
pancreatolysis	destruction of pancreatic tissue
pancreatopathy	any disease of the pancreas
proctoclysis	irrigation of the rectum and anus
proctologist	physician specialist in diseases of the anus and rectum
proctopexy	fixation of a prolapsed anus and rectum (synonyn: rectopexy)
proctoplegia	paralysis of the rectum and anus
proctorrhaphy	suture of the anus and rectum
proctoscope	instrument for examining the anus and rectum
proctoscopy	process of using a proctoscope
rectocele	herniation of the rectum
rectoclysis	irrigation of the rectum
rectocystotomy	incision into the urinary bladder through the rectum
rectoplasty	surgical repair of the rectum
rectorrhaphy	suturing of the rectum

▶ GLOSSARY

rectoscope	instrument used to examine the rectum	splenorrhagia	hemorrhage of the spleen
rectoscopy	process of using a rectoscope (adjective: rectoscopic)	splenorrhaphy	suturing of the spleen
rectourethral	pertaining to the rectum and urethra	stomatalgia	mouth pain
sigmoidoscope	instrument for examining the sigmoid and large colon	stomatitis	inflammation of the mouth
splenectomy	excision of the spleen	stomatomycosis	fungal condition of the mouth
splenomegaly	enlarged spleen	stomatopathy	any disease of the mouth
splenopathy	any spleen disease	stomatoplasty	surgical repair of the mouth
splenopexy	fixation of a prolapsed spleen	stomatorrhagia	hemorrhage of the mouth
splenoptosis	prolapsed spleen	stomatoscope	instrument used to examine the mouth
		stomatoscopy	process of using a stomatoscope

The
Lovely
Bones
Alice Seabold

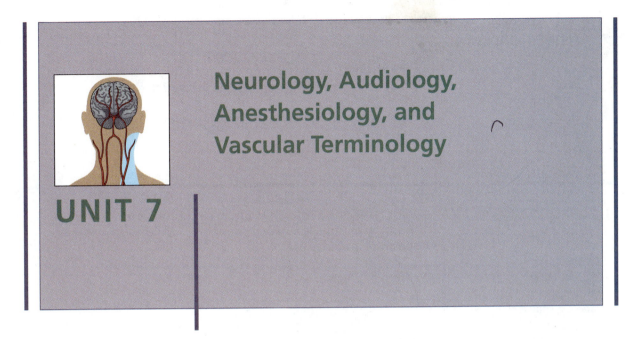

UNIT 7

Neurology, Audiology, Anesthesiology, and Vascular Terminology

Read through the list of word parts in the table below. Then work the frames in the first part of this unit. Refer back to this list when necessary.

Combining Form	Combining Form	Suffix
neur/o (nerve or neuron)	**blast/o** (germ or embryonic; gives rise to something else)	-blast (word itself)
angi/o (vessel)		-spasm (word itself)
my/o (muscle)	**spasm/o** (involuntary contraction)	-osis (use with **scler/o**)
arteri/o (artery)	**scler/o** (hard)	-lysis (use with all)
thromb/o (clot)	**lys/o** (breaking down, destruction)	-oma (use with **fibr/o**)
phleb/o (vein)	**fibr/o** (fibrous, fiber)	-pathy, noun suffix (use with first column)
hem/o, hemat/o (blood)		-genesis, noun suffix (use with **my/o, thromb/o, neur/o**)
ather/o (fatty or porridgelike)		-ectasia (use with **angi/o, arteri/o, phleb/o**)
ven/i (vein)		-rrhexis (use with **angi/o, arteri/o, phleb/o**)

223

ANSWER COLUMN	
	7.1 An embryonic (germ) cell from which a muscle cell develops is a my/o/blast. A germ cell from which a nerve cell develops is a _____ /_____ /_____. A germ cell from which vessels develop is an _____ /_____ /_____.
neur/o/blast **nōōr´** ō blast angi/o/blast **an´** jē o blast	
	7.2 A spasm is an involuntary twitching or contraction. A spasm of a nerve is a neur/o/spasm. A spasm of a muscle is a _____ /_____ /_____. A spasm of a vessel is an _____ /_____ /_____.
my/o/spasm **mī´** ō spaz əm angi/o/spasm **an´** jē ō spaz əm	

	7.3
	Give the words for
	  arterial spasm
	  _____ /_____ /_____;
	  gastric spasm
	  _____ /_____ /_____;
	  softening of the stomach walls
	  _____ /_____ /_____ /_____.

arteri/o/spasm är **tir´** ē ō spaz əm gastr/o/spasm **gas´** trō spaz əm gastr/o/malac/ia gas´ trō mə **lā´** shə	

	7.4
	==My/o/pathy means a generalized disease condition of the muscles.==
	Build words meaning
	  a generalized disease condition of the vessels
	  _____ /_____ /_____;
	  a generalized disease condition of the nerves
	  _____ /_____ /_____.

angi/o/pathy an jē op´ ath ē neur/o/pathy nōōr op´ ath ē	
	7.5 ==A (condition of) hardening of nerve tissue is neur/o/scler/osis.== A hardening of a vessel is _____ /_____ /_____ /_____. A hardening of muscle tissue is _____ /_____ /_____ /_____.
angi/o/scler/osis an´ jē ō sklə **rō´** sis my/o/scler/osis mī´ ō sklə **rō´** sis	

ANSWER COLUMN

neur/o/logist
nōōr ol′ ō jist
neur/o/logy
nōōr ol′ ō gē
neur/itis
nōōr ī′ tis

7.6
Use **neur/o** plus suffixes you have already learned in previous units to build words meaning
  a specialist who studies nervous system disorders
  _____ /_____ /_____;
  the study of the nervous system
  _____ /_____ /_____;
  inflammation of a nerve
  _____ /_____.

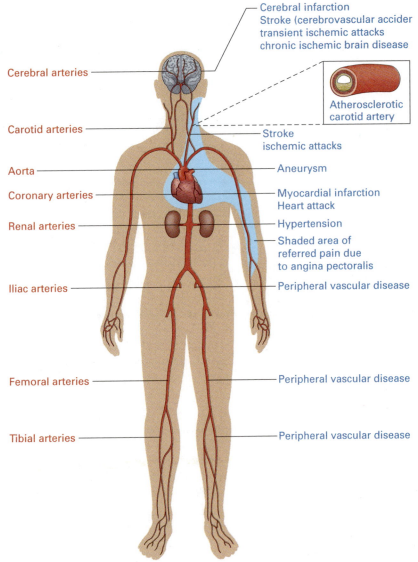

Affected site

Complication

Cerebral infarction
Stroke (cerebrovascular accider
transient ischemic attacks
chronic ischemic brain disease

Cerebral arteries

Atherosclerotic
carotid artery

Carotid arteries

Stroke
ischemic attacks

Aorta — Aneurysm

Coronary arteries — Myocardial infarction
Heart attack

Renal arteries — Hypertension

Shaded area of
referred pain due
to angina pectoralis

Iliac arteries — Peripheral vascular disease

Femoral arteries — Peripheral vascular disease

Tibial arteries — Peripheral vascular disease

Arteries affected by atherosclerosis and possible complications

▶ **ANSWER COLUMN**

eeee   *TAKE A CLOSER LOOK*

7.7
Look up neur/o/logist and neur/o/surgeon in your dictionary and read the definitions of both. Write the distinction below:
** _____
_____

7.8
A muscle tumor is a my/oma.
A nerve tumor is a
_____ /_____.
A vessel tumor is an
_____ /_____.
A fibrous tumor is a
_____ /_____.

neur/oma
nōōr **ō′** mə
angi/oma
an jē **ō′** mə
fibr/oma
fī **brō′** mə

7.9
The destruction of muscle tissue is my/o/lysis.
The destruction of nerve tissue is
_____ /_____ /_____.
The destruction or breaking down of vessels is
_____ /_____ /_____.

neur/o/lysis
nōō **rol′** ə sis
angi/o/lysis
an′ jē **ol′** ə sis

7.10
Build words meaning
    destruction (breakdown) of fat (lipids)
    _____ /_____ /_____;
    destruction (breakdown) of cells
    _____ /_____ /_____.

lip/o/lysis
li **pol′** ə sis
cyt/o/lysis
sī **tol′** ə sis

7.11
arteri/o is used in words about the arteries. Arteries are blood vessels that carry blood away from the heart. A word meaning hardening of the arteries is
_____ /_____ /_____ /_____ (AS).

arteri/o/scler/osis
är tir′ ē ō sklə **rō′** sis

7.12
Arteri/o/scler/osis means hardening of the arteries.
Build words meaning
    a fibrous condition of the arteries
    _____ /_____ /_____ /_____;
    a softening of the arteries
    _____ /_____ /_____.

arteri/o/fibr/osis
är tir′ ē ō fī **brō′** sis
arteri/o/malacia
är tir′ ē ō mə **lā′** shə

▶ **ANSWER COLUMN**

ather/o/scler/osis
a´ ther ō skler ō´ sis

7.13
Refer to the diagram of atherosclerosis on page 225. Recall that **ather/o** means fatty or porridgelike. Hardening of the blood vessels (arteries) caused by a fatty substance (atheroma) is a condition called _____ /____ /_____ /_____.

---

ather/o/scler/osis
a´ ther ō skler ō´ sis

7.14
Atherosclerosis occurs primariy in medium to large blood vessels and can decrease vascular supply causing ischemia and necrosis. This leads to myocardial infarction (heart attack) or cerebral infarction (stroke). Fatty streaks inside the carotid arteries is an indication of _____ /____ /_____ /_____.
NOTE: Look up ischemia and necrosis in your dictionary.

---

ather/ectomy
a´ ther **ek**´ tō mē
end/arter/ectomy
end är´ ter **ek**´ tō mē

7.15
If a large ather/oma develops from the fatty streak an ather/ectomy may be performed. Excision of an ather/oma is called _____ /_____ or
_____ /_____ /_____. This is most commonly performed on the carotid artery.

---

atherosclerosis

7.16
Nonsurgical treatment of atherosclerosis includes bringing cholesterol to normal levels, increasing the high-density lipoproteins (HDL), decreasing the low-density lipoproteins (LDL), and stopping smoking. Diet, exercise, and lifestyle changes can help reduce the risk of death from _____.

---

angina pectoris
an **ji**´ na pek **tor**´ is   or
an´ ji na pek **tor**´ is

7.17
Ather/o/scler/o/tic coronary artery disease is the most common cause of angina pectoris. If the oxygen demand is higher than that supplied to the heart muscle, *_____ can occur.
NOTE: Look up angina pectoris in your dictionary.

---

hem/angi/o/blast
hēm **an**´ gē ō blast
hem/arthr/osis
hēm är **thrō**´ sis

7.18
hem/o refers to blood. A benign tumor of a blood vessel is a hem/angi/oma. (Note dropped o.)
An embryonic blood vessel cell is a
_____ /_____ /____ /_____.
A condition of blood in a joint is
_____ /_____ /_____.

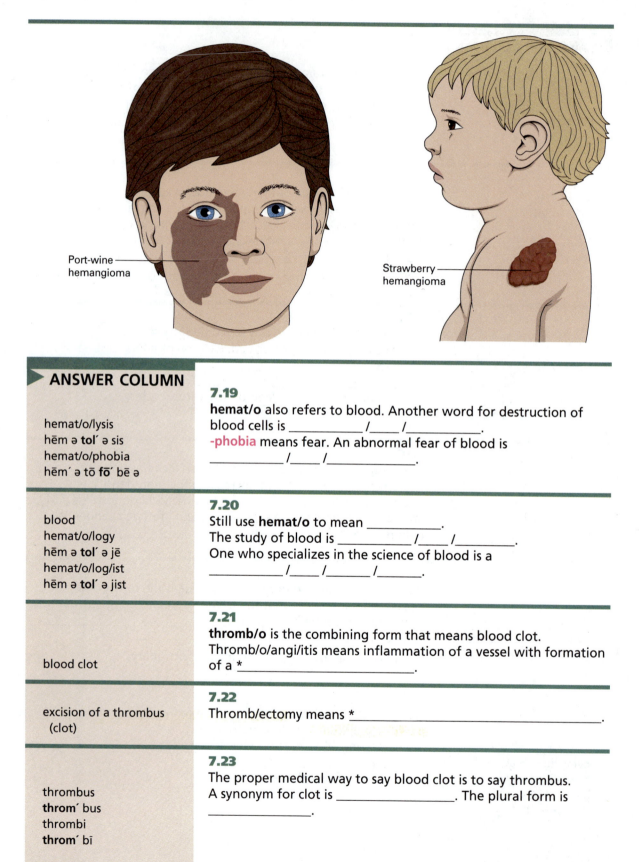

Port-wine hemangioma

Strawberry hemangioma

ANSWER COLUMN	
hemat/o/lysis hēm ə **tol**′ ə sis hemat/o/phobia hēm′ ə tō **fō**′ bē ə	**7.19** **hemat/o** also refers to blood. Another word for destruction of blood cells is _____ /____ /_____. **-phobia** means fear. An abnormal fear of blood is _____ /____ /_____.
blood hemat/o/logy hēm ə **tol**′ ə jē hemat/o/log/ist hēm ə **tol**′ ə jist	**7.20** Still use **hemat/o** to mean _____. The study of blood is _____ /____ /_____. One who specializes in the science of blood is a _____ /____ /_____ /_____.
blood clot	**7.21** **thromb/o** is the combining form that means blood clot. Thromb/o/angi/itis means inflammation of a vessel with formation of a *_____.
excision of a thrombus (clot)	**7.22** Thromb/ectomy means *_____.
thrombus **throm**′ bus thrombi **throm**′ bī	**7.23** The proper medical way to say blood clot is to say thrombus. A synonym for clot is _____. The plural form is _____.

ANSWER COLUMN

inflammation of a lymph vessel with formation of a thrombus (clot) or condition of this	**7.24** Recall **lymph/o** means lymphatic tissue. Thromb/o/lymph/ang/itis means *_____ _____.
inflammation of a vein with thrombus formation	**7.25** **phleb/o** is a combining form for vein. Thromb/o/phleb/itis means *_____ _____.

thromb/osis
throm **bō´** sis
thromb/o/cyte
throm´ bō sīt
thromb/oid
throm´ boid
	7.26
	See, you are great at figuring out meanings. Now, using **thromb/o**, build words meaning
	   a condition of forming a thrombus
	   _____ /_____;
	   a cell that aids clotting
	   _____ /_____ /_____;
	   resembling a thrombus
	   _____ /_____.

thromb/o/gen/ic
throm´ bō **jen´** ik
thromb/o/lysis
throm **bol´** ə sis
thromb/o/cyt/o/penia
throm´ bō sī´ tō **pē´** nē ə
	7.27
	Build words meaning
	   pertaining to the formation of a thrombus
	   _____ /_____ /_____ /_____;
	   destruction of a thrombus
	   _____ /_____ /_____;
	   lack of cells that aid in clotting (platelets)
	   _____ /_____ /_____ /_____ /_____.
	Great! You are good at word building, too.

INFORMATION FRAME	**7.28** A thrombus may block or "occlude" a vessel. This occlusion may cause ischemia, stopping blood supply to the tissues, producing an infarct (necrosis of tissue). If this happens in the heart muscle, the condition is called myocardial infarction (MI).
eeee *TAKE A CLOSER LOOK*	**7.29** Look up the following terms in your medical dictionary and write their definitions: occlusion *_____ _____; infarct *_____ _____; myocardial *_____ _____.

ANSWER COLUMN	
	7.30 A thrombus or piece of a thrombus may move through blood vessels to another part of the body. This moving thrombus is called an embolus. An embolus may cause a block in a vessel called an
occlusion ō klōō′ shun	_____.
	7.31 If an artery of the heart muscle is occluded and an area of tissue
my/o/cardi/al in/farct/ion mī ō kär′ dē əl in fark′ shun	has no blood supply, a *____ /____ /_____ /____ ____ /_____ /_____ (MI) may occur.
	7.32 If an artery supplying the cerebrum (brain) is occluded,
cerebr/al in/farct/ion se rē′bral in fark′ shun	a *_____ /____ ____ /_____ /_____ (CVA, cerebrovascular accident, stroke) could occur.
	7.33 Recall that arteries (**arteri/o**) are vessels that carry blood away from the heart. Veins (**phleb/o**) are vessels that carry blood back to
heart	the _____.
	7.34 One combining form for vein is **phleb/o**. Arteriosclerosis is
arteries phleb/o/scler/osis fleb′ ō sklə rō′ sis	hardening of the _____. Hardening of veins is called _____ /____ /_____ /_____.
	7.35 Build words meaning
	excision of a vein

phleb/ectomy
fli bek′ tə mē
phleb/o/pexy
fleb′ ō pek sē
	_____ /_____;
	   surgical fixation of a vein
	   _____ /____ /_____.

	7.36 Dilation and dilatation are synonyms for stretching or increase in diameter. **-ectasia** is also used as a suffix for dilatation. Build words meaning
	venous dilatation (stretching)

phleb/ectasia
fleb′ ek tā′ shə
arteri/ectasia
är tir′ ē ek tā′ shə
angi/ectasia
an′ jē ek tā′ shə
	_____ /_____;
	   arterial dilatation
	   _____ /_____;
	   vessel dilatation
	   _____ /_____.

▶ **ANSWER COLUMN**

7.37
Phleb/o/plasty means

surgical repair of a vein   * _____ .

Phleb/o/tomy means

incision into a vein or
  venipuncture
  vēn´ i punk tyo͞or   * _____ .

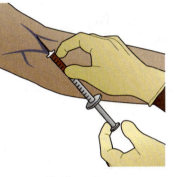

Venipuncture

7.38
ven/i/puncture   **ven/o** and **ven/i** are also combining forms for vein. To obtain a
vēn´ i punk tyo͞or   ven/ous blood sample, a _____ /_____ /_____ is
                      performed.

7.39
ven/ous   Venous blood is the dark blood in the veins. Blood flow through
vēn´ us   the veins back to the heart is called _____ /_____ return.
ven/ous   Administering medication within a vein is an
                   intra/_____ /_____ injection.

7.40
                   -rrhexis is a suffix meaning rupture. Hyster/o/rrhexis means
rupture of the uterus   * _____ .

7.41
                   With **-rrhexis** you learn the last of the Greek "rrh" forms. **-rrhea, -**
suffixes   **rrhagia, -rrhaphy,** and **-rrhexis** are _____ .

7.42
                   Cyst/o/rrhexis means
rupture of the bladder   * _____ .

                   Enter/o/rrhexis means
rupture of the small   * _____ .
  intestine

ANSWER COLUMN

-rrhea, discharge or flow -rrhagia, hemorrhage -rrhaphy, suture -rrhexis, rupture	**7.43** To summarize, the four "rrh" suffixes you have learned are _____ , meaning _____ _____ , meaning _____ _____ , meaning _____ _____ , meaning _____

cardi/o/rrhexis
kär´ dē ō **rek**´ sis
angi/o/rrhexis
an´ jē ō **rek**´ sis
	7.44
	Build words meaning
	   rupture of the heart
	   _____ / _____ / _____ ;
	   rupture of a vessel
	   _____ / _____ / _____ .

arteri/o/rrhexis
är tir´ ē ō **rek**´ sis
phleb/o/rrhexis
fleb´ ō **rek**´ sis
	7.45
	Build words meaning
	   rupture of an artery
	   _____ / _____ / _____ ;
	   rupture of a vein
	   _____ / _____ / _____ .

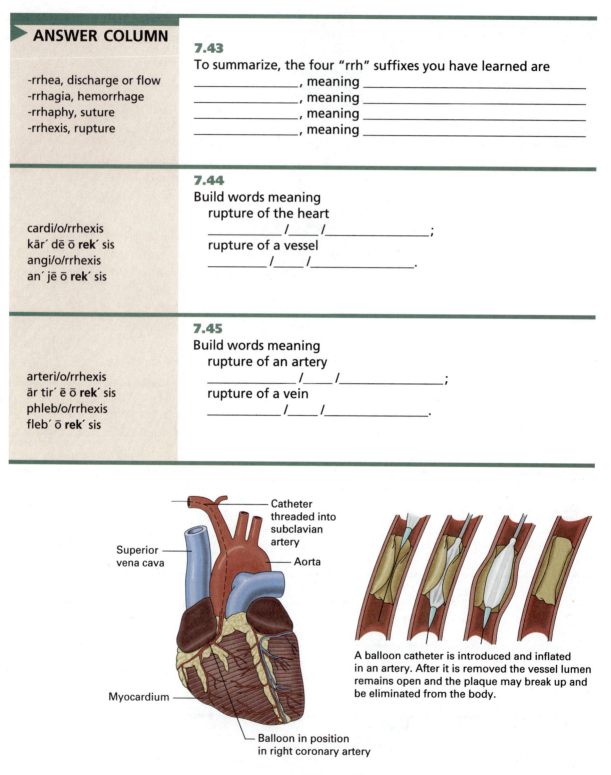

Catheter threaded into subclavian artery

Superior vena cava

Aorta

Myocardium

Balloon in position in right coronary artery

A balloon catheter is introduced and inflated in an artery. After it is removed the vessel lumen remains open and the plaque may break up and be eliminated from the body.

Balloon angioplasty

▶ **ANSWER COLUMN**

7.46
Build terms that mean
   repair of a vessel

angi/o/plasty
an´ jē ō plas tē
angi/o/graphy
an jē **og**´ raf ē
angi/o/scopy
an jē **os**´ kō pē

_____ /____ /_____;
   process of obtaining an x-ray of a vessel
_____ /____ /_____;
   process of using a looking device to examine a vessel
_____ /____ /_____.

7.47
Give the meaning of the following terms:
phleb/o/plasty

repair of a vein

*_____;

phleb/o/graphy (ven/o/graphy)

process of obtaining an
 x-ray of a vein

*_____.

7.48
Rupture of the tissues of the uterus is called

metr/o/rrhexis or
mē trō **rek**´ sis
hyster/o/rrhexis
his´ ter ō **rek**´ sis

_____ /____ /_____.

7.49
Build words meaning
   rupture of the liver

hepat/o/rrhexis
hep at ōr **eks**´ is
hepat/o/rrhaphy
hep at **ōr**´ a fē
hepat/o/rrhea
hep at ō **rē**´ ə

_____ /____ /_____;
   suturing of the liver (wound)
_____ /____ /_____;
   excessive discharge of bile from the liver
_____ /____ /_____.

7.50
Build words meaning
   rupture of the bladder

cyst/o/rrhexis
sis´ tō **reks**´ is
cyst/o/rrhagia
sis´ tō **rā**´ jē ə
cyst/o/rrhea
sis tō **rē**´ ə
cyst/o/rrhaphy
sis **tōr**´ a fē

_____ /____ /_____;
   hemorrhage from the bladder
_____ /____ /_____;
   discharge from the bladder
_____ /____ /_____;
   suturing of the bladder
_____ /____ /_____.

Good!

► **ANSWER COLUMN**

INFORMATION FRAME

7.51
Esthesia is a word meaning feeling or sensation. Think of the English word aesthetics, meaning that which we perceive or sense. an- is a form of the prefix a-. an- means without (e.g., anemia, lack of blood; anorexia, lack of appetite).

7.52
Recall that a- and an- are prefixes meaning without or lack of. Analyze the following words by dividing them into their word parts. Look up the meanings in your dictionary:

esthesiometer

_____ /_____ /_____

esthesi/o/meter
es thēs´ ē om´ ə ter
an/esthesi/a
an es **thēs´** ē ə
an/esthesi/o/logy
an es thēs´ ē **ol´** o jē
an/esthet/ist
an **es´** the tist

anesthesia

_____ /_____ /_____

anesthesiology

_____ /_____ /_____ /_____

anesthetist

_____ /_____ /_____

7.53
Build words that mean
without or lack of sensation

anesthesia

_____;

a person who administers anesthetic agents

anesthetist

_____;

a physician specialist in anesthesia

anesthesiologist

_____.

7.54
Novocaine is used to remove sensation in a specific area. It is a

an/esthet/ic
an es **the´** tik

local _____ /_____ /_____.

7.55
Think of the meaning as you analyze the following words:
dysesthesia

dys/esthesi/a
dis es thēs´ ē ə
hypo/esthesi/a
hī´ pō es **thēs´** ē ə

_____ /_____ /_____;

hypoesthesia

_____ /_____ /_____.

7.56
Algesia is a noun meaning oversensitivity to pain. Hyper/esthesi/a is a synonym for algesia. Algesia means

oversensitivity to pain or
   hyperesthesia

* _____.

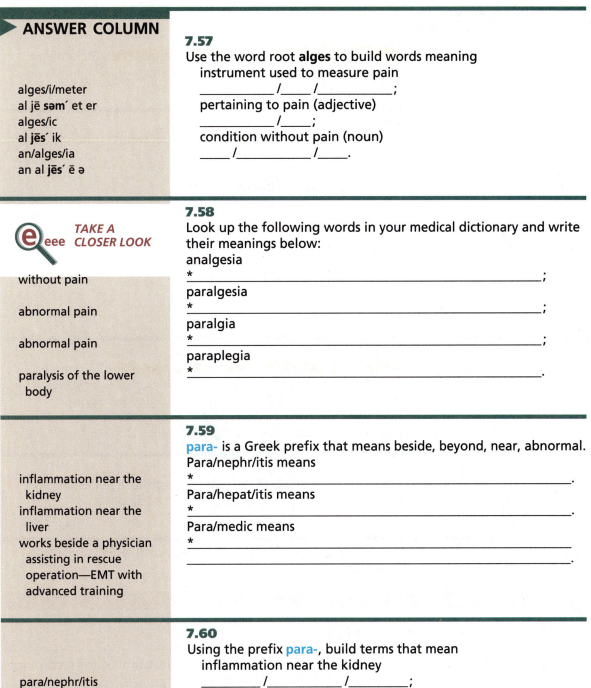

ANSWER COLUMN

7.57

Use the word root **alges** to build words meaning
instrument used to measure pain
__________ /____ /__________;
pertaining to pain (adjective)
__________ /____;
condition without pain (noun)
____ /__________ /____.

alges/i/meter
al jē **səm**′ et er
alges/ic
al **jēs**′ ik
an/alges/ia
an al **jēs**′ ē ə

7.58

TAKE A CLOSER LOOK

Look up the following words in your medical dictionary and write their meanings below:
analgesia
* ____;
paralgesia
* ____;
paralgia
* ____;
paraplegia
* ____.

without pain

abnormal pain

abnormal pain

paralysis of the lower body

7.59

para- is a Greek prefix that means beside, beyond, near, abnormal.
Para/nephr/itis means
* ____.
Para/hepat/itis means
* ____.
Para/medic means
* ____
____.

inflammation near the kidney
inflammation near the liver
works beside a physician assisting in rescue operation—EMT with advanced training

7.60

Using the prefix para-, build terms that mean
inflammation near the kidney
________ /__________ /________;
inflammation near the fallopian tubes
________ /______________ /________;
inflammation near the liver
________ /__________ /________;
disease near a bone and joint
________ /________ /____ /______________ /____ /__________.

para/nephr/itis
par′ ə nef **rī**′ tis
para/salping/itis
par′ ə sal pin **jī**′ tis
para/hepat/itis
par′ ə hep at **ī**′ tis
para/oste/o/arthr/o/pathy
par′ ə os′ tē ō är **throp**′ ə thē

para/lysis
par **al**′ ə sis

7.61
Paralysis is a loss of muscle function and sensation. Para/plegia is
_____ / _____ of the lower body.

---

para/phasia
par ə **fā**′ sē ə
a/phasia
ā **fā**′ sē ə
brady/phasia
brad i **fā**′ sē ə
tachy/phasia
tak i **fā**′ sē ə
dys/phasia
dis **fā**′ sē ə

7.62
phas/o means speech. Build the following terms related to speech:
    abnormal speech (dysfunction)
    _____ / _____;
    unable to speak (without speech)
    _____ / _____;
    slow speech
    _____ / _____;
    fast speech
    _____ / _____;
    difficulty speaking
    _____ / _____.

**INFORMATION
FRAME**

7.63
Paroxysmos is a Greek word meaning an irritation. A symptom
that comes upon someone suddenly, for example, difficulty
breathing in the middle of the night, is called paroxysm.
Paroxysmal nocturnal dyspnea (PND) is a sudden onset of
shortness of breath (SOB) at night.

---

paroxysm/al
par oks **iz**′ mal

7.64
Waking in the middle of the night with difficulty breathing is
called _____ / _____ nocturnal dyspnea.

Use the following combining forms and suffixes in Frames
7.65–7.83.

Combining Form	Meaning	Suffix
my/o	muscle	-graph (instrument for recording)
audi/o	hearing	-gram (record, picture)
phon/o	voice, vocal sounds	-algia (pain)
phas/o	speech	-logy (study of)
kinesi/o	movement	

ANSWER COLUMN	
	7.65 **phon/o** means voice or vocal sounds. A/phonia means
unable to make sounds	*_____.
	Dys/phonia means
weak voice (poor, etc.)	*_____.

	7.66
	Brady/phasia means
slow speech	*_____.
	A/phasia means
absence of speech	*_____.
	Phon/ic means
pertaining to the voice	*_____.
	A phon/o/meter is

an instrument for
  measuring intensity of
  vocal sounds
	*_____.

	7.67 Build terms that mean the study of: voice or vocal sounds
phon/o/logy fon **ol′** ō jē audi/o/logy aw de **ol′** ō jē phas/o/logy fās **ol′** ō jē	_____ /_____ /_____; hearing _____ /_____ /_____; speech _____ /_____ /_____.

	7.68 *Myon* is a Greek word meaning muscle. Myocarditis means inflammation of the heart muscle. **my/o** is used in words referring
muscles	to the _____.

	7.69
INFORMATION FRAME	There are three main types of muscle found throughout the body. Study the table that follows to discover each type, its location, and main function.

► **ANSWER COLUMN**

Muscle Type	Location	Function
striated (skeletal, voluntary) **rhabdomy/o**	covers skeleton Example: rhabdomyosarcoma	skeletal movement
smooth (visceral, involuntary) **leiomy/o**	organs, vessels Example: leiomyofibroma	movement of liquids, gases, and solids
cardiac **myocardi/o**	heart Example: myocardiopathy	maintain heartbeat

7.70
Using the words my/o/gram, my/o/graph, and my/o/graphy, fill in the blanks:

myogram _____ the chart;
myograph _____ the instrument;
myography _____ the process.

7.71
muscles   My/asthenia gravis is a condition of the _____.

7.72
Using **my/o**, **fibr/o**, and **-oma**, build a term meaning a fibrous
my/o/fibr/oma   muscle tumor: ____ /____ /_____ /_____. This is also called a
mī ō fib **rō´** mə   lei/o/my/oma uteri or fibroid tumor of the uterine _____
muscle   or my/o/metr/ium.

7.73
Build words meaning
    resembling muscle
my/oid   ____ /_____;
mī´ oid   muscle tumor containing fatty elements
my/o/lip/oma   ____ /____ /_____ /_____;
mī ō lip **ō´** mə   muscle disease
my/o/pathy   ____ /____ /_____;
mī **op´** ath ē   heart muscle disease
cardi/o/my/o/pathy or   _____ /____ /_____ /____ /_____.
kär´ dē ō mī **op´** ə thē
my/o/cardi/o/pathy
mī´ ō kär dē **op´** ə thē

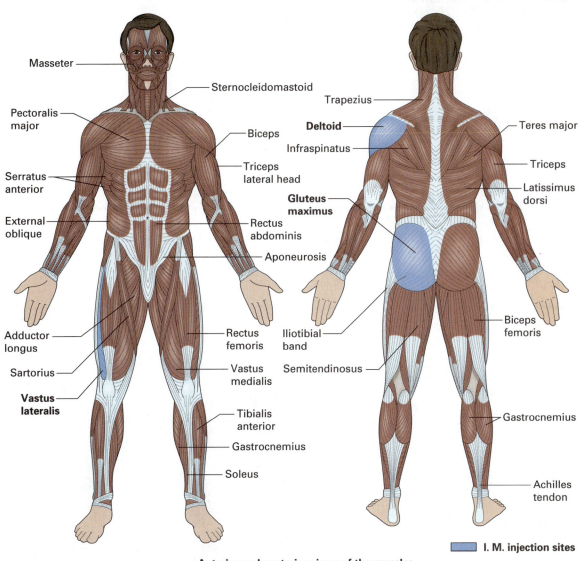

Masseter

Sternocleidomastoid

Trapezius

Pectoralis major

Biceps

Deltoid

Infraspinatus

Teres major

Serratus anterior

Triceps lateral head

Triceps

External oblique

Gluteus maximus

Latissimus dorsi

Rectus abdominis

Aponeurosis

Adductor longus

Rectus femoris

Iliotibial band

Biceps femoris

Sartorius

Vastus medialis

Semitendinosus

Vastus lateralis

Tibialis anterior

Gastrocnemius

Gastrocnemius

Soleus

Achilles tendon

I. M. injection sites

Anterior and posterior views of the muscles

ANSWER COLUMN

eee *TAKE A CLOSER LOOK*

more than 60

7.74
Look up words beginning with **my/o** in your dictionary.
Count how many of the words you know.
Write the number here:
* _____ .

muscles

smooth muscle

heart muscle

7.75
When you see **my/o**, you will think of _____ .
When you see **leiomy/o**, you will think of
* _____ .

When you see **myocardi/o**, you will think of
* _____ .

ANSWER COLUMN	
slowness of movement	**7.76** The main function of muscles is movement. **kinesi/o** is used in words to mean movement or motion. Brady/kinesia means * _____.
pain on movement or movement pain	**7.77** Kinesi/algia means * _____.
kinesi/algia ki nē′ sē **al**′ jē ə	**7.78** Kinesi/algia occurs when you have to move any sore or injured part of the body. Moving a broken arm causes _____ / _____.

Professional Profiles ◀◀◀◀◀◀◀◀◀◀◀◀◀◀◀◀◀◀◀◀◀◀◀◀◀◀◀◀

Physical therapists (PTs) assess, prevent, and treat movement dysfunction and physical disabilities by using technological interventions as well as personal contact. In addition to patient care, the physical therapist may consult, supervise, administer, research, and provide community service through private practice or employment within an in-patient facility or clinic. **Physical therapy assistants** are supervised by the physical therapist and may administer physical therapy treatments as well as help with record keeping, billing, and reception. There are several professional organizations involved with education and credentialling of physical therapists. They include the American Association of Rehabilitation Therapy (AART), the American Physical Therapy Association (APTA), and the American Congress of Physical Medicine and Rehabilitation (ACPMR).

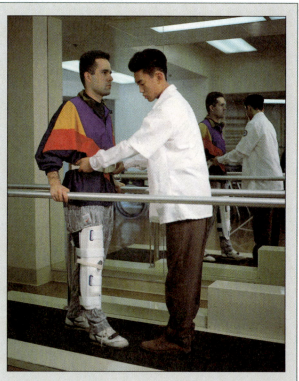

Physical therapist

ANSWER COLUMN	
	7.79 After one's first ride on horseback, almost any movement causes
kinesialgia	_____.
	7.80 -logy is used like a suffix to mean study of. (Remember -logist?) The study of muscular body movements is
kinesi/o/logy ki nē′ sē **ol**′ ə jē	_____ /_____ /_____.
	7.81 Kinesi/o/logy is the study of movement. The study of muscular movement during exercise would be done in the field of
kinesiology	_____.
	7.82 An exercise physiologist studies the science of how the body moves, called _____.
kinesiology	
	7.83 Recall brady- is the prefix for slow. Slowness of movement is called _____ /_____.
brady/kinesia brād′ i ki **nē**′ sē ə or brād′ ē ki **nē**′ sē ə	

Abbreviation	Meaning	Abbreviation	Meaning
AANA	American Association of Nurse Anesthetists	CAD	coronary artery disease
AART	American Association of Rehabilitation Therapy	CRNA	certified registered nurse anesthetist
		C-Section	cesarean section
ACPMR	American Congress of Physical Medicine and Rehabilitation	EMG	electromyogram
		HA	hearing aid, headache
		HDL	high-density lipoproteins
ADL	activities of daily living	IV	intravenous
		LDL	low-density lipoproteins
AE	above the elbow		
AK	above the knee	MD	muscular dystrophy, myocardial disease
AOD	arterial occlusive disease	MFT	muscle function test
APTA	American Physical Therapy Association	MHz	megahertz
		MI	myocardial infarction
AS	arteriosclerosis, left ear	MS	multiple sclerosis
ASCVD	arteriosclerotic cardiovascular disease	PND	paroxysmal nocturnal dyspnea
		PT, protime	prothrombin time
ASHD	arteriosclerotic heart disease	PT	physical therapy (therapist)
BE	below the elbow, barium enema	PTT	partial thromboplastin time
BK	below the knee	ROM	range of motion
CABG	coronary artery bypass graft	SOB	short of breath
		TENS	transcutaneous electric nerve stimulation

To complete your study of this unit, work the review activities on the next pages. Also, listen to the audiotapes that accompany *Medical Terminology: A Programmed Text,* 8th edition, and practice your pronunciation.

Additional practice exercises for this unit are available on the Student Practice disk found in the back of the textbook.

▶ **REVIEW ACTIVITIES**

Circle and Correct
Circle the correct answer for each question. Then, check your answers in Appendix A.

1. Suffix for surgical fixation:
    a. -ptosis   b. -plasty
    c. -pexy   d. -ectasia

2. Combining form for vein:
    a. phlebo   b. ven
    c. venous   d. thrombo

3. Suffix for rupture:
    a. -ptosis   b. -ectasis
    c. -rrhaphy   d. -rrhexis

4. Suffix for most x-ray procedures:
    a. -graphy   b. -electric
    c. -Roentgen   d. -graph

5. Prefix for without:
    a. not-   b. inter-
    c. an-   d. dys-

6. Word root for oversensitivity to pain:
    a. alges   b. analgia
    c. esthesia   d. algia

7. Prefix for abnormal, near, or beyond:
    a. meta-   b. para-
    c. ultra-   d. ab-

8. Combining form for voice:
    a. phago   b. phono
    c. plaso   d. phaso

9. Suffix for speech:
    a. -phasia   b. -plasia
    c. -phonia   -d. phagia

10. Combining form for hearing:
    a. phono   b. phaso
    c. oto   d. audio

11. Word root for movement:
    a. my   b. esthesi
    c. kinesi   d. motor

12. Suffix for tumor:
    a. -algia   b. -itis
    c. -genic   d. -oma

13. Combining form for hard:
    a. cranio   b. skullo
    c. osteo   d. sclero

14. Word root for vessel:
    a. arterio   b. arter
    c. angi   d. vesic

15. Suffix for destruction:
    a. -plasty   b. -rrhexis
    c. -lysis   d. -malacia

16. Word root for blood clot:
    a. thromb   b. hem
    c. hemat   d. embolism

17. Combining form for blood:
    a. hemato   b. penia
    c. emia   d. thrombo

▶ REVIEW ACTIVITIES

Select and Construct

Select the correct word parts from the list below and construct medical terms that represent the given meaning.

a	algeso(ic)	algia(esic)	an	analg
angio	arterio	ather/o	audio	brady
cardio	dynia	dys	echo	ectasia
entero	esthesi/o(a)	fibr/o	gram	graph(y)
hepato	ist	itis	kinesi/o(a)	logist
logy	ma	meter	myo	neur/o
o(sis)	para	pathy	phaso(ia)(ic)	phlebo
phono(ia)(ic)	plasty	plegia(ic)	rrhexis(ia)	sclero
scopy	spasm	tachy	thromb/o	veno

1. hardening of an artery _____
2. dilation of a vein _____
3. rupture of the intestine _____
4. x-ray of a vessel _____
5. instrument for measuring touch _____
6. physician specialist who prepares patients for painless surgery _____
7. pain-relieving medication (adjective) _____
8. inflammation near the liver _____
9. unable to make sounds (with voice) _____
10. instrument for measuring muscle function _____
11. difficult or painful movement _____
12. instrument for measuring hearing function _____
13. difficulty speaking _____
14. paralysis of the lower body _____
15. fibrous and muscle tumor _____
16. large vessel hardening due to fatty streaks _____
17. repair of a vessel _____
18. condition of blood clots _____
19. abnormal muscle contraction _____
20. tumor of fiber and nerve _____
21. inflammation of vein caused by clots _____
22. specialist in nerve disorders _____
23. heart muscle disease _____

Define and Dissect

► **REVIEW ACTIVITIES**

Give a brief definition and dissect each term listed into its word parts in the space provided on the right. Check your answers by referring to the frame listed in parentheses and your medical dictionary. Then, listen to the audiotapes to practice pronunciation.

1. neuroblast (7.1)

   _____ / ____ / _____
   rt   v   rt

   _____
   definition

2. myosclerosis (7.5)

   ____ / ____ / _____ / _____
   rt   v   rt   suffix

3. arteriofibrosis (7.12)

   _____ / ____ / _____ / _____
   rt   v   rt   suffix

4. hematolysis (7.19)

   _____ / ____ / _____
   rt   v   suffix

5. thrombogenic (7.27)

   _____ / ____ / _____ / ____
   rt   v   rt   suffix

6. occlusion (7.28)

   _____ / _____
   rt   suffix

7. neurologist (7.6)

   _____ / ____ / _____
   rt   v   suffix

8. myocardial (7.31)

   ____ / ____ / _____ / _____
   rt   v   rt   suffix

9. hemangioblast (7.18)

   _____ / _____ / ____ / _____
   rt   rt   v   suffix

10. phlebosclerosis (7.34)

    _____ / ____ / _____ / ____
    rt   v   rt   suffix

11. arteriectasia (7.36)

    _____ / _____
    rt   suffix

12. cystorrhexis (7.50)

    _____ / ____ / _____
    rt   v   suffix

▶ REVIEW ACTIVITIES

13. angioplasty (7.46)

_____ / ___ / _____
rt   v   suffix

14. phlebography (7.47)

_____ / ___ / _____
rt   v   suffix

15. anesthetist (7.52)

____ / _____ / _____
pre   rt   suffix

16. dysesthesia (7.55)

_____ / _____ / ____
pre   rt   suffix

17. analgesia (7.57)

____ / _____ / ____
pre   rt   suffix

18. paranephritis (7.59)

_____ / _____ / ____
pre   rt   suffix

19. bradyphasia (7.62)

_____ / _____ / ____
pre   rt   suffix

20. aphonia (7.65)

____ / _____
pre   rt/suffix

21. phasology (7.67)

_____ / ___ / _____
rt   v   suffix

22. myography (7.70)

____ / ___ / _____
rt   v   suffix

23. audiology (7.67)

_____ / ___ / _____
rt   v   suffix

24. kinesiology (7.80)

_____ / ___ / _____
rt   v   suffix

25. bradykinesia (7.76)

_____ / _____ / ____
pre   rt   suffix

26. phlebotomy (7.37)
　　　　　　　/_____/_____
　　　　　rt　　　v　　suffix

27. anesthesiologist (7.53)
_____/_____/____/_____
　pre　　　rt　　　v　　suffix

28. hepatorrhea (7.49)
_____/____/_____
　　　rt　　　v　　suffix

29. tachyphasia (7.62)
_____/_____
　　pre　　　suffix

30. paralysis (7.61)
_____/_____
　　pre　　　suffix

31. phonometer (7.66)
_____/____/_____
　　rt　　　v　　suffix

32. myofibroma (7.72)
____/____/_____/_____
rt　　v　　　rt　　suffix

33. paraplegia (7.61)
_____/_____
　　pre　　　suffix

34. angiorrhexis (7.44)
_____/____/_____
　rt　　　v　　suffix

35. ischemia (7.28)
_____/_____
　　　rt　　suffix

36. infarction (7.28)
____/_____/_____
　pre　　　rt　　suffix

37. paroxysmal (7.64)
_____/_____
　　　rt　　suffix

► **REVIEW ACTIVITIES**

Abbreviation Matching
Match the following abbreviations with their definition.

_____ 1. MHz

_____ 2. MS

_____ 3. EMG

_____ 4. HA

_____ 5. AANA

_____ 6. ASHD

_____ 7. BE

_____ 8. MFT

_____ 9. ROM

_____ 10. ADL

a. muscular dystrophy
b. milliamperes
c. arteriosclerotic heart disease
d. range of motion
e. arteriosclerotic cardiovascular disease
f. multiple fracture test
g. American Association of Nurse Anesthetists
h. electroencephalogram
i. American Association of Naturopaths
j. hearing aid
k. megahertz
l. electromyogram
m. heartache
n. muscle function test
o. ad lib
p. below the ear
q. above the elbow
r. activities of daily living
s. below the elbow, barium enema
t. multiple sclerosis

Abbreviation Fill-ins
Fill in the blanks with the correct abbreviations

11. high-density lipoproteins _____

12. myocardial infarction _____

13. prothrombin time _____

14. coronary artery bypass graft _____

15. intravenous _____

16. below the knee _____

17. muscular dystrophy _____

18. transcutaneous electrical nerve stimulation _____

19. paroxysmal nocturnal dyspnea _____

20. short of breath _____

▶ CASE STUDIES

Write the term next to its meaning given below. Then, draw slashes to analyze the word parts. Note the use of medical abbreviations. Look these up in your dictionary or find them in Appendix B. If you have any questions about the answers, refer to your medical dictionary or check with your instructor for the answers in Appendix A.

CASE STUDY 7-1
DISCHARGE SUMMARY

Pt: female, age 36, gravida II, para II

Dx: 1. Intrauterine pregnancy—term

2. Previous myomectomy

3. Uterine leiomyomata

4. Fertility

Operations: 1. Primary low vertical cesarean section

2. Incidental appendectomy

3. Bilateral partial salpingectomy

Ms. Cecilia Julius has had a previous myomectomy with invasion of the intrauterine cavity. Therefore, she is going to have a primary C-Section for delivery with this neonate. She developed another large myoma during this pregnancy, but it has not been a problem until this point. On the same day of admission she underwent a primary low vertical cesarean section with an estimated blood loss of 700 cc. There was delivery of a 7 lb 11 oz female with Apgars of 8 and 9. Her postoperative course was basically unremarkable and she remained afebrile. Postoperative hemoglobin: 13.4 gm. The bladder and bowel habits were normal by her fourth postoperative day, and Ms. Julius was ready for discharge.

1. excision of the appendix _____

2. Hgb or Hb, in RBCs _____

3. cubic centimeters _____

4. pound, ounce _____

5. adm, entering the hospital _____

6. cesarean section delivery _____

7. two sides _____

8. excision of the uterine tubes _____

9. excision of a muscle tumor _____

10. fibroid tumors of the uterus _____

11. newborn infant _____

12. gram _____

► CROSSWORD PUZZLE

Check your answers by going back through the frames or checking the solution in Appendix C.

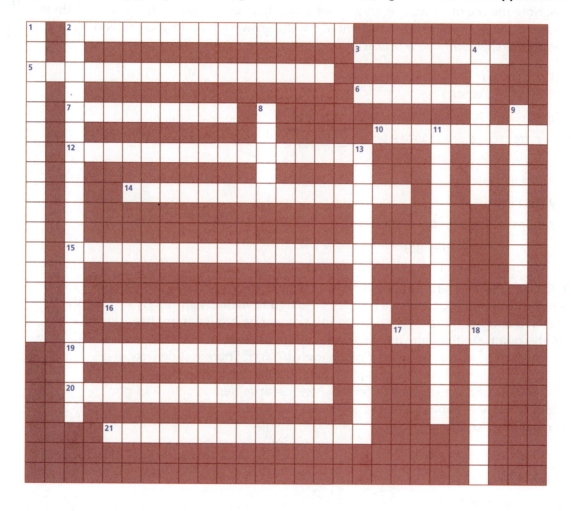

Across

2. inflammation near the fallopian tubes
3. muscle tissue destruction
5. inflammation of a vein caused by a clot
6. pertaining to pain (adj.)
7. blockage
10. emergency technician with advanced training
12. lack of platelets
14. blood clot in a vessel causing inflammation
15. inflammation of a lymph vessel caused by a clot
16. hardening of a vein
17. blood clot
19. science studying administration of anesthetics
20. rupture of the uterus
21. rupture of an artery

Down

1. hardening of the arteries
2. disease near the bone and joint
4. condition stopping blood supply
8. muscle tumor
9. lipid destruction
11. fatty deposits on medium to large vessels, causing hardening
13. condition of fibrous growth in the arteries (plural)
18. instrument used to make a picture of muscle function

▶ GLOSSARY

algesia	condition of pain sensitivity
algesic	pertaining to algesia
algesimeter	instrument for measuring level of pain
analgesia	condition without pain
anesthesia	condition of no sensation
anesthesiology	science of studying the administration of anesthetics
anesthetic	agent that produces loss of sensation
angiectasia	dilation of a vessel
angioblast	immature vessel cell
angiogram	x-ray of a vessel
angiolysis	vessel destruction
angioma	vessel tumor
angiopathy	vessel disease
angioplasty	surgical repair of a vessel
angiorrhexis	rupture of a blood vessel
angiosclerosis	hardening of a vessel
angioscopy	process of looking into a vessel using a scope
angiospasm	vessel spasm
aphasia	unable to speak
aphonia	unable to make sounds with the voice
arteriectasia	dilation of an artery
arteriofibrosis	condition of fibrous growth in the arteries
arteriomalacia	softening of the arteries
arteriorrhexis	rupture of an artery
arteriosclerosis	hardening of the arteries
arteriospasm	spasm of an artery
atherectomy	excision of an atheroma
atheroma	fatty tissue tumor inside a large vessel

atherosclerosis	fatty deposits on medium to large vessels, causing hardening
audiology	the science studying hearing
bradyphasia	slow speech
cardiorrhexis	rupture of the heart
cystorrhexis	rupture of the bladder
cytolysis	cell destruction
dysesthesia	difficult or painful sensation
dysphasia	difficulty speaking (garbled speech)
dysphonia	difficulty making sounds with the voice
enterorrhexis	rupture of the small intestine
esthesiometer	instrument used to measure the amount of sensation
fibroma	fibrous tumor
gastromalacia	softening of the stomach
gastrospasm	stomach spasm
hemangioblast	immature blood vessel cell
hemarthrosis	blood in a joint
hematologist	physician specialist in blood disorders
hematology	specialty of studying the blood
hematolysis	destruction of blood (hemolysis)
hematophobia	abnormal fear of blood
hepatorrhexis	rupture of the liver
hyperesthesia	oversensitivity to touch (may be painful)
hypoesthesia	below normal ability to feel (touch)
hysterorrhexis	rupture of the uterus
infarction	necrosis of tissue due to ischemia
ischemia	condition of stopping blood supply
lipolysis	lipid destruction
metrorrhexis	rupture of uterine tissues
myoblast	immature muscle cell

► GLOSSARY

myocardial	pertaining to the heart muscle (myocardium)
myocarditis	inflammation of the myocardium
myofibroma	fibrous muscle tumor
myogram	picture of muscle function
myograph	instrument used to make a picture of muscle function
myography	the process of using a myograph
myolysis	muscle tissue destruction
myoma	muscle tumor
myopathy	muscle disease
myosclerosis	hardening of a muscle
myospasm	muscle spasm
neuroblast	immature nerve cell
neurologist	physician specialist in nervous system disorders
neurolysis	nerve destruction
neuroma	nerve tumor
neuropathy	nerve disease
neurospasm	nerve spasm
neurosurgeon	physician who performs surgery on or near nerves
parahepatitis	inflammation near the liver
paralgesia	pain in the lower body
paralgia	abnormal pain
paralysis	loss of muscle function and sensation
paramedic	emergency technician with advanced training
paranephritis	inflammation near the kidney
paraosteo-arthropathy	disease near the bone and joint
paraphasia	abnormal speech

paraplegia	paralysis in the lower body
parasalpingitis	inflammation near the fallopian tubes
paroxysmal	pertaining to a sudden onset of an attack, symptoms, or emotion
phasology	the science of studying speech
phlebectasia	dilation of a vein
phlebectomy	excision of a vein
phlebography	x-ray process
phlebopexy	fixation of a prolapsed vein
phleboplasty	surgical repair of a vein
phleborrhexis	rupture of a vein
phlebosclerosis	hardening of a vein
phlebotomy	venipuncture
phonic	pertaining to voice (sound)
phonology	the study of the voice (sound)
thrombectomy	excision of a clot
thromboangiitis	blood clot in a vessel causing inflammation
thrombocyte	blood clotting cell (platelet)
thrombocytopenia	lack of platelets
thrombogenic	pertaining to producing clots
thromboid	resembling a clot
thrombolymph-angitis	inflammation of a lymph vessel caused by a clot
thrombolysis	clot destruction
thrombophlebitis	inflammation of a vein caused by a clot
thrombosis	condition of forming clots
thrombus	blood clot
venipuncture	incision into a vein with a needle to remove a venous blood sample (synonym: phlebotomy)
venous	pertaining to veins

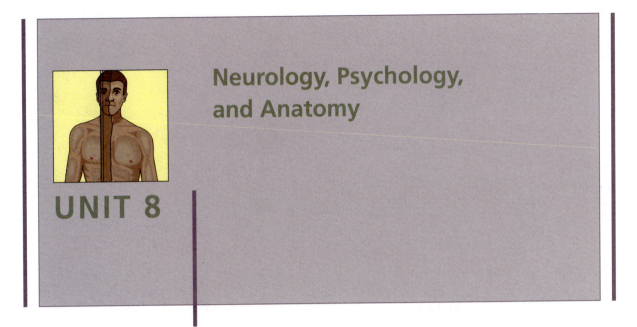

Neurology, Psychology, and Anatomy

UNIT 8

8.1
Recall that **neur/o** is used in words that refer to nerves. Neur/algia means pain along the course of a _____.
Neuropathy refers to any disease of the _____.

nerve
nerves

8.2
Neur/o/arthr/o/pathy is a disease of _____ and
_____.

nerves
joints

8.3
Neur/o/logy is the medical specialty that deals with the nervous system. A physician who specializes in diseases of the nervous system is a _____ /_____ /_____.
Refer to the illustration of the nerves on page 254.

neur/o/logist
nōō rol′ ə jist

8.4
Build words meaning
    inflammation of a nerve
    _____ /_____;
    destruction of nerve tissue
    _____ /_____ /_____;
    surgical repair of nerves
    _____ /_____ /_____;
    nervous system surgeon
    _____ /_____ /_____.

neur/itis
nōō rī′ tis
neur/o/lysis
nōō rol′ ə sis
neur/o/plasty
nōō′ rō plas tē
neur/o/surgeon
nōō′ rō **sur**′ jən

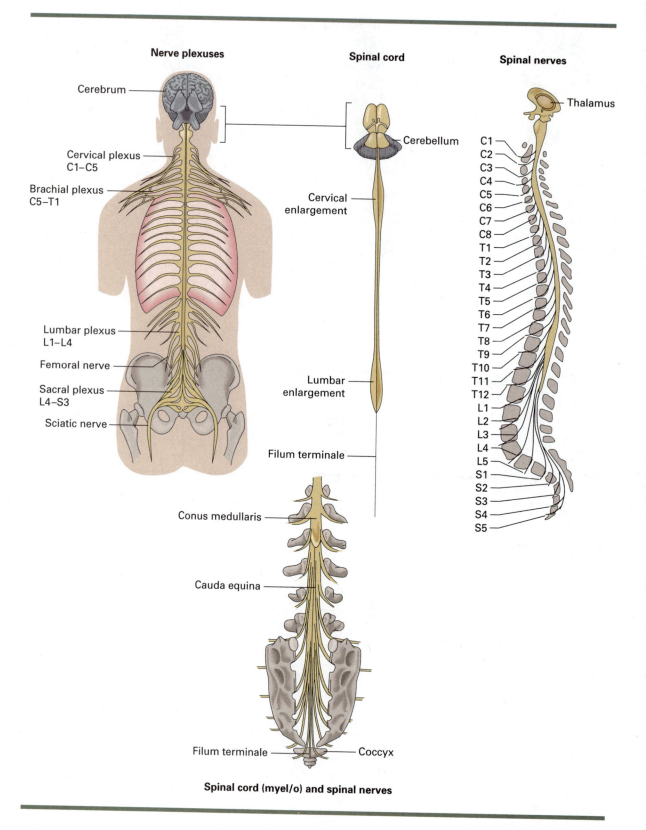

Nerve plexuses

Cerebrum

Cervical plexus
C1–C5

Brachial plexus
C5–T1

Lumbar plexus
L1–L4

Femoral nerve

Sacral plexus
L4–S3

Sciatic nerve

Spinal cord

Cerebellum

Cervical
enlargement

Lumbar
enlargement

Filum terminale

Conus medullaris

Cauda equina

Filum terminale — Coccyx

Spinal nerves

Thalamus

C1
C2
C3
C4
C5
C6
C7
C8
T1
T2
T3
T4
T5
T6
T7
T8
T9
T10
T11
T12
L1
L2
L3
L4
L5
S1
S2
S3
S4
S5

Spinal cord (myel/o) and spinal nerves

▶ **ANSWER COLUMN**

trips

8.5
Neur/o/tripsy means surgical crushing of a nerve. The word root for crushing (usually by rubbing or grinding) is _____.

---

neur/o/tripsy
noo´ rō trip sē

8.6
Tripsis, from which we get -tripsy, is a Greek word that means rubbing or massage. *Tripsis* can be carried to the point of crushing or grinding. Surgical crushing of a nerve is
_____ /_____ /_____.

---

lith/o/tripsy
lith´ ō trip sē

8.7
In some cases of lith/iasis, it may be necessary to crush calculi so they may be passed. A word that means surgical crushing of stones as in the bladder or ureters is _____ /_____ /_____.

---

lithotripsy

8.8
Therapeutic ultrasound (high-frequency sound waves) can be used to fragment stones in the kidney. This is ultrasonic
_____.

ⓔeee *TAKE A*
CLOSER LOOK

8.9
Look up myel/itis in your dictionary. From the definition, you conclude that **myel** is the word root for spinal cord or bone marrow. Write two words for spinal cord and two words for bone marrow using **myel**:

_____
_____
_____
_____

---

bone marrow germ cell
myel/o

8.10
Find the word myeloblast in your dictionary. Write the meaning:
* _____.
The combining form of **myel** is _____ /_____.

---

myel/o/cyt/ic
mī´ el ō **sit´** ik
myel/o/cele
mī´ el ō sēl

8.11
Find words meaning
  pertaining to myelocytes
_____ /_____ /_____ /_____;
  herniation of the spinal cord
_____ /_____ /_____.

ANSWER COLUMN	
defective (poor or abnormal) formation	**8.12** -plasia means formation or change in development of the sense of molding and numbers of cells. This kind of formation occurs naturally instead of being done by a plastic surgeon. Dys/plasia means *_____.
myel/o/dys/plasia mī el ō dis **plā´** zhə	**8.13** Build a term that means defective (poor or bad) formation of the spinal cord: _____ /____ /_____ /_____ (body part) + (disorder)
hyper/plasia hī pər **plā´** zhə or hī pər **plā´** zē ə	**8.14** A/plasia means failure of an organ to develop properly. A word that means overgrowth or too many cells is _____ /_____.
hypo/plasia hī pō **plā´** zhə or hī pō **plā´** zē ə	**8.15** If growth of too many cells is hyper/plasia, underdevelopment or not enough cells is expressed as _____ /_____. **NOTE:** Review the text and illustrations in Unit 2 for information on hypertrophy and hypotrophy. The terms hyperplasia and hypoplasia mean something different.

chondr/o/dys/plasia
kon´ drō dis **plā´** zhə
oste/o/chondr/o/dys/plasia
os´ tē ō kon´ drō dis **plā´** zhə
	8.16
	Using myel/o/dys/plasia as a model, build words meaning
	    defective formation of cartilage
	_____ /____ /_____ /_____;
	    defective formation of bone and cartilage
	_____ /____ /_____ /____ /_____ /_____.
	NOTE: -plasia may also be pronounced **plā´** zē ə.

neur/o/myel/itis nōō´ rō mī´ ə **lī´** tis	**8.17** Form a word meaning inflammation of nerves and spinal cord: _____ /____ /_____ /_____.
✔ SPELL CHECK	**8.18** **psych/o** (sī´ kō) refers to the mind. Look up **psych/o** in your dictionary and read the definition. See how many everyday terms begin with the word root **psych**. Be sure to watch your spelling on this one. The p is silent and the y is like an i.

> **ANSWER COLUMN**

psych/o/logy
sī **kol**´ ō jē

8.19
The study of the mind, mental processes, and human behavior is
_____ /_____ /_____.

---

psych/o/analysis
sī´ kō a **nal**´ ə sis
psych/o/somatic
sī´ kō sō **mat**´ ik
psych/o/sexual
sī´ kō **sex**´ ū əl

8.20
Using your dictionary, analyze and read the meanings of
psychoanalysis _____ /_____ /_____,
** _____;
psychosomatic _____ /_____ /_____,
** _____;
psychosexual _____ /_____ /_____,
** _____;

---

psych/iatrist
sī **kī**´ ə trist
psych/iatry
sī **kī**´ ə trē

8.21
Psychiatry is the field of medicine that studies and deals with
mental and neurotic disorders. The physician who specializes in
this field of medicine is called a _____ /_____.
The treatment of mental disorders by a psychiatrist is called
_____ /_____.

🏛 **WORD ORIGINS**

8.22
In Greek mythology Psyche was Cupid's lover. She was the
beautiful daughter of a king and personification of fervent
emotion. After many difficult trials Psyche was made a goddess by
Zeus and was united with Cupid on Mount Olympus. *Psyche* in
Greek refers to the soul, spirit, or breath that creates life as
distinguished from the physical aspects.

---

psych/o/logist
sī **kol**´ ə jist

8.23
Psych/o/logy is the science that studies human behavior. The
scientist or therapist who works in this field is called a
_____ /_____ /_____.

---

psych/o/therapy
sī´ kō **thair**´ ə pē

8.24
Psych/o/therapy is a process of healing mental disorders using
words, art, drama, or movement to express feelings. A clinical
psych/o/logist helps clients with mental disorders by using
_____ /_____ /_____.

---

psych/osis
sī **kō**´ sis

8.25
Psych/o/genesis means the formation of mental characteristics. A
severe mental condition marked by loss of contact with reality,
delusions, or hallucinations is _____ /_____.

> ► **ANSWER COLUMN**

8.26

Psych/o/neurosis (neur/o/sis), an emotional and behavioral disorder, is manifested by anxiety. A psych/o/neur/o/tic person is one who suffers from a _____ /_____ /_____ /_____ or _____ /_____.

psych/o/neur/osis
sī′ kō nōō rō′ sis
neur/osis
nōō rō′ sis

8.27

The patient suffering from a neurosis knows the real from the unreal and only exaggerates reality. Individuals who will not touch others because they fear contact with germs may suffer from _____.

neurosis

8.28

ⓔeee TAKE A CLOSER LOOK

Obsessive-compulsive disorder (OCD) is a neurosis characterized by repeated distressing thoughts that produce anxiety and uncontrollable repeated actions that must be done to relieve the anxiety. A person may fear illness and think that they are being constantly exposed to germs. They may refuse to leave the house without wearing gloves and a mask, only eat boiled food, clean their house compulsively, and exclude social contact. OCD is a type of _____ /_____ . Look up OCD and other neuroses in your dictionary.

neurosis
nōō rō′ sis

8.29

INFORMATION FRAME

Psych/o/trop/ic (*trope*, **Greek** for turn) medications may be used to alter emotions or behavior.

8.30

A patient with a psychoneurosis may be given a _____ /_____ /_____ /_____ medication to lower anxiety.

psych/o/trop/ic
sī′ kō trō′ pik

8.31

Use **psych/o** to build words meaning
medication that alters mind and emotions
_____ /_____ /_____ /_____;
severe mental condition (delusional)
_____ /_____;
mental processes that cause movement
_____ /_____ /_____;
mental disorder related to sexual function
_____ /_____ /_____ /_____.

psych/o/trop/ic
sī′ kō trō′ pik
psych/osis
sī kō′ sis
psych/o/motor
sī′ kō mō′ ter
psych/o/sexu/al
sī′ kō seks′ yōō al

ANSWER COLUMN

neuroses or
psychoneuroses

8.32
Psychoneuroses (neuroses, plural) take many forms. Obsessive-compulsive reaction, conversion reaction, and phobias are forms of _____ (plural form).

8.33
In your dictionary read about the psychopath and the psychopathic personality. Also read the definition of psychopathy.

psych/o/motor
sī´ kō **mō´** ter

8.34
motor is a word root referring to movement. Mental processes that cause movement are _____ /_____ /_____ functions.

motor

8.35
A neuron that innervates a muscle causes movement. It is called a _____ neuron.

TAKE A CLOSER LOOK

mental processes
(mind or soul)

8.36
Let your eye wander down the columns of **psych** words in the dictionary. Read about any that interest you. Note the information following the words psychiatric and psychoanalysis. All **psych/o** words refer to *_____.

psych/o/pharmac/o/logy
sī´ kō fär ma **kol´** ō jē

8.37
pharmac/o (as in pharmacy) means drugs or medicine. Neur/o/pharmacology is the study of drugs that affect the nervous system. The study of drugs that act on the mind and emotions is _____ /_____ /_____ /_____ /_____.

INFORMATION FRAME

8.38
Psych/o/pharmac/o/logy includes the study of using medications to treat mental illness. The following are all examples of psychotropic medications: antidepressants (prozac), tranquilizers (thorazine), neuroleptics, sedatives, and anticonvulsants (dilantin).

pharmac/o/logy
fär´ ma **kol´** ō jē

8.39
A pharmac/ist is licensed to dispense prescription and non-prescription medications from a pharmacy. To become a pharmacist, a person must study _____ /_____ /_____.

► **ANSWER COLUMN**

💡 INFORMATION
FRAME

8.40
In your dictionary look at the words beginning with **gnos**. They come from the Greek word meaning knowledge.

---

knowledge

8.41
The words gnosia and gnosis are medical words built from the Greek word meaning _____.

---

pro

8.42
pro- is a prefix meaning in front of; pro/gnos/is means foreknowledge or predicting the outcome of a disease. The prefix that means before or in front of is _____.

---

pro/gnos/is
prog **nō**′ sis

8.43
Leukemia is a serious disease associated with leukocytes. The _____ /_____ /_____ for acute leukemia is grave.

Professional Profiles ◄◄◄◄◄◄◄◄◄◄◄◄◄◄◄◄◄◄◄◄◄◄◄◄◄◄◄◄◄◄

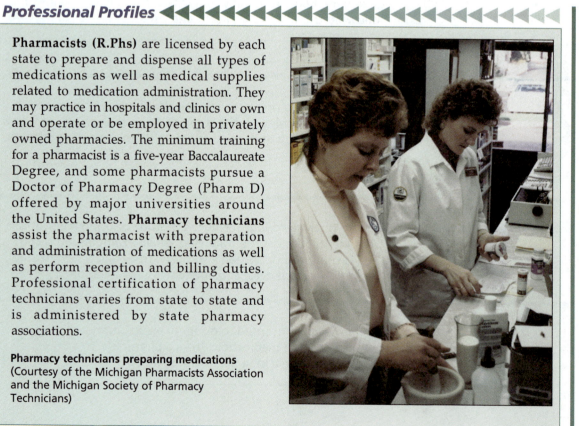

Pharmacists (R.Phs) are licensed by each state to prepare and dispense all types of medications as well as medical supplies related to medication administration. They may practice in hospitals and clinics or own and operate or be employed in privately owned pharmacies. The minimum training for a pharmacist is a five-year Baccalaureate Degree, and some pharmacists pursue a Doctor of Pharmacy Degree (Pharm D) offered by major universities around the United States. **Pharmacy technicians** assist the pharmacist with preparation and administration of medications as well as perform reception and billing duties. Professional certification of pharmacy technicians varies from state to state and is administered by state pharmacy associations.

Pharmacy technicians preparing medications
(Courtesy of the Michigan Pharmacists Association and the Michigan Society of Pharmacy Technicians)

ANSWER COLUMN	**8.44** Procephalic means in the front of the head. Analyze procephalic: _____ /_____ /_____. Prognostic means giving an indication concerning the outcome of a disease. Analyze prognostic: _____ /_____ /_____.
pro/cephal/ic prō sə **fal**´ ik pro/gnos/tic prog **nos**´ tik	
knowing through or know through	**8.45** dia- means through or complete. Dia/gnos/is literally means *_____. (Identification of a disease through signs and symptoms)
dia/gnos/tic dī ag **nos**´ tik dia/gnos/e **dī**´ ag nōs	**8.46** Dia/gnos/tic is the adjectival form of diagnosis and dia/gnos/e is the verb. When the results of the _____ /_____ /_____ (adjective) tests are complete, the physician will _____ /_____ /_____ (verb) the condition of the patient.
dia/gnos/is dī əg **nō**´ sis	**8.47** A diagnosis (identification of a disease) is made by studying through its symptoms. When a patient tells of having chills, hot spells, and a runny nose, the physician may make the _____ /_____ /_____: viral syndrome.
diagnosis	**8.48** Nurses observe patients for signs and symptoms of conditions that require treatment. After careful observation, a nurse will summarize these findings by writing a nursing _____.
flowing through	**8.49** The literal meaning of dia/rrhea (watery stool) is *_____.
INFORMATION FRAME	**8.50** Dia/lysis is the separation of substances in a solution. Hem/o/dia/lysis removes waste from the blood by using an artificial kidney machine.
dia/lysis dī **al**´ i sis	**8.51** Dialysis is a process of destroying waste products in the blood by diffusion through a membrane. People with kidney failure (ESRD, end-stage renal disease) may need _____ /_____ to remove waste from their blood.

dialysis

8.52

Peritoneal dialysis and hemodialysis are two types of

_____.

dia

8.53

A diascope is placed on the skin, and the skin is looked at *through* the instrument to see superficial surface lesions, and other things. The word part for through is _____.

When studying anatomy we use many directional words. The following table is to help you understand the use of 14 of them. Use this table while working Frames 8.54–8.73.

Directional Word	Combining Form	Meaning
dorsal	dors/o	near or on the back
ventral	ventr/o	near or on the belly side of the body
anterior (ant)	anter/o	toward the front or in front of
posterior (post)	poster/o	following or located behind
cephalic	cephal/o	upward, toward the head
caudal, caudad	caud/o	downward, toward the tail
medial	medi/o	toward the midline
lateral	later/o	toward the side, away from the midline
superior	super-	above
inferior	sub- or infra-	below
proximal	proxim/o	near the point of origin
distal	dist/o	away from the point of origin
sagittal	sagitt/o	vertical, anteroposterior direction or plane dividing into left and right
coronal	coron/o	resembling a crown or encircling

▶ **ANSWER COLUMN**

anter/o/later/al
an ter ō **lat´** er al
anter/o/medi/al
an ter ō **mēd´** ē al
anter/o/super/ior
an ter ō sup **ēr´** ē or

8.54
The combining forms for anterior and posterior do not include the i. They are **anter/o** and **poster/o**. Using the information about directional terms in the table, build terms that mean pertaining to the
    front and side
    _____ /____ /_____ /____;
    front and middle
    _____ /____ /_____ /____;
    front and top
    _____ /____ /_____ /_____.

poster/o/later/al
pōst´ er ō **lat´** er al
poster/o/extern/al
pōst´ er ō eks **tern´** al
poster/o/intern/al
pōst er ō in **tern´** al

8.55
Build terms that mean pertaining to the
    back and side
    _____ /____ /_____ /____;
    back and outside of the body
    _____ /____ /_____ /____;
    back and inside of the body
    _____ /____ /_____ /____.

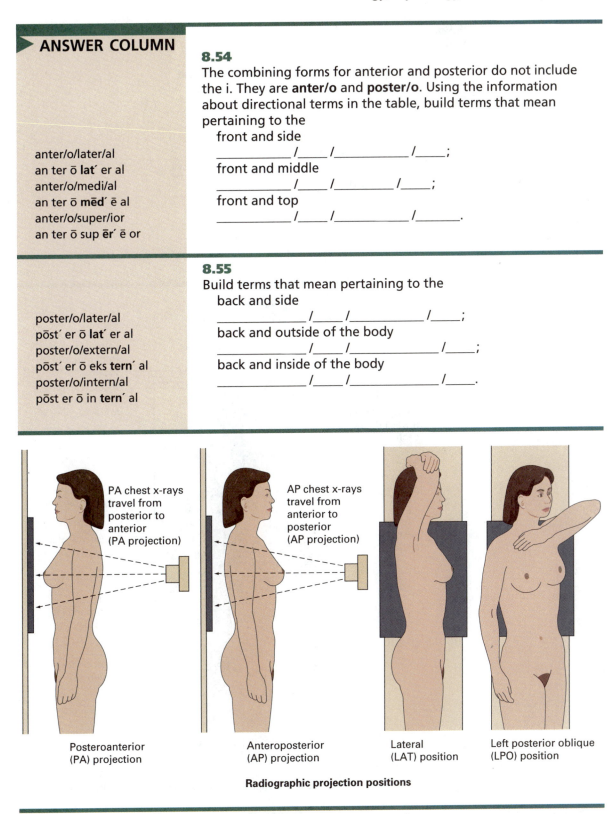

PA chest x-rays travel from posterior to anterior (PA projection)

AP chest x-rays travel from anterior to posterior (AP projection)

Posteroanterior (PA) projection

Anteroposterior (AP) projection

Lateral (LAT) position

Left posterior oblique (LPO) position

Radiographic projection positions

ANSWER COLUMN

anter/o/poster/ior or
an´ ter ō pōst ēr´ ē
ventr/o/dorsal
vent rō **dor**´ sal
dors/o/cephal/ad
dor sō **sef**´ əl ad
ventr/ad (ventral) or
vent´ rad (**ven**´ trəl)
anter/ior
an **tēr**´ ē or

8.56

Build terms that mean pertaining to the
front and back (from front to back)

_____ /_____ /_____ /_____ (AP)
or
_____ /_____ /_____;
toward the back of the head
_____ /_____ /_____ /_____;
toward the front
_____ /_____.

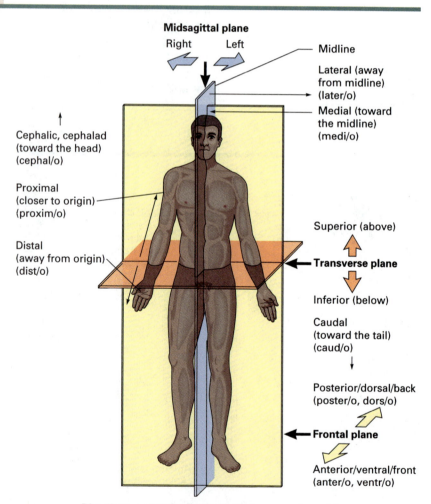

Midsagittal plane

Right   Left

Midline

Lateral (away
from midline)
(later/o)

Medial (toward
the midline)
(medi/o)

Cephalic, cephalad
(toward the head)
(cephal/o)

Proximal
(closer to origin)
(proxim/o)

Distal
(away from origin)
(dist/o)

Superior (above)

Transverse plane

Inferior (below)

Caudal
(toward the tail)
(caud/o)

Posterior/dorsal/back
(poster/o, dors/o)

Frontal plane

Anterior/ventral/front
(anter/o, ventr/o)

Directions and planes of the body in anatomic position

► **ANSWER COLUMN**

8.57
Proximal (**proxim/o**) means closer to a designated point (like the origin of a muscle or limb), and distal (**dist/o**) means further from a designated point. Because the elbow is closer to the shoulder than the hand is, the elbow is _____ /_____ to the shoulder. Because the ankle is further from the hip than the knee, the ankle is _____ /_____ to the hip.

proxim/al
proks´ i mal
dist/al
dis´ tal

8.58
A fracture in the upper part (closer to the hip) of the femur (thigh bone) is a fracture of the _____ end of the femur.
A fracture in the lower part of the femur is a fracture of the _____ end.

proximal

distal

8.59
The bone in the tip of a finger (phalanx) is the _____ phalanx, because it is farther from the origin of the finger.
The phalanx close to the palm is the _____ phalanx.

distal

proximal

8.60
After studying the table on page 262, provide the meaning for the following terms:
medi/o/later/al *_____;
super/o/later/al *_____;
cephal/o/caud/al *_____.

middle and side
above and to the side
head to tail

8.61
It is often necessary to look at anatomy by taking views of planes or slices of the body. This happens when using tomography and sonography. A sagittal cut is made in a vertical, anteroposterior direction. Such a cut made at the midline to divide the body into equal right and left halves is called the _____ /_____ plane.

mid/sagitt/al
mid **saj´ i tal**

8.62
Any vertical slice from front to back is a _____ /_____ view.

sagitt/al
saj´ i tal

🏛 *WORD ORIGINS*

8.63
In Latin *sagittalis* means arrowlike. The constellation and astrological sign Sagittarius is the shape of a mythological character, a Centaur, that is half man, half horse drawing a bow with a star for its arrow point. It is as if to say if struck with an arrow a person would be cut into halves.

> ANSWER COLUMN

8.64
The coron/al suture line of the skull sits at the crown of the skull.
Coron/al comes from a Greek word root meaning crown or circle.
The corona dentis is the _____ of a tooth. The coron/ary
arteries _____ the heart to supply the muscle with blood.

crown
circle (encircle)

8.65
The arteries encircling the heart are the _____ / _____
arteries.
The veins encircling the heart are the _____ / _____
veins.

coron/ary
kor´ ən air ē
coron/ary

INFORMATION FRAME

8.66
To find a word root for navel, look up navel in the dictionary. A
synonym for navel is a Latin word, *umbilicus*. The Greek combining
form **omphal/o** comes from *omphalos*.

8.67
Inflammation of the umbilicus is _____ / _____.

omphal/itis
om fəl ī´ tis

8.68
In the dictionary, turn to words beginning with **omphal/o**. The
combining form for navel is _____ / ____.

omphal/o

8.69
Using **omphal/o**, build words meaning
  pertaining to the navel
  _____ / ____;
  excision of the umbilicus
  _____ / _____;
  herniation of the navel (umbilical hernia)
  _____ / ____ / _____.

omphal/ic
om **fal´** ik
omphal/ectomy
om fə **lek´** tə mē
omphal/o/cele or
om´ fə lō sēl, om **fal´** ō sēl
umbilico/o/cele
um bil´ **i k**ō sēl

8.70
Build words meaning
  umbilical hemorrhage
  _____ / ____ / _____;
  discharge flowing from the navel
  _____ / ____ / _____;
  rupture of the navel
  _____ / ____ / _____.

omphal/o/rrhagia
om´ fâ lō **rāj´** ē ə
omphal/o/rrhea
om´ fâ lō **rē´** ə
omphal/o/rrhexis
om´ fəl ō **reks´** is

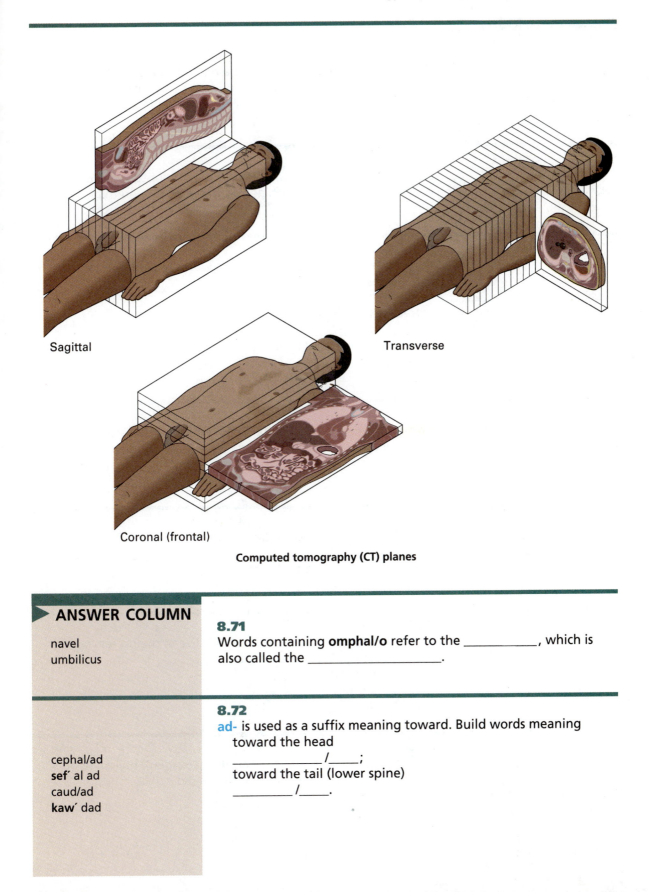

Sagittal

Transverse

Coronal (frontal)

Computed tomography (CT) planes

ANSWER COLUMN	
navel umbilicus	**8.71** Words containing **omphal/o** refer to the _____, which is also called the _____.

cephal/ad
sef´ al ad
caud/ad
kaw´ dad
	8.72
	ad- is used as a suffix meaning toward. Build words meaning
	  toward the head
	  _____ /_____;
	  toward the tail (lower spine)
	  _____ /_____.

ANSWER COLUMN	
	8.73 Human development is usually in a head-to-body (tail) direction. (The structures of the head develop first.) This is called
cephal/o/caud/al sef´ al ō **kaw**´ dal	_____ /____ /_____ /____ development.
	8.74 **aer/o** is used in words to mean air. You undoubtedly know the words aer/ial, and aer/ialist. **aer/o** always makes you think of
air	_____.
	8.75 Using what you need of **aer/o**, build words meaning abnormal fear of air
aer/o/phobia air´ ō **fō**´ bē ə aer/o/therapy air´ ō **ther**´ ə pē aer/o/cele **air**´ ō sēl	_____ /____ /_____; treatment with air _____ /____ /_____; herniation containing air _____ /____ /_____.
	8.76 *Bios* is the Greek word for life. Bi/o/chemistry is the study of chemical changes in living things. The science (study of) living things is ____ /____ /_____.
bi/o/logy bī **o**´ lə jē	
	8.77 A bi/o/logist is one who studies * _____. Bi/o/genesis is the formation of * _____.
living things or life living things	

	8.78
	An an/aer/o/bic plant or animal cannot live in the presence of air (an-—without). Analyze anaerobic:
	    prefix (without) ____;
	    combining form (air)_____ /____;
	    suffix (life) _____.

an aer/o bic	
	8.79 If anaerobic means existing without air (oxygen), build a word that means needing air (oxygen) to live (adjective): _____ /____ /_____.
aer/o/bic air ō´ bik	

ANSWER COLUMN	
	8.80 Use aerobic or anaerobic in Frames 8.80–8.82. The bacterium that causes pneumonia requires air to live. These bacteria are considered _____ bacteria.
aerobic	
an/aer/o/bic an ə **rō**′ bik	**8.81** The tetanus bacillus causes lockjaw. Lockjaw can develop only in closed wounds where air does not penetrate (e.g., stepping on an old nail). The tetanus bacillus is an ____ /_____ /____ /_____ bacterium. Read about tetanus in your medical dictionary.
anaerobic	**8.82** Botulism is a serious type of food poisoning. It occurs from eating improperly canned meats and vegetables. Cans do not admit air. The bacillus that causes botulism is _____.
living or live	**8.83** A bi/o/psy is an excision of tissue for examination of * _____ tissue.
color	**8.84** A combining form that means color is **chrom/o**. The Greek word for a color is *chroma*. There are English words chroma and chrome. **chrom/o** makes you think of _____.
chrom/o/blast **krō**′ mō blast	**8.85** A chrom/o/cyte is any colored cell. An embryonic color (pigment) cell is called a _____ /____ /_____.

chrom/o/lysis
krō **mol**′ ə sis
chrom/o/gen/esis
krō′ mō **jen**′ ə sis
chrom/o/meter
krō **mom**′ ə ter
	8.86
	Build words meaning
	    destruction of color (in a cell)
	    _____ /____ /_____;
	    formation of pigment (color)
	    _____ /____ /_____ /_____;
	    instrument for measuring amount of color in a substance
	    _____ /____ /_____.

chrom/o/philic krō′ mō **fil**′ ik	**8.87** **phil** is a word root meaning attracted to or loves. A chrom/o/philic cell is one that takes a stain easily (attracts stain). Some leukocytes stain deeper than others. They are more _____ /____ /_____ than the less easily stained leukocytes.

► **ANSWER COLUMN**

chromophilic

8.88
Some cells are chrom/o/phobic and will not stain at all. They are
not _____.

EXAMPLE: Gram-negative bacteria will not attract color from the
gram stain.

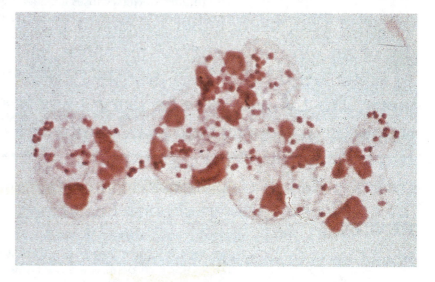

Neisseria gonorrhoeae in synovial fluid

---

staining easily

a/chrom/o/philic
ā′ krō mō **fil**′ ik

8.89
Chromophilic means *_____.
The word that means something does not (without) stain easily is
_____ /_____ /_____ /_____.

---

bad, painful, or difficult

well or easy

8.90
dys- means *_____.
The opposite of **dys-** is **eu-**. **eu-** means
*_____.

---

eu/pepsia
yōō **pep**′ sē ə
eu/peptic
yōō **pep**′ tik
eu/pnea
yōōp **nē**′ ə or
yōōp′ nē ə

8.91
Form the word that means the opposite of
   dys/pepsia
   _____ /_____;
   dys/peptic
   _____ /_____;
   dys/pnea
   _____ /_____.

ANSWER COLUMN	
	8.92 Form the opposite of dys/kines/ia _____ /_____ /_____; dys/esthes/ia _____ /_____ /_____; dys/phor/ia _____ /_____ /_____.

eu/kinesi/a
yo͞o ki **nē**´ zhə
eu/esthesi/a
yo͞o es **thē**´ zhə
eu/phor/ia
yo͞o **fôr**´ ē ə

8.93
-tocia is a suffix meaning labor. Dys/tocia (dis **tō**´ shə) means difficult labor. Eu/tocia (ū **tō**´ shə) means
* _____.

easy or normal labor
and childbirth

Think

8.94
If you work a frame and have forgotten what the word root means, look it up in your medical dictionary. Use this frame to take a breath and _____.

8.95
Thanatos is a Greek word meaning death. The word root for death is **than**. When someone has an easy or peaceful death, it is called _____ /_____ /_____. Many ethical medical questions surround the subject of _____. If this interests you, you may want to learn about active and passive euthanasia.

eu/than/asia
yo͞o than **ā**´ zhə
euthanasia

8.96
Another area of ethics is the study of eu/gen/ics (good development). Researchers are working on ways of improving humans through genetic engineering. Look up eugenic in your dictionary and analyze the word parts:
eu- _____;
gen * _____;
-ic * _____.

good
form or produce
adjective ending

8.97
Eugenic sterilization is selective sterilization of individuals that society says have undesirable traits or would be unable to be good parents. One controversial topic of bi/o/ethics is whether or not severely mentally impaired adult patients may be selected for _____ /_____ /_____ sterilization.

eu/gen/ic
yo͞o **jen**´ ik

INFORMATION FRAME

8.98
Bi/o/ethics and medical ethics are topics that deal with decisions about life and medical treatments that concern right and wrong as seen by society and individuals.

ANSWER COLUMN	
bi/o/ethics bī ō **eth**´ iks	**8.99** Euthanasia and eugenics are both controversial topics concerning _____ /_____ /_____.
dys/entery **dis**´ en tair ē	**8.100** Recall that **enter/o** is the combining form for intestine. Infections of the intestine can be viral, bacterial, or parasitic and cause pain and diarrhea. This painful or difficult small intestinal condition is called _____ /_____. **NOTE: enter/o** is used more with words about the small intestine and **col/o** is used for large intestine.
dysentery	**8.101** Travelers are cautioned not to drink water in countries with poor sanitation systems to avoid contracting amebic _____.
men/ses or **men**´ sis men/struation men strōō **ā**´ shun	**8.102** **men/o** is used in words referring to the menses. In Latin *mensis* means month. Men/ses is another way of saying men/struation, which occurs at monthly cycles. **men/o** in any word should make you think of _____ /_____.
✔ SPELL CHECK	**8.103** Watch the spelling and pronunciation of menstruation. There is a "u" after the "str" and it is pronounced with a long "u" sound.
men/o/rrhea men ə **rē**´ ə dys/men/o/rrhea dis´ men ə **rē**´ ə	**8.104** Men/arche (men **ar**´ kē) comes from the Greek words *men* for month and *arche* for beginning. Menarche refers to a female's first menstrual period. Build words meaning flow of menses _____ /_____ /_____; painful (bad or difficult) menstrual flow _____ /_____ /_____ /_____.
menstruation or menses excessive menstruation or menstrual hemorrhage	**8.105** Men/o/pause (**men**´ ō paws) means permanent cessation of *_____. Men/o/rrhagia (men ō **rā**´ jē ə) means *_____.

▶ **ANSWER COLUMN**	**8.106** Build words meaning 　　absence (without) menstrual flow 　　_____ /_____ /_____ /_____; stopping menstrual flow 　　_____ /_____ /_____.

a/men/o/rrhea
ā men ə **rē´** ə
men/o/stasis
mə **nos´** te sis

---

act of controlling
　blood flow
phleb/o/stasis or
fli **bos´** tə sis
ven/o/stasis
vē **nos´** tə sis

8.107
-stasis means the act or condition of stopping or controlling.
Hem/o/stasis means *_____.
A word meaning control of blood flow in veins is
_____ /_____ /_____.

---

arteri/o/stasis
är tir´ ē **os´** tə sis
lymph/o/stasis
lim **fos´** tə sis

8.108
Build words meaning
　　control of flow in arteries
　　_____ /_____ /_____;
control of lymph flow
　　_____ /_____ /_____.

PRONUNCIATION NOTE

8.109
Medical terms ending in -stasis are formally pronounced as
indicated in Frames 8.107 and 8.108. In practice you will probably
hear the following instead:
　　phlebostasis—flē bō **stā´** sis
　　venostasis—vē nō **stā´** sis
　　arteriostasis—är tir ē ō **stā´** sis
　　hemostasis—hē mō **stā´** sis

---

syphil/o

8.110
Syphilis is a sexually transmitted disease (STD). Read about the
disease in your dictionary. Note the origin of the word. Look at
the words beginning with **syphil**. The combining form used in
words referring to this disease is _____ /_____.

---

syphil/o/psych/osis
sif´ il ō sī **kō´** sis
syphil/o/phobia
sif´ il ō **fōb´** ē ə
syphil/o/therapy
sif´ il ō **ther´** a pē

8.111
Using **syphil**, build terms that mean
　　mental condition caused by syphilis
　　_____ /_____ /_____ /_____;
fear of contracting syphilis
　　_____ /_____ /_____;
therapy for syphilis
　　_____ /_____ /_____.

ANSWER COLUMN	

8.112
Build words meaning
   a syphilitic tumor

syphil/oma

_____ /_____;
   any syphilitic disease

syphil/o/pathy
(You pronounce)

_____ /_____ /_____.

8.113
-cyesis comes from the Greek word *kyesis* meaning pregnancy.
pseudo- means false. A pseud/o/cyesis (soo dō sī ē´ sis) or
pseud/o/pregnancy is a false pregnancy. A pseud/o/science is a

false science

*_____.

8.114
Pseud/o/mania is a psychosis in which patients have a false
or pretended mental disorder. Pseud/o/paralysis means

false paralysis
  (paralysis not due
  to nerve damage)

*_____.

8.115
Build words meaning
   a false cyst

pseud/o/cyst
soo´ dō sist
pseud/o/edema
soo´ dō ə **dē**´ mə
pseud/o/esthesi/a
soo´ dō es **thē**´ zhə

_____ /_____ /_____;
   false edema

_____ /_____ /_____;
   false or imaginary sensation

_____ /_____ /_____ /_____.
Look up and learn the meaning of edema.

8.116
Build words meaning
   false hypertrophy

pseud/o/hyper/trophy

_____ /_____ /_____ /_____;
   false tuberculosis (TB)

pseud/o/tubercul/osis

_____ /_____ /_____ /_____;
   false nerve tumor

pseud/o/neur/oma
(You pronounce)

_____ /_____ /_____ /_____.

8.117
✓ SPELL CHECK

Words built with **pseud/o** often give students spelling and
pronunciation problems. Remember, the "p" is silent and the "eu"
is like a "u".

ANSWER COLUMN	
viscer/o	**8.118** The viscera (singular: viscus) are the internal organs of the body. Viscer/ad means toward the viscera. Viscer/o/genic means development of organs. The combining form for viscera is _____ /____.
organs (internal)	**8.119** In the words viscer/o/motor, viscer/o/pariet/al, and viscer/o/pleur/al, **viscer/o** refers to _____.
periton/eum per i tō **nē´** um	**8.120** Locate the peritoneum below. The membrane that lines the abdominal cavity is the _____ /_____.

Parietal pleura — Lungs
Visceral pleura
Parietal peritoneum
Visceral peritoneum (on top of each organ)
Intestine

Ventral cavity membranes

> **ANSWER COLUMN**

pleur/al
pl͞oor´ əl

8.121
Locate the pleura on page 275. The membrane that covers the lungs is the visceral _____ /_____ membrane.

🔆 *INFORMATION FRAME*

8.122
pariet/o is the combining form for wall. Uses of visceral (**vis´** er əl) and parietal (pa **rī´** ə təl):

visceral pleura   (membrane on the surface of the lung)
parietal pleura   (membrane on chest cavity wall)
visceral peritoneum (membrane on the surface of the organs of the abdominal cavity)
parietal peritoneum (membrane on the abdominal cavity wall)

---

viscer/al
vis´ er əl
pariet/al
pa **rī´** ə təl

8.123
Name the membrane that
    covers the surface of the lungs
    _____ /_____ pleura;
    is on the thoracic cavity wall
    _____ /_____ pleura.

---

viscer/o/ptosis
vis´ ər op **tō´** sis
viscer/algia
vis´ ər **al´** jē ə
viscer/al
vis´ ər əl

8.124
Build words meaning
    prolapse of organs
    _____ /_____ /_____;
    pain in organs
    _____ /_____;
    pertaining to organs
    _____ /_____.

---

viscer/o/sensor/y
vis´ er ō **sens´** ôr ē
viscer/o/skelet/al
vis´ er ō **skel´** e tal
viscer/o/gen/ic
vis´ er ō **jen´** ik

8.125
Build words beginning with **viscer/o** that mean
    sensory function of organs
    _____ /_____ /_____ /_____;
    pertaining to organs and the skeleton
    _____ /_____ /_____ /_____;
    pertaining to the development of organs
    _____ /_____ /_____ /_____.

Abbreviation	Meaning	Abbreviation	Meaning
ant	anterior	ou	both eyes
AP	anteroposterior to posterior	PA	posteroanterior to anterior
APA	American Psychiatric Association	PDR	*Physician's Desk Reference*
Bx, Bl	biopsy	Pharm D	doctor of pharmacy
D	diopter	PT	physical therapy
DRG	diagnosis-related group	Px	prognosis
Dx	diagnosis	ROP	right occiput posterior
ESRD	end-stage renal disease	R.Ph	registered pharmacist
EST	electroshock therapy	RPR, VDRL	syphilis tests (blood serum)
Hx	history	Rx	take, prescribe, prescription
LAT	lateral		
LMP	last menstrual period	STD	sexually transmitted disease
LOA	left occiput anterior	TB	tuberculosis
NIMH	National Institute of Mental Health	Tx	treatment
OCD	obsessive-compulsive disorder	USP	*United States Pharmacopeia*
OT	occupational therapy	VD	venereal disease (old terminology)

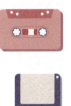

To complete your study of this unit, work the review activities on the next pages. Also, listen to the audiotapes that accompany *Medical Terminology: A Programmed Text,* 8th edition, and practice your pronunciation.

Additional practice exercises for this unit are available on the Student Practice disk found in the back of the textbook.

▶ **REVIEW ACTIVITIES**

Circle and Correct

Circle the correct answer for each question. Then, check your answers in Appendix A.

1. Combining form for nerve:
    a. myo   b. neuro
    c. psycho   d. phreno

2. Word root for surgical crushing:
    a. clysis   b. lithy
    c. lysis   d. trips

3. Combining form for spinal cord:
    a. myelo   b. myo
    c. mylo   d. milo

4. Word root for mind:
    a. mento   b. pysch
    c. psych   d. pyscho

5. Combining form for drugs:
    a. psycho   b. pharmacy
    c. pharmaco d. narco

6. Prefix for in front of:
    a. sub-   b. pro-
    c. post-   d. an-

7. Prefix for through:
    a. gnosis-   b. pre-
    c. pro-   d. dia-

8. Suffix for substance that affects:
    a. -pathic   b. -tropic
    c. -trophic d. -phobic

9. Word root for front:
    a. frontal   b. post
    c. ante   d. anter

10. Combining form for back:
    a. posto   b. posterio
    c. ventr   d. postero

11. Adjectival form for side:
    a. anterial b. dorsal
    c. lateral   d. laterial

12. Combining form for umbilicus:
    a. omphalo   b. onycho
    c. umbilical d. omphalic

13. Combining form for without air:
    a. pneumo   b. apnea
    c. anaero   d. aerobic

14. Suffix for attraction to:
    a. -philic   b. -phobic
    c. -phagic   d. -appeal

15. Prefix for false:
    a. fraud-   b. psycho-
    c. pseudo-   d. mal-

16. Prefix for easy or good:
    a. a-   b. eu-
    c. dys-   d. eas-

17. Prefix or suffix for toward:
    a. rrhexis   b. al
    c. ad   d. to

18. Word root for color:
    a. chrom   b. chlor
    c. xanth   d. philic

19. Combining form for menstruation:
    a. metro   b. metrio
    c. orrhea   d. meno

20. Suffix for controlling or stopping:
    a. -rrhagia b. -centesis
    c. -stasis   d. -dilation

21. Combining form for wall:
    a. peritoneo b. parieto
    c. viscero   d. septum

▶ REVIEW ACTIVITIES

Select and Construct—Part I

Select the correct word parts from the list below and construct medical terms that represent the given meaning.

blast	cephal/o/ic	chondro	dextr/o/ous	dia
dys	gnosis	hyper	itis	lateral
litho	logist	logy	lysis	motor
myelo	neuro	pariet/o/al	pathy	periton/eum
pharmaco	plasia	pro	psycho	tripsy
tropic				

1. embryonic spinal cord cell _____

2. any disease of the nerves _____

3. filtering blood through a membrane (artificial kidney) _____

4. surgical crushing of a stone _____

5. poor development of cartilage _____

6. mind-altering drugs _____

7. study of drug therapy _____

8. in front of the head _____

9. recognition of a disease through its symptoms and signs _____

10. mental processes that cause movement _____

11. overdevelopment (number of cells) _____

12. defective development of the spinal cord _____

Now, on your own, use the word parts list above to build a medical term and give its meaning.

13. _____   _____
            word   meaning

14. _____   _____
            word   meaning

15. _____   _____
            word   meaning

16. _____   _____
            word   meaning

► REVIEW ACTIVITIES

Select and Construct—Part II

Select the correct word parts from the list below and construct medical terms that represent the given meaning.

a	aero	an	antero(ior)	arterio
bio (bic)	caud(al)	cephal/o	chromo	dys
edema	eu	hemo	intern	kinesia
latero(al)	lysis	medio	men/o	omphalo
osis	pariet(al)	pepsia	periton(eum)	philic
phobia	phoria	pleura	pnea	poster(ior)
pseudo	ptosis	rrhea	stasis	syphilo
thanas/ia	trophy	tubercul	ventro	viscero(al)

1. from front to back _____

2. from head to tail _____

3. including the front and side _____

4. poor digestion _____

5. good feeling (well-being) _____

6. easily stained _____

7. control of flow of blood _____

8. false TB _____

9. metabolism with air _____

10. membrane of the lung cavity wall _____

11. membrane on the abdominal organs _____

12. discharge from the navel _____

13. easy (peaceful) death _____

14. difficult (painful) menstruation _____

15. easy breathing _____

Now, on your own, use the word parts list above to build a medical term and give its meaning.

16. _____   _____
            word   meaning

17. _____   _____
            word   meaning

18. _____   _____
            word   meaning

19. _____   _____
            word   meaning

20. _____   _____
            word   meaning

► REVIEW ACTIVITIES

Define and Dissect

Give a brief definition and dissect each term listed into its word parts in the space provided on the right. Check your answers by referring to the frame listed in parentheses and your medical dictionary. Then, listen to the audiotapes to practice pronunciation.

1. neurologist (8.3)

   _____ / ___ / _____
   rt   v   suffix

   _____
            definition

2. neurosurgeon (8.4)

   _____ / ___ / _____
   rt   v   rt/suffix

   _____

3. psychologist (8.23)

   _____ / ___ / _____
   rt   v   suffix

   _____

4. neurotripsy (8.6)

   _____ / ___ / _____
   rt   v   suffix

   _____

5. myelocytic (8.11)

   _____ / ___ / _____ / _____
   rt   v   rt   suffix

   _____

6. psychosomatic (8.20)

   _____ / ___ / _____
   rt   v   rt/suffix

   _____

7. psychiatrist (8.21)

   _____ / _____
   rt   suffix

   _____

8. psychopharmacology (8.37)

   _____ / ___ / _____ / ___ / _____
   rt   v   rt   v   suffix

   _____

9. prognostic (8.44)

   _____ / _____ / _____
   pre   rt   suffix

   _____

10. hemodialysis (8.50)

   _____ / ___ / _____ / _____
   rt   v   pre/rt   suffix

   _____

11. psychoneurosis (8.26)

   _____ / ___ / _____ / _____
   rt   v   pre/rt   suffix

   _____

12. myelodysplasia (8.13)

   _____ / ___ / _____ / _____
   rt   v   pre/rt   suffix

   _____

▶ **REVIEW ACTIVITIES**

13. lithotripsy (8.7)

_____ / ____ / _____
    rt   v   suffix

_____

14. proximal (8.57)

_____ / ____
         rt   suffix

_____

15. dorsocephalad (8.56)

_____ / ___ / _____ / _____
    rt   v   rt   suffix

_____

16. posterolateral (8.55)

_____ / ____ / _____ / _____
    rt   v   rt   suffix

_____

17. omphalocele (8.69)

_____ / ____ / _____
      rt   v   suffix

_____

18. aerotherapy (8.75)

_____ / ____ / _____
    rt   v   rt/suffix

_____

19. anaerobic (8.81)

_____ / _____ / ____ / _____
   pre   rt   v   suffix

_____

20. biopsy (8.83)

_____ / ____ / _____
   rt   v   suffix

_____

21. chromolysis (8.86)

_____ / ____ / _____
    rt   v   suffix

_____

22. eukinesia (8.92)

_____ / _____ / _____
   pre   rt   suffix

_____

23. euthanasia (8.95)

_____ / _____ / _____
   pre   rt   suffix

_____

24. dysmenorrhea (8.104)

_____ / _____ / ____ / _____
    pre   rt   v   suffix

_____

25. syphilopsychosis (8.111)

_____ / ___ / _____ / _____
    rt   v   rt   suffix

_____

▶ **REVIEW ACTIVITIES**

26. pseudocyesis (8.113)

_____ / ____ / _____
          rt   v   rt/suffix

_____

27. pseudoneuroma (8.116)

_____ / ____ / _____ / _____
          rt   v   rt   suffix

_____

28. visceroptosis (8.124)

_____ / ____ / _____
          rt   v   suffix

_____

29. visceropleural (8.119)

_____ / ____ / _____ / _____
          rt   v   rt   suffix

_____

30. distal (8.57)

_____ / _____
          rt   suffix

_____

31. mediolateral (8.60)

_____ / ____ / _____ / _____
          rt   v   rt   suffix

_____

32. omphalorrhagia (8.70)

_____ / ____ / _____
          rt   v   suffix

_____

33. dyspnea (8.91)

_____ / _____
          pre   suffix

_____

34. cephalocaudal (8.73)

_____ / ____ / _____ / _____
          rt   v   rt   suffix

_____

35. achromophilic (8.89)

____ / _____ / ____ / _____
pre   rt   v   suffix

_____

36. phlebostasis (8.107)

_____ / ____ / _____
          rt   v   suffix

_____

37. visceromotor (8.119)

_____ / ____ / _____
          rt   v   rt/suffix

_____

38. chromophobic (8.89)

_____ / ____ / _____
          rt   v   suffix

_____

▶ REVIEW ACTIVITIES

Diagram Labels

From what you have learned about directional terms, complete the diagram below by labeling the blanks with the proper direction term or word part.

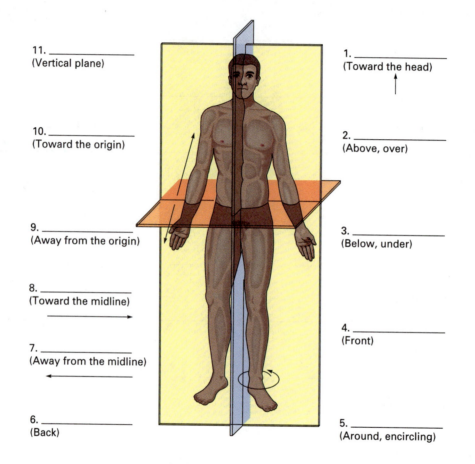

11. _____
(Vertical plane)

10. _____
(Toward the origin)

9. _____
(Away from the origin)

8. _____
(Toward the midline)

7. _____
(Away from the midline)

6. _____
(Back)

1. _____
(Toward the head)

2. _____
(Above, over)

3. _____
(Below, under)

4. _____
(Front)

5. _____
(Around, encircling)

▶ REVIEW ACTIVITIES

Abbreviation Matching
Match the following abbreviations with their definition.

_____ 1. Dx

_____ 2. Rx

_____ 3. Hx

_____ 4. D

_____ 5. PT

_____ 6. ESRD

_____ 7. R.Ph

_____ 8. PDR

_____ 9. DRG

_____ 10. OCD

a. treatment

b. prescribe

c. diagnosis-related group

d. diopter

e. drugstore

f. registered pharmacist

g. certified pharmacy technician

h. diagnosis

i. esophagogastric disease

j. physician's assistant

k. history

l. *Physician's Desk Reference*

m. physical therapy

n. end-stage renal disease

o. both eyes

p. *Drug Reference Guide*

q. obsessive-compulsive disorder

Abbreviation Fill-ins
Fill in the blanks with the correct abbreviations.

11. left occiput anterior _____

12. sexually transmitted disease _____

13. syphilis test _____

14. lateral _____

15. last menstrual period _____

16. posteroanterior _____

17. biopsy _____

18. tuberculosis _____

▶ **CASE STUDIES**

Write the term next to its meaning given below. Then, draw slashes to analyze the word parts. Note the use of medical abbreviations. Look these up in your dictionary or find them in Appendix B. If you have any questions about the answers, refer to your medical dictionary or check with your instructor for the answers in Appendix A.

CASE STUDY 8-1
SUMMARY

Pt: 83-year-old single women, Ht: 5'2", Wt: 110, BP104/60, T98.9. R20

Dx: 1. **Obsessive-compulsive disorder**
    2. **Hypothyroidism**
    3. **Incontinence**

This 83-year-old, single, woman presented in the emergency room with complaints of anxiety, fear of impending death, panic, fatigue, and **diarrhea**. She has had a history of hospitalization for obsessive-compulsive disorder between the ages of 35 and 55 where she was treated with EST, **psychotropic** medication, and **psychotherapy**. She was released to an adult foster care home where she lived for approximately 10 years moving from home to home with difficulty conforming to house rules about bathroom privileges and **paranoia**. She is currently living in an apartment. Although fully aware of her condition and has been advised of new treatments for **OCD**, she has refused medication and continues her daily routine of hand washing for as long as 30 minutes at a time several times a day. She explains that she is afraid people have entered her apartment and touched her bag of soaps and towels and that she had to throw it all away. She also states that the women in her building have tried to have her evicted because she looks so young for her age and does not go out at night for fear of being raped. **Psychiatric** referral and 50 mg Melaril tid is recommended. Physical examination does not reveal any significant abnormality and she appears in remarkably good cardiovascular health. She states that she walks the equivalent of two miles a day from her apartment to the store or restaurant. The skin on her hands is thin, pink, and dry from hand washing. She does feel fatigued and has a history of hypothyroidism and has not taken medication for several weeks since her prescription ran out. RX: 200 mcg Synthroid is recommended after lab results called. She has occasional accidents from incontinence and diarrhea. She was advised of the use of incontinence garments and will be assessed for **UTI**. Lab order: T3, T4, CBC, Ua with C&S if necessary, OB stool. Psychiatric consult ordered.

1. abnormally slow acting thyroid   _____
2. uncontrolled bowel movement or urination   _____
3. pertaining to psychiatry   _____
4. neurosis characterized by anxiety and ritual behavior   _____
5. urinary tract infection   _____
6. electroshock therapy   _____
7. watery stool   _____
8. blood pressure, temperature, pulse, respiration   _____
9. urinalysis with culture and sensitivity   _____
10. delusions of persecution and grandeur   _____

▶ CROSSWORD PUZZLE

Check your answers by going back through the frames or checking the solution in Appendix C.

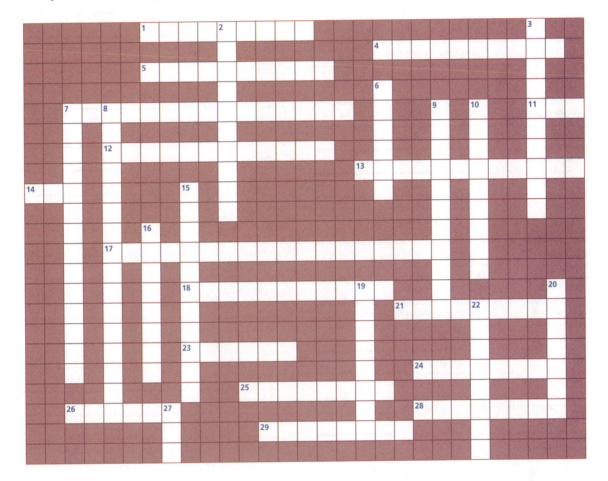

Across

1. permanent cessation of menses
4. membrane of the abdomen
5. pertaining to the bone marrow cell
7. back to front
11. direction from front to back (abbreviation)
12. mental processes that affect sexual response
13. surgical crushing of a nerve
14. obsessive-compulsive disorder (abbreviation)
17. study of mind-altering drugs
18. stone crushing
21. poor digestion
23. easy breathing
24. below
25. treatment used for ESRD
26. away from a designated point or point of origin
28. anteroposterior vertical cut
29. pertaining to organ

Down

2. pertaining to prognosis
3. easy death
6. monthly endometrial bleeding (period)
7. false sensation
8. mental condition caused by untreated syphilis
9. destruction of color
10. nerve pain
15. umbilicocele (synonym)
16. difficult labor
19. above
20. side
22. selection of good genes
27. direction to the side (abbreviation)

► GLOSSARY

achromophilic	resisting color (stain)
aerobic	requiring air to live
aerocele	herniation containing air
aerophobia	abnormal fear of air
aerotherapy	treatment using air (respiratory therapy)
amenorrhea	cessation of menstruation
anaerobic	able to live without air
anterolateral	front and side
anteromedial	front and middle
anteroposterior	from front to back
anterosuperior	front and top
arteriostasis	control of flow through arteries
bioethics	study of what is good and bad for living things
biology	science studying living things
caudad	toward the tail (sacrum)
cephalad	toward the head
cephalocaudal	from head to tail
chondrodysplasia	defective development of cartilage
chromogenesis	formation of color
chromolysis	destruction of color
chromometer	measuring color
chromophilic	attracting color (stain)
coronal	pertaining to the crown or encircling
coronary	pertaining to the crown or encircling (reference to around the heart)
diagnosis	identifying a disease
dialysis	separating of substances in a solution (filtration)
diarrhea	abnormally loose watery bowel movement
distal	away from a point of origin or designated point

dorsal	back (posterior)
dorsocephalad	from back toward the head
dysentery	inflammation of the intestine
dysmenorrhea	difficult or painful menstruation
dyspepsia	poor digestion
dyspnea	difficulty breathing
dystocia	difficulty in labor
eugenics	choosing good genetic trait to propagate
eupepsia	good digestion
eupnea	easy breathing
euthanasia	easy death
eutocia	easy labor
hyperplasia	overdevelopment (too many cells)
hypoplasia	underdevelopment (too few cells)
inferior	below
lateral	side
lithotripsy	surgical crushing of a stone
lymphostasis	control of lymph flow
medial	middle
menopause	cessation of menstruation, ovulation, and atrophy of female reproductive system
menorrhagia	hemorrhage during menstruation
menses	menstruation (menorrhea), menses
midsagittal	the plane dividing the body into equal right and left halves
myelocele	herniation of the spinal cord
myelocytic	pertaining to bone marrow (or spinal cord) cells
myelodysplasia	defective development of the spinal cord or bone marrow
neuralgia	nerve pain
neuritis	nerve inflammation

► GLOSSARY

neuroarthropathy	any disease of the nerves and joints
neurologist	physician specialist in nervous system disorders
neurolysis	nerve destruction
neuroplasty	surgical repair of the nerves
neurosurgeon	physician who performs surgery of the nervous system
neurotripsy	surgical crushing of a nerve
omphalectomy	excision of the umbilicus
omphalic	pertaining to the umbilicus
omphalitis	inflammation of the umbilicus
omphalocele	umbilical hernia (umbilicocele)
omphalorrhagia	hemorrhage of the umbilicus
omphalorrhea	discharge from the umbilicus
omphalorrhexis	rupture of the umbilicus
osteochondro-dysplasia	defective development of bone and cartilage
parietal	pertaining to the wall
peritoneum	membrane of the abdomen
phlebostasis	control of flow through a vein (venostasis)
pleura	membrane of the lungs
posteroanterior	from back to front
posteroexternal	back and outside
posterointernal	back and inside
posterolateral	back and side
procephalic	in front of the head
prognosis	predicting the outcome of a disease
prognostic	pertaining to a prognosis
proximal	near the point of origin or a designated point
pseudocyesis	false pregnancy (pseudopregnancy)
pseudocyst	false cyst
pseudoedema	false swelling
pseudoesthesia	false sensation (i.e., phantom limb)
psychiatrist	physician specialist in mental disorders
psychiatry	the practice of treating mental disorders by a psychiatrist
psychoanalysis	method of psychotherapy which includes obtaining as thorough mental, social, and emotional history to uncover subconscious conflicts
psychologist	scientist who researches or therapist who treats individuals for mental disorders
psychology	the study of the mind and mental processes
psychomotor	mental processes that produce movement
psychoneurosis	affective disorder including abnormal anxiety that may be accompanied by compulsive disorder, depression, or dissociation (neurosis)
psychopathic	pertaining to one with a defective character or personality, or pertaining to the treatment of mental disorders
psycho-pharmacology	the science studying medications that effect mental processes and emotions
psychosexual	thoughts and emotions that affect sexual function
psychosis	severe mental condition marked by loss of reality
psychosomatic	physical ailment with mental or emotional origin
psychotropic	medication used to alter mental processes and emotional states
sagittal	vertical in an anteroposterior direction or plane
superior	above
syphilophobia	abnormal fear of syphilis
syphilopsychosis	severe mental condition caused by untreated syphilis
syphilotherapy	treatment for syphilis

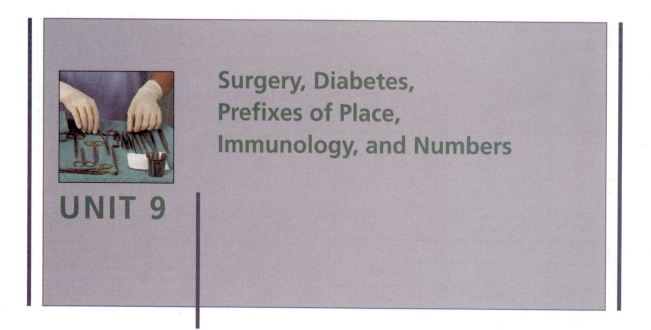

Surgery, Diabetes, Prefixes of Place, Immunology, and Numbers

UNIT 9

9.1
lapar/o means abdominal wall. A laparectomy is an excision of part of the *_____.

abdominal wall

9.2
The process of examining the abdominal cavity with a scope is called _____ /_____ /_____.

lapar/o/scopy
lap ə **ros**´ kō pē

💡 **INFORMATION FRAME**

9.3
A lapar/o/scope is a special instrument that allows a physician to view the inside of the abdominal cavity and its organs. Surgery can also be performed while using a laparoscope (usually attached to a video screen). See the illustration on page 291.

9.4
Lapar/o/scop/ically assisted vaginal hyster/ectomy (LAVH) is actually the removal of the uterus through the vagina assisted by looking through the _____ /_____ /_____ from within the abdominal cavity.

lapar/o/scope
lap´ är ō skōp

290

ANSWER COLUMN	
	9.5 Chole/cyst/ectomy can also be performed with the assistance of the laparoscope. This would be called
lapar/o/scop/ic lap´ är ō **skō´** pik	_____ /____ /_____ /____ cholecystectomy.
	9.6 An incision into the abdominal wall is a
lapar/o/tomy lap´ ə **rot´** ə mē lapar/o/rrhaphy lap´ ə **rôr´** ə fē	_____ /____ /_____. A suturing of the abdominal wall is _____ /____ /_____.
	9.7 Give the meaning for the following words about the abdomen (use your dictionary if needed): laparohepatotomy

incision into the liver
  through the abdomen
new opening in the colon
  through the abdomen
incision into the stomach
  through the abdomen
	*_____;
	laparocolostomy
	*_____;
	laparogastrotomy
	*_____.

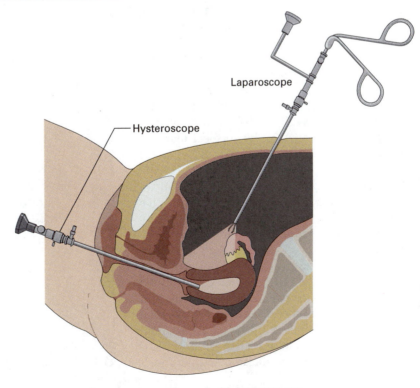

Laparoscopy performed with hysteroscopy

ANSWER COLUMN	
	9.8 There may be longer words than this. If there are, there are not many. Analyze it for fun. Think of the word parts. Laparohysterosalpingo-oophorectomy * _____

abdomen, uterus,
  fallopian tubes,
  ovaries, excision
	_____.

	9.9 **pyr/o** is used in words to mean heat or fever or fire. The early Greeks and Romans burned their dead on funeral pyres. A pyr/o/maniac is one who has a madness (excessive preoccupation) for starting or seeing _____.
fires	
	9.10 Pyr/exia means fever. A condition of heat (heartburn) is _____ / _____. A condition of high fever (over 102°F) is _____ / _____.
pyr/osis pī **rō**′ sis hyper/pyrexia hī′ per pī **reks**′ ē ə	

Professional Profiles ◄◄◄◄◄◄◄◄◄◄◄◄◄◄◄◄◄◄◄◄◄◄◄◄◄◄◄◄

Certified Surgical Technologists (CSTs) are an integral part of a surgical team. They prepare the operating room by selecting and opening sterile supplies; assembling, adjusting, and checking nonsterile equipment; and operating sterilizers, lights, suction machines, electrosurgical units, and diagnostic equipment. The CST most often functions as a member of the surgical team by passing instruments, sutures, and sponges during surgery, holding retractors, receiving specimens, as well as assisting other team members in gowning and gloving. They give preoperative care to surgical patients by providing physical and emotional support, checking charts, and observing vital signs. The Accreditation Review Committee on Education in Surgical Technology (ARC-ST) recommends educational standards and accredits programs. Voluntary professional certification is obtained from the Association of Surgical Technologists (AST) upon passing a CST national certification examination.

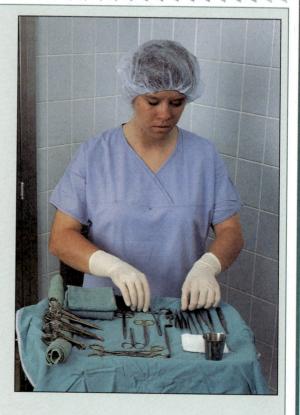

ANSWER COLUMN

9.11
Build words meaning
    instrument for measuring heat (thermometer)

pyr/o/meter
_____ /_____ /_____;
destruction by fever

pyr/o/lysis
_____ /_____ /_____;
abnormal fear of fire

pyr/o/phobia
_____ /_____ /_____;
madness (obsession) for setting fires

pyr/o/mania
(You pronounce)
_____ /_____ /_____.

9.12
A pyr/o/toxin is a toxin (poison) produced by

fever or high body
  temperature, etc.
*_____.

9.13
hydro- (a combining form and prefix) means water or fluid. hidro-
(from the Greek *hidros*) means sweat. A hidro/cyst/aden/oma is a

sweat
cystic tumor of a _____ gland.

9.14
inflammation of sweat
  glands
Hidr/aden/itis means *_____
_____.

9.15
The three words below mean sweating; define and divide them
into their word parts.

hidr/osis
condition of sweating
hyper/hidr/osis
profuse sweating
hidr/o/rrhea
flow of sweat
(You pronounce)
hidrosis _____ /_____,
*_____;
hyperhidrosis _____ /_____ /_____,
*_____;
hidrorrhea _____ /_____ /_____,
*_____.

9.16
The word an/hidr/osis means

absence of sweat
*_____.

9.17
Both hydro- and hidro- are pronounced alike.

water or fluid
sweat
Hydro, with a y, means *_____.
Hidro, with an i, means _____.

▶ **ANSWER COLUMN**

eeee *TAKE A CLOSER LOOK*

9.18

glyc/o (glycos) and **gluc/o (glucos)** are different translations of Greek word parts meaning sweet or sugar. Here are some examples of sweet words:

glycogenesis/glucogenesis: formation of sugar
glycoprotein/glucoprotein: substance made of sugar and protein
glycosuria/glucosuria: **(glycos/glucos)** sugar in the urine

Look up terms beginning with **gluco** and **glyco** in your dictionary. They are interchangeable in some words, but notice many in which they have a unique use.

9.19

Glycogen is "animal starch" formed from simple sugars and stored as reserve fuel. The cells of the body use a simple sugar, glucose, to release energy. To use its reserve fuel supply of animal starch, the body must convert _____ /_____ /_____ to glucose.

glyc/o/gen
glī´ kō jen

9.20

gluc/o is a combining form for glucose. The formation of glucose from glycogen stores is called _____ /_____ /_____ /_____ or _____ /_____ /_____ /_____.

gluc/o/gen/esis
glōō´ kō **jen´** ə sis
glyc/o/gen/esis
glī´ kō **jen´** ə sis

9.21

Glucose is used by the muscles to release energy. Glycogen is the reserve food supply of glucose. Glucose is the usable form of stored _____.

glycogen

9.22

Glycogen is potential sugar. Glucose is usable sugar. In words, **glyc/o** should make you think of

* _____.

sugar or sweet

Glucose tolerance test (GTT) graph

▶ **ANSWER COLUMN**

TAKE A CLOSER LOOK
e̯eee

9.23
Diabetes mellitus has many forms, all of which are characterized by hyperglycemia and other metabolic disturbances. Listed below are three types of diabetes mellitus and their characteristics.

Type I (Insulin-dependent diabetes mellitus [IDDM])
IDDM is characterized by onset in youth, exogenous insulin dependency, tendency to ketoacidosis, viral etiology, autoimmune basis, and genetic predisposition.

Type II (Non–insulin-dependent diabetes mellitus [NIDDM])
NIDDM is characterized by onset in adults over 40, some endogenous insulin production, obesity or normal weight, and can be treated with diet modification and oral hypoglycemic agents.

Gestational diabetes mellitus (GDM)
GDM occurs in individuals not previously diabetic who develop hyperglycemia during pregnancy. These women may progress to other diabetes mellitus or return to normal glucose levels postpartum.

too much sugar in the blood (high blood sugar)	**9.24** Recall that **-emia** means condition in the blood. Glyc/emia means sugar in the blood. A symptom of diabetes is hyper/glyc/emia. This means *_____ _____.
hypo/glyc/emia hī′ pō glī **sē**′ mē ə	**9.25** Hyper/glyc/emia means high blood sugar. The word that means low blood sugar is _____ /_____ /_____.
hypoglycemia	**9.26** When a person produces too much insulin, the blood glucose level may decrease to below normal. This is called _____.
glyc/o/gen/esis glī′ kō **jen**′ ə sis	**9.27** If glucogenesis is the formation of glucose, then the formation of glycogen from food is _____ /____ / _____ /_____.
glyc/o/lysis glī **kol**′ ə sis glyc/o/rrhea glī′ kō **rē**′ ə	**9.28** The breakdown (destruction) of sugar is _____ /____ /_____. The discharge (flow) of sugar from the body is _____ /____ /_____.
sugar fat	**9.29** Glyc/o/lipid should make you think of two foods: _____ and _____.

▶ **ANSWER COLUMN**

The following table is for use in building words for Frames 9.30–9.62.

Prefix of Location	Meaning
ecto-	outer-outside
endo-	inner-inside
meso-	middle
retro-	backward-behind
para-	near

---

endo/derm
en´ dō dûrm

9.30
The blast/o/derm is an embryonic disk of cells that gives rise to the three main layers of tissue in humans. The outer germ layer is called the ecto/derm. The inner germ layer is called the _____ /_____.

---

meso/derm
mez´ ō dûrm

9.31
Between the ectoderm and endoderm is a middle germ layer called the _____ /_____.

---

ecto/derm
ek´ tō dûrm

9.32
The ectoderm forms the skin. The nervous system arises from the same layer as the skin. This layer is the _____ /_____.

---

ectoderm

9.33
Sense organs and some glands are also formed from the _____.

---

endoderm

9.34
The endo/derm forms organs inside the body. The stomach and small intestine arise from the _____.

---

mesoderm

9.35
The mesoderm forms the organs that arise between the ectoderm and endoderm. Muscles are formed by the _____.

---

ectoderm
mesoderm
endoderm

9.36
The blastoderm gives rise to the three germ layers. They are
outer _____;
middle _____;
inner _____.

ANSWER COLUMN	

9.37
ecto- is a Latin prefix for outside. exo- is a Greek prefix for outside. Something produced within an organism is said to be endo/gen/ous. Something produced outside an organism is _____ /_____ or _____ /_____.

ecto/genous
ek **toj´** ə nəs
exo/genous
eks **oj´** ə nəs

9.38
Type I diabetics (IDDM) produce very little endogenous insulin. Therefore, they must take _____ (from an outside source) insulin.

ectogenous or
exogenous

9.39
People with IDDM have hyperglycemia and no insulin to carry the glucose into the cells. Therefore they exhibit the three "P's" as classic symptoms. Recall the prefix poly- and build words that represent these symptoms:
excessive urination _____ /____ /____;
excessive thirst   _____ /_____ /____;
excessive hunger _____ /_____ /____.

poly/ur/ia
poly/dips/ia
poly/phag/ia

9.40
Ecto/cyt/ic is an adjective meaning outside a cell. An adjective meaning inside a bladder is _____ /_____ /____.

endo/cyst/ic
en´ dō **sis´** tik

9.41
-plasm is used as a suffix in words about the substance of cells (cyt/o/plasm). proto- means first. Think of prot/o/type. Prot/o/plasm is the substance of life. The protoplasm that forms the outer membrane of the cell is called _____ /_____. The protoplasm within the cell is called _____ /_____.

ecto/plasm
endo/plasm or
  cyt/o/plasm
(You pronounce)

9.42
Endo/crani/al is an adjective meaning within the cranium. An adjective meaning within cartilage is
_____ /_____ /____.

endo/chondr/al
en´ dō **kon´** drəl

ANSWER COLUMN	
	9.43 Endo/enter/itis means inflammation of the lining of the small intestine. Build words meaning pertaining to the lining of the heart (adjective)
endo/cardial or endo/cardiac endo/colitis (You pronounce)	_____ / _____ ; inflammation of the lining of the colon _____ / _____ .
	9.44 An endo/scope is an instrument used to look into a hollow organ or cavity of the body, as in viewing the stomach. The process of viewing the stomach through an instrument is called
endo/scopy en´ **dos**´ kō pē gastr/o/scopy gas **tros**´ kō pē	_____ / _____ or _____ / ____ / _____ .
	9.45 Esophag/o/gastr/o/duoden/o/scopy (EGD) is one type of
endoscopy	_____ .

WORD BUILDING

ESOPHAG/O	+	GASTR/O	+	DUODEN/O	+	SCOPY
combining form		combining form		combining form		suffix

	9.46 Using what you know about endo-, **arter**, and -ectomy, complete the definition of this term: end/arter/ectomy—removal of a substance (usually an atheroma)
inside	from the _____ of an artery.
💡 INFORMATION FRAME	**9.47** Note the involved development of the word ectopic (out of place): **ect/o**—outside **top/os**—place (Greek word) **-ic**—adjectival suffix
	9.48 An ectopic pregnancy occurs outside of the uterus (usually in a fallopian tube). A salpingectomy may be required after the rupture of an ____ / _____ pregnancy.
ec/topic ek **top**´ ik	
	9.49 If endometrial tissue occurs in the fallopian tubes, a fertilized egg can lodge in it, thus causing pregnancy. This is an
ectopic	_____ pregnancy.

► **ANSWER COLUMN**

9.50

An embryo's development in the abdominal cavity is also an
_____ pregnancy.

ectopic

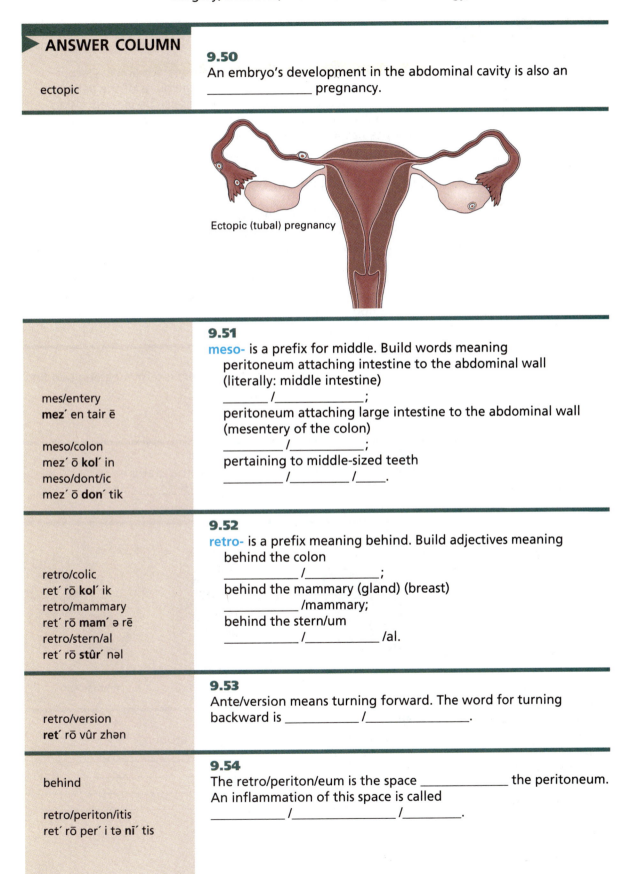

Ectopic (tubal) pregnancy

9.51

meso- is a prefix for middle. Build words meaning
    peritoneum attaching intestine to the abdominal wall
    (literally: middle intestine)

mes/entery
mez´ en tair ē

_____ / _____ ;
peritoneum attaching large intestine to the abdominal wall
(mesentery of the colon)

meso/colon
mez´ ō **kol´** in

_____ / _____ ;
pertaining to middle-sized teeth

meso/dont/ic
mez´ ō **don´** tik

_____ / _____ / ____ .

9.52

retro- is a prefix meaning behind. Build adjectives meaning
    behind the colon

retro/colic
ret´ rō **kol´** ik

_____ / _____ ;
behind the mammary (gland) (breast)

retro/mammary
ret´ rō **mam´** ə rē

_____ /mammary;
behind the stern/um

retro/stern/al
ret´ rō **stûr´** nəl

_____ / _____ /al.

9.53

Ante/version means turning forward. The word for turning
backward is _____ / _____ .

retro/version
ret´ rō vûr zhən

9.54

The retro/periton/eum is the space _____ the peritoneum.
An inflammation of this space is called

behind

_____ / _____ / _____ .

retro/periton/itis
ret´ rō per´ i tə **nī´** tis

ANSWER COLUMN	
	9.55 Recall that ERCP is an x-ray procedure in which an endo/scope is used to inject a contrast medium into the ducts of the pancreas and gallbladder so that any obstructions can be viewed. Using what you know about the word parts you have already learned, draw the slashes for the ERCP terms:
endo/scop/ic retro/grade chol/angi/o/pancreat/o/- graphy	endoscopic _____ ; retrograde _____ ; cholangiopancreatography _____. Refer to the illustration on page 209.
bending forward	**9.56** Flex/ion is bending or shortening of a body part (usually at a joint). **ante-** is the prefix for front or forward. Therefore, the word ante/flexion means *_____.
retro/flexion **re´ trō flek shən**	**9.57** **retro-** means behind (or backward). Build a term meaning bending backward: _____ / _____.
bending backward	**9.58** Retro/flexion of the uterus means that the uterus is *_____.

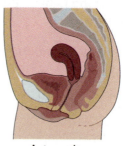 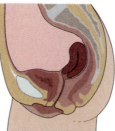 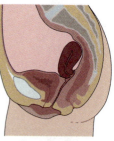

Anteversion   Marked retroversion   Retroflexion

near the center or
  around the center
inflammation around
  the appendix
	9.59
	para- as a prefix means near, beside, or around.
	Para/centr/al means *_____
	
	_____.
	
	Para-/appendic/itis means *_____
	
	_____.

ANSWER COLUMN	

9.60
Build words meaning
inflammation around (near) the bladder
_____ /_____ /_____;
inflammation of tissues around (near) the vagina
_____ /_____ /_____.

para/cyst/itis
par´ ə sis **tī´** tis
para/colp/itis
par´ ə kol **pī´** tis

9.61
Build words meaning inflammation of tissues
near the liver
_____ /_____ /_____;
near the kidney
_____ /_____ /_____.

para/hepat/itis

para/nephr/itis
(You pronounce)

9.62
ecto- means _____.
endo- means _____.
meso- means _____.
para- means _____.
retro- means _____.

outer
inner
middle
around (near)
behind

9.63
immun/o is the combining form for immune. Immun/ity is one of the body's protections from diseases. The study of the function of the immune system is called _____ /_____ /_____.

immun/o/logy
im´ yōō **nol´** ō jē

9.64
Immun/ization injections and oral preparations are given so that a person may develop an immune response to certain diseases. The process is known as immun/o/therapy. DPT (diphtheria, pertussis, tetanus) and OPV (oral polio vaccine) are two types of
_____ /_____ /_____
or
_____ /_____ /_____.

immun/o/therapy
im´ yōō nō **ther´** a pē
immun/i/zations
im´ yōō nə **zā´** shunz

9.65
Immun/o/logists are studying HIV (human immun/o/deficiency virus), which causes AIDS (acquired immunodeficiency syndrome). Because it is characterized by inability to fight off diseases, AIDS is a type of _____ /_____/_____ disease.

immun/o/deficiency
im´ yōō nō de **fish´** en cē

9.66
INFORMATION FRAME
When an antigen (like a foreign protein) invades the body, special leukocytes (lymphocytes) produce antibodies to disable the invader. This antigen-antibody reaction is called the immune response.

ANSWER COLUMN

immun/ity
im **y o͞o**´ ni tē

9.67
Chickenpox is caused by the virus *Varicella zoster*. When first infected, the person becomes ill. If infected again, the person will most likely not become ill due to acquired active _____ /_____.

---

immunity

9.68
An infant being breast fed receives antibodies from its mother's body through the breast milk. This type of immunity is called passive _____.

🏛 **WORD ORIGINS**

vaccin/ation
vak sin ā´ shun

9.69
Vaccines (immunizations) are usually given by injection to stimulate the body's natural immune response. This allows us to resist an infection when exposed to that specific organism in the future. The word vaccine comes from the Latin word for cow, *vacca*. Edward Jenner first innoculated a young boy with a substance from the sore of a milkmaid infected with cowpox. At a later time, he exposed the boy to smallpox and the boy resisted the disease. This was the first vaccination (immunization).

---

vaccin/e
vak **sēn**´

9.70
The oral polio _____ (OPV) stimulates resistance to polio.

TYPICAL IMMUNIZATIONS (VACCINES)

DPT	diphtheria, pertussis, tetanus
OPV	oral polio vaccine
HBV	hepatitis B virus
MMRV	measles, mumps, rubella
Hib	*Haemophilus influenzae b* (for meningitis)
Td	tetanus
Var	chicken pox (Varicella zoster)

---

self

9.71
aut/o is a combining form that means self. You already recognize **auto** in such ordinary English words as aut/o/mobile (a self-propelled vehicle) and aut/o/bi/o/graphy. **aut/o** means _____.

---

one's own skin

9.72
Aut/o/di/a/gnos/is means diagnosing one's own diseases.
Aut/o/derm/ic pertains to dermat/o/plasty with
*_____.

ANSWER COLUMN	**9.73** Aut/o/nom/ic (aw´ tō **nom**´ ik) means self-controlling, as in the nervous system. Aut/o/lysis (aw **tol**´ ə sis) means
self-destruction or self-destroying	*_____.
aut/o/immun/ity aw´ tō im **yōō**´ ni tē	**9.74** If one's own body produces antibodies to one's own tissues (like being allergic to yourself), _____ /____ /_____ /_____ has occurred. **EXAMPLE:** Rh factor reactions during some pregnancies and rheumatoid arthritis.
aut/o/phobia aw tō **fō**´ bē ə	**9.75** Aut/o/phagia means biting one's self. A word that means abnormal fear of being alone is _____ /____ /_____.

aut/o/hem/o/therapy
aw´ tō hēm´ ō **ther**´ a pē
aut/o/plasty
aw´ tō plas tē
	9.76
	Build terms that mean
	    therapy with one's own blood (transfusion)
	    _____ /____ /_____ /____ /_____;
	    surgery using grafts from one's own body
	    _____ /____ /_____.

aut/o/logous aw **tol**´ ō gus	**9.77** Aut/o/logous is an adjective meaning originating in itself or coming from one's own body. Persons anticipating surgery can have blood taken and saved for their own use if needed. This would be an _____ /____ /_____ blood transfusion.
aut/o/graft **aw**´ tō graft	**9.78** Keeping the previous frame in mind, think of what an aut/o/graft might be. A burn victim needing a skin graft may use his or her own healthy skin as an _____ /____ /_____.
aut/o/gen/ous aw **to**´ jen us	**9.79** The term aut/o/genous has a similar meaning to aut/o/logous. If a vaccine is made from a culture of the patient's own bacteria, this is called an _____ /____ /_____ /_____ vaccine.

ANSWER COLUMN

aut/o/phobia
  abnormal fear of one's
  self or being alone

aut/o/phagia
  biting one's self

9.80
Great! When you analyze a word, think of its meaning. If you have forgotten a part of the word, look it up. Analyze:

autophobia _____ /_____ /_____,

_____ ;
meaning

autophagia _____ /_____ /_____,

_____ .
meaning

Study this table. Notice the specific use of each prefix.

NUMERICAL PREFIXES			
Greek	**Latin**	**Meaning**	**Examples**
hemi-	semi-	half	hemiplegia, semiconscious
mono-	uni-	one	monocyte, uniparous
prot-	prim-	first	protozoan, primigravida
di(plo)-	bi-	two	diplococci, bifurcation
tri-	tri-	three	triglyceride, triceps
tetra-	quadr-	four	tetramastia, quadriplegia
penta-	quint-	five	pentadactyl, quintuplets
hexa-	sexta-	six	hexapodia, sexagenarian
hepta-	septa-	seven	heptachromic, septuplet
octa-	oct-	eight	octodont, octogenarian
enne(a)-	non(i)-	nine	ennead, nonipara
deca-	dec(i)-	ten, tenth	decaliter, deciliter
hecto- (100)	cent(i)- (0.01)	one hundred, one hundredth	hectogram, centigram
kilo- (1,000)	mill(i)- (0.001)	one thousand, one thousandth	kilometer, millimeter

Then use this knowledge to work the rest of the frames in this unit.

one

9.81
mono- means one or single. You know it in the ordinary English words monorail, monopoly, and monogamy. Whenever you see mono-, you think of _____.

▶ **ANSWER COLUMN**	
one	**9.82** A mono/graph deals with a single subject. A mono/nucle/ar cell has _____ nucleus.

mono/cyte
mon/oma
(You pronounce)
	9.83
	Mono/mania is an abnormal preoccupation with one subject only.
	Build words meaning
	   one cell _____ /_____ (a type of leukocyte);
	   one tumor _____ /_____.

mono/my/o/plegia
mon′ ō mī ō **plē**′ jē ə
mono/neur/al
mon ō **nōōr**′ əl
mono/cyt/osis
mon′ ō sī **tō**′ sis
	9.84
	Build words that begin with mono-.
	   paralysis of one muscle
	   _____ /_____ /_____ /_____;
	   pertaining to one nerve
	   _____ /_____ /_____;
	   condition of increase in monocytes
	   _____ /_____ /_____.

mono/nucle/osis mon′ ō nōō klē **ō**′ sis	**9.85** Mono/nucle/osis (mono) is a condition caused by a viral infection that can damage the liver. One of the signs is an abnormally high monocyte count. Mono/cyt/osis may be an indication of _____ /_____ /_____.
many or more than one	**9.86** multi- means the opposite of mono-. multi- (as in multiply) means * _____.
many	**9.87** In ordinary English, you are acquainted with multi- in the words multiply and multitude. Something composed of multiple parts has _____ parts.
many capsules	**9.88** Something that is multi/capsular has * _____.
many glands many cells many nuclei	**9.89** Multi/glandular is an adjective meaning * _____. Multi/cellular is an adjective meaning * _____. Multi/nuclear is an adjective meaning * _____.

▶ **ANSWER COLUMN**

9.90
A multi/para is a woman who has brought forth (borne) more than one child. **par** is one word root meaning to bear.
Multi/par/ous is the adjectival form of _____ /_____.

multi/para
mul **tip´** ə rə

9.91
Multi/para always refers to the mother. Multi/par/ous may refer to the mother or may mean multiple birth (twins or triplets). When desiring to indicate that a woman has borne more than one child, use the noun _____.

multipara

9.92
Multi/par/ous is the adjectival form of _____ /_____. To indicate that twins are born, say _____ /_____ /_____ birth.

multi/para
multi/par/ous
mul **tip´** ər əs

9.93
To indicate that triplets are born, say _____ birth. If ten children were born, you would still use the adjective _____.

multiparous

multiparous

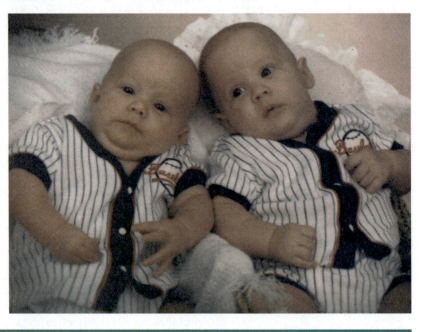

Identical twins: Multiparous (refers to a woman who has given birth to more than one child)

9.94
nulli- means *none*. To nullify something is to bring it to nothing. There are not many medical words using **nulli-**; but when you do see it, it means _____.

> **ANSWER COLUMN**

a woman who has never borne a child primi/para prī **mip′** ər ə	**9.95** A nulli/para is *_____. primi- means first. A woman who is having her first child is a _____ /_____ (noun).

primi/gravida prim′ i **grav′** i da	**9.96** *Gravida* is a Latin word meaning heavy or weighted down. In medical terms it is used to mean pregnant. A woman experiencing her first pregnancy is called a _____ /_____.

💡 **INFORMATION FRAME**	**9.97** **gravida** refers to pregnancies, whereas **para** refers to live births. A woman who has been pregnant four times and had two spontaneous abortions (miscarriages) and two live births would be described on the chart as grav IV, ab II, para II.

nulli/para nu **lip′** ar ə no live births nulli/par/ous nu **lip′** ar us pertaining to no live births primi/para prī **mip′** ar ə first live birth	**9.98** Analyze the following and define: nullipara _____ /_____ (noun), *_____; nulliparous _____ /_____ /_____ (adjective), *_____; primipara _____ /_____ (noun), *_____.

nulli-
mono-
multi-
para-
primi-
	9.99
	Give the prefix for
	  none _____;
	  one (single) _____;
	  many _____;
	  bear _____;
	  first _____.

ten tenth	**9.100** deca- and deci- both mean ten but are used differently. deca- is used in words meaning the whole number ten. deci- is used in words meaning the fraction one tenth. A decaliter (dal) is _____ liters. A deciliter (dl) is one _____ of a liter.

ANSWER COLUMN	

9.101
Build words that mean
   ten grams

deca/gram
de´ ka gram
deci/gram
de´ si gram

_____ /_____ (dag);
one tenth of a gram
_____ /_____ (dg).

9.102
kilo- and milli- both refer to thousand but are used differently.
kilo- is used in words to mean one thousand. milli- is used in
words to mean one thousandth. A kilometer (km) is one

thousand
thousandth

_____ meters. A millimeter (mm) is one
_____ of a meter.

9.103
Build words that mean
   one thousand grams

kilo/gram
ki´ lo gram
milli/gram
mi´ li gram

_____ /_____ (kg);
one thousandth of a gram
_____ /_____ (mg).

9.104
A volume measurement that is frequently used when giving
injections is the cubic centimeter (cc). It is the amount of fluid in
one centimeter cubed. If the physician writes an order to give 0.5 cc
of Tetanus Toxoid, the medical assistant will inject one half of a

cubic centimeter

*_____ of insulin.

9.105
Do the work on this frame using the table on page 304.
Build words that mean
   one hundred meters

hecto/meter
hek **tom´** ə ter
centi/meter
sen´ ti mē ter
hecto/gram
hek´ to gram
centi/gram
sen´ ti gram

_____ /_____ (hm);
one hundredth of a meter
_____ /_____ (cm);
one hundred grams
_____ /_____ (hg);
one hundredth of a gram
_____ /_____ (cg).

Good work!

Abbreviation	Meaning
2 h pc, 2°pc	two hours postcibal (after meal)
2 h pp, 2°pp	two hours postprandial (after meal)
2 h pg, 2°pg	two hours post–glucose test (after drinking glucose)
$C_6H_{12}O_6$	glucose
ab (I, II, III)	abortion (spontaneous or induced) number
AIDS	acquired immunodeficiency syndrome
ARC	AIDS-related complex
CST	certified surgical technologist
DPT or DTP	diphtheria, pertussis, tetanus
EGD	esophagogastroduodenoscopy
ERCP	endoscopic retrograde cholangiopancreatography
FBS	fasting blood sugar
grav (I, II, III)	number of pregnancies
GTT	glucose tolerance test (3 h, 5 h)
HB	hepatitis virus
hBv	hepatitis B vaccine
Hib	*Haemophilus influenzae* vaccine
HIV	human immunodeficiency virus
IDDM (Type I diabetes)	insulin-dependent diabetes mellitus
LAVH	laparoscopically assisted vaginal hysterectomy
mg/dL	milligrams per deciliter
MMRV	measles, mumps, rubella
mono	mononucleosis
NIDDM (Type II diabetes)	noninsulin-dependent diabetes mellitus
OPV	oral poliovirus vaccine
para (I, II, III)	number of live births
S/A, S&A	sugar and acetone
Td	tetanus
Var	chicken pox vaccine (*Varicella zoster*)

Also, study the weights and measures abbeviations in Appendix A. To complete your study of this unit, work the review activities on the next pages. Also, listen to the audiotapes that accompany *Medical Terminology: A Programmed Text,* 8th edition, and practice your pronunciation.

Additional practice exercises for this unit are available on the Student Practice disk found in the back of the textbook.

► REVIEW ACTIVITIES

Circle and Correct
Circle the correct answer for each question. Then, check your answers in Appendix A.

1. Word root for abdominal wall:
   a. abdomeno   b. lapar
   c. hepar   d. hyster

2. Suffix for destruction:
   a. -tripsy   b. -stasis
   c. -pexy   d. -lysis

3. Combining form for sweat:
   a. hidro   b. hydro
   c. sudoriferous   d. hyper

4. Suffix meaning in the urine:
   a. -urea   b. -uria
   c. -uric   d. -uro

5. Prefix for inner or inside:
   a. inter-   b. infra-
   c. meso-   d. endo-

6. Prefix for behind or in back of:
   a. meso-   b. retro-
   c. ante-   d. posterior-

7. Combining form for sugar:
   a. glyco   b. glucos
   c. glycemia   d. galactose

8. Prefix for outer:
   a. exto-   b. ecto-
   c. endo-   d. external-

9. Word for turning:
   a. retro   b. flexion
   c. strepto   d. version

10. Prefix for middle:
   a. endo-   b. inter-
   c. meso-   d. medi-

Count and write the prefix. Then, build a word using that prefix.

Prefix			Word
_____	1. none	no pregnancies	_____
_____	2. first	first live birth	_____
_____	3. one	one cell	_____
_____	4. two	two branches (use your dictionary)	_____
_____	5. three	three sided	_____
_____	6. four	paralysis, four limbs	_____
_____	7. five	five infants born at the same time (use your dictionary)	_____
_____	8. six	sixth pregnancy	_____
_____	9. seven	seventh live birth	_____
_____	10. eight	person 80 years old (use your dictionary)	_____
_____	11. nine	ninth pregnancy	_____
_____	12. ten	ten liters	_____
_____	13. one hundred(th)	1/100th of a meter	_____
_____	14. one thousand(th)	1000 calories	_____
_____	15. many	many glands	_____

▶ REVIEW ACTIVITIES

Select and Construct
Select the correct word parts from the list below and construct medical terms that represent the given meaning.

aden	ante	cardial	colo	cystic
deca	deci	derm	ecto	emia
endo	enter(o)(y)	flexion	gen(esis)ous	gluco
glyco	gram	hecto	hepat	hidro
hyper	hypo	itis	kilo	laparo
lipid	lysis	mammary	mes(o)	meter
milli	(o)sis	ous	para	peritoneal
phobia	pic	plasm	pyro	retro
rrhea	scope (ic)	stomy	tomy	version

1. instrument for looking into the abdomen
2. developed within
3. condition of heat
4. excessive sweating
5. peritoneum attaching intestine to the abdominal wall
6. behind the abdominal membrane
7. breakdown of sugar
8. pertaining to the heart lining
9. outside of its place example: pregnancy (adjective)
10. inflammation around the bladder
11. bending forward (bowing)
12. twisting (turning) backward
13. instrument used to look inside
14. high blood sugar
15. containing sugar and fat
16. ten grams
17. one thousandth of a meter

▶ REVIEW ACTIVITIES

Define and Dissect
Give a brief definition and dissect each term listed into its word parts in the space provided on the right. Check your answers by referring to the frame listed in parentheses and your medical dictionary. Then, listen to the audiotapes to practice pronunciation.

1. laparotomy (9.6)

_____ / _____ / _____
rt   v   suffix

_____
definition

2. laparohepatotomy (9.7)

_____ / ___ / _____ / ___ / _____
rt   v   rt   v   suffix

3. pyrolysis (9.11)

_____ / _____ / _____
rt   v   suffix

4. pyrexia (9.10)

_____ / _____
rt   suffix

5. glucogenesis (9.20)

_____ / _____ / _____ / _____
rt   v   rt   suffix

6. glycogenesis (9.27)

_____ / _____ / _____ / _____
rt   v   rt   suffix

7. ectoderm (9.32)

_____ / _____
pre   rt

8. endoscopy (9.44)

_____ / _____
pre   suffix

9. mesentery (9.51)

_____ / _____
pre   rt/suffix

10. retromammary (9.52)

_____ / _____
pre   rt/suffix

11. retroperitonitis (9.54)

_____ / _____ / _____
pre   rt   suffix

12. paracolpitis (9.60)

_____ / _____ / _____
pre   rt   suffix

13. retroflexion (9.57)   _____ / _____
                          pre   rt/suffix

14. anteversion (9.53)   _____ / _____
                          pre   rt/suffix

15. hypoglycemia (9.26)   _____ / _____ / _____
                          pre   rt   suffix

16. glucosuria (9.18)   _____ / ___ / _____
                          rt   v   rt/suffix

17. laparoscopic (9.5)   _____ / ___ / _____ / _____
                          rt   v   rt   suffix

18. glycoprotein (9.18)   _____ / ___ / _____
                          rt   v   rt

19. mesodontic (9.51)   _____ / _____ / _____
                          pre   rt   suffix

20. cholangiopancreatography (9.55) _____ / _____ / __ / _____ / __ / _____
                                     rt   rt   v   rt   v   suffix

21. immunology (9.63)   _____ / ___ / _____
                          rt   v   suffix

22. immunodeficiency (9.65) _____ / ___ / _____
                             rt   v   rt/suffix

23. autoimmunity (9.74)   _____ / ___ / _____ / _____
                          pre   v   rt   suffix

24. autophagia (9.80)   _____ / ___ / _____
                          pre   v   rt/suffix

25. mononucleosis (9.85) _____ / _____ / _____
                          pre   rt   suffix

26. multiparous (9.92)   _____ / _____ / _____
                          pre   rt   suffix

▶ REVIEW ACTIVITIES

27. primigravida (9.96)

_____ / _____
       pre   rt/suffix

_____

28. kilometer (table)

_____ / _____
       pre   suffix

_____

29. centigram (table)

_____ / _____
       pre   rt

_____

30. quadriplegia (table)

_____ / _____
       pre   rt/suffix

_____

31. sextagenarian (table)

_____ / _____
       pre   rt/suffix

_____

32. septuplets (table)

_____ / _____
       pre   rt/suffix

_____

33. immunization (9.64)

_____ / _____ / _____
       rt   v   suffix

_____

34. autohemotherapy (9.76)

_____ / _____ / _____ / _____ / _____
   pre   v   rt   v   suffix

_____

35. monocytosis (9.84)

_____ / _____ / _____
       pre   rt   suffix

_____

36. hemiplegia (table)

_____ / _____
       pre   suffix

_____

37. deciliter (table)

_____ / _____
       pre   rt

_____

38. nullipara (9.98)

_____ / _____
       pre   rt/suffix

_____

39. bifurcation (table)

_____ / _____ / _____
   pre   rt   suffix

_____

▶ REVIEW ACTIVITIES

Abbreviation Matching—Part I
Match the following abbreviations with their definition.

_____ 1. 2 h pc

_____ 2. GTT

_____ 3. FBS

_____ 4. Type II diabetes

_____ 5. S&A

_____ 6. $C_6H_{12}O_6$

_____ 7. EGD

_____ 8. IDDM

a. glucose
b. sugar and acetone
c. NIDDM
d. IDDM
e. two hours after meal
f. acid fast bacillus
g. endoscopic exam of the pancreas
h. fasting blood sugar
i. glucose tolerance test
j. carbon dioxide
k. esophagogastroduodenoscopy
l. Type I diabetes mellitus

Abbreviation Matching—Part II
Match the following abbreviations with their definition.

_____ 1. ab II

_____ 2. OPV

_____ 3. mono

_____ 4. HBV

_____ 5. AIDS

_____ 6. HIV

_____ 7. para II

_____ 8. DPT

a. human immunodeficiency virus
b. diphtheria, pertussis, tetanus
c. one
d. oral poliovirus vaccine
e. acute autoimmune disease
f. herpes influenza virus
g. two abortions
h. acquired immunodeficiency syndrome
i. two abscesses
j. mononucleosis
k. hepatitis B vaccine
l. two live births (viable)
m. diplococcus per throat

Abbreviations—Weights and Measures
State the correct abbreviation for the following weights and measures.

_____ 1. kilogram

_____ 2. ounce

_____ 3. cubic centimeter

_____ 4. megahertz

_____ 5. teaspoon

_____ 6. pound

_____ 7. dram

_____ 8. one and one half

_____ 9. units

_____ 10. drops

► **CASE STUDIES**

Write the term next to its meaning given below. Then, draw slashes to analyze the word parts. Note the use of medical abbreviations. Look these up in your dictionary or find them in Appendix B. If you have any questions about the answers, refer to your medical dictionary or check with your instructor for the answers in Appendix A.

CASE STUDY 9-1
CONSULTATION NOTE

Pt: female, age 34

Dx: 1. Obesity **hypoventilation syndrome**

2. Diabetes mellitus, **IDDM**

Ms. Betty Sweet presented with a history of morbid obesity and previous admission for respiratory insufficiency. She entered the emergency room complaining of progressive fatigue, sleepiness, **cephalalgia**, **narcolepsy**, general weakness, and **dyspnea**. She admits to a dry nonproductive cough without congestion, **URI symptoms**, recent fevers, sweats, or chills. For her headache she had been taking an occasional nonprescription **analgesic** only amounting to 2 aspirins/week and denied any other drug use. Ms. Sweet has a history of IDDM and had been maintained on 25 **U** of insulin until August 11th when she was increased to 40 units. A urinary tract infection was an incidental finding. She has not checked her blood sugars at home and does not know whether or not she has had any **hypoglycemic** reactions. Ms. Sweet has progressive increasing lethargy and feeling unrested. Past history is also significant for a hospitalization in 1988 for which she required **ventilatory** support for obstructive **apnea**. She was discharged home on nasal **CPAP** and was able to lose 20–30 pounds with marked improvement in her symptoms. She has since gained the weight back over the last 6 months or so and is dieting again. Of note at that time was Swan-Ganz **catheterization**, which revealed elevated pulmonary artery pressures.

1. introduction of a tube to evacuate or irrigate a body cavity   _____

2. cessation of breathing   _____

3. insulin-dependent diabetes mellitus   _____

4. upper respiratory infection   _____

5. sleep seizures   _____

6. continuous positive air pressure   _____

7. reduced depth of breaths   _____

8. symptoms that run together   _____

9. how the patient feels   _____

10. units   _____

11. low blood sugar (adjective)   _____

12. pain reliever   _____

13. headache   _____

14. difficulty breathing   _____

15. getting air in lungs (adjective)   _____

▶ CROSSWORD PUZZLE

Check your answers by going back through the frames or checking the solutions in Appendix C.

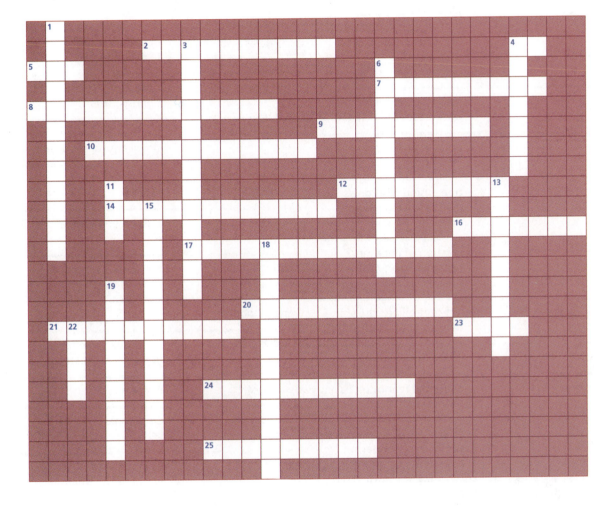

Across

2. no sweat
4. after meal (abbreviation)
5. glucose tolerance test (abbreviation)
7. no live births
8. a symptom is monocytosis
9. give yourself tissue
10. first pregnancy
12. stuff inside the cell
14. inflammation near the vagina
16. lack of this hormone causes diabetes
17. many glands
20. five born at the same time
21. sugar breakdown
23. measles, mumps, rubella vaccine (abbreviation)
24. scoping the abdominal cavity
25. likes to set fires (compulsion)

Down

1. behind the sternum
3. opposite of low blood sugar
4. synonym for hyperthermia
6. lining of the uterus
11. diphtheria, pertussis, tetanus (abbreviation)
13. the middle of the intestine
15. bend back
18. vaccine
19. one tenth of a liter
22. laparoscopically assisted vaginal hysterectomy (abbreviation)

▶ GLOSSARY

anhidrosis	absence of sweating
autodermic	plastic surgery and grafting using one's own skin (dermatoplasty)
autodiagnosis	diagnosing one's self
autogenous	made by or from one's own tissues (adjective)
autograft	graft of tissue from one's own body
autohemotherapy	transfusion with one's own blood (autologous donor)
autoimmunity	reaction of immune response to one's own tissues
autonomic	self-controlling part of the nervous system (adjective)
autophagia	biting one's self
autophobia	abnormal fear of one's self, being alone
blastoderm	embryonic disk that gives rise to the endoderm, mesoderm, ectoderm
centigram	one hundredth of a gram (0.01 g)
centimeter	one hundredth of a meter (0.01 m)
choleangiopancreato-graphy	x-ray of bile ducts and pancreatic ducts using contrast medium
cytoplasm	substance within the cell (endoplasm)
decagram	ten grams
decaliter	ten liters
decigram	one tenth of a gram (0.1 g)
deciliter	one tenth of a liter (0.1 L)
ectocytic	outside the cell (extracellular)
ectoderm	outer germ layer (embryonic)
ectogenous	made outside the body (from another source)
ectopic	outside of normal location
ectoplasm	outer membrane of the cell
endocardium	the inner membrane layer of the heart
endochondral	within cartilage
endocolitis	inflammation of the lining of the colon
endocystic	inside a cyst
endoderm	embryonic inner germ layer
endoenteritis	inflammation of the lining of the small intestine
endogenous	manufactured within the body
endometrium	inner layer of the uterus
endoscopy	use of a scope to look into the body (especially hollow organs)
millimeter	one thousandth of a meter (0.001 m)
monocyte	one cell (type of leukocyte)

▶ GLOSSARY

monocytosis	increase in the number of monocytes
monoma	a single tumor
monomyoplegia	paralysis of one muscle
mononeural	involving one nerve
mononuclear	having one nucleus
mononucleosis	viral infection causing monocytosis
multicapsular	having more than one capsule (adjective)
multicellular	having or involving many cells (adjective)
multiglandular	having or involving many glands (adjective)
multinuclear	a cell having more than one nucleus (adjective)
multipara	having many live births (born in third trimester)
nullipara	having no pregnancies carried to the third trimester live births
para-appendicitis	inflammation near the appendix
paracentral	near the center
paracolpitis	inflammation around the vagina
paracystitis	inflammation near the urinary bladder
parahepatitis	inflammation near the liver
paranephritis	inflammation near the kidney
primigravida	first pregnancy
primipara	first live birth
pyrexia	fever (hyperthermia)
pyrolysis	destruction of tissue caused by fever
pyromania	compulsion (madness) for setting fires
pyrometer	thermometer
pyrophobia	abnormal fear of fire
pyrosis	heartburn
pyrotoxin	poisonous by-product of metabolism created during fever
retrocolic	behind the colon (adjective)
retroflexion	bending backward
retromammary	behind the breast (adjective)
retroperitoneum	area behind the peritoneum
retroperitonitis	inflammation behind the peritoneum
retrosternal	behind the sternum (adjective)
retroversion	turning backward (twisting back)
vaccine	substance used to stimulate an immune response

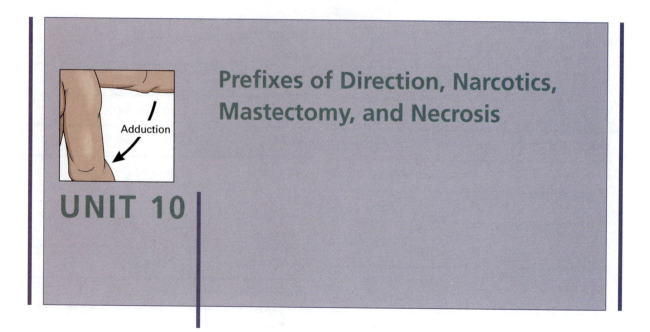

UNIT 10

Prefixes of Direction, Narcotics, Mastectomy, and Necrosis

Adduction

Prefixes representing place often cause difficulty in word building because of their similarity. Use this information carefully while working through Frames 10.1–10.32.

PREFIX	MEANING	SENSE OF MEANING
ab	from	away from
de	from	down from or from—resulting in less than
ex	from	out from

10.1

Recall ab/duction and ad/duction. You have already learned ab- is the opposite of ad-. ad- means toward. ab- means _____.

from

10.2

Ab/duct/ion (ab **duk´** shun) means moving away from the midline. Ab/norm/al means going *_____ normal.

away from

10.3

Ab/or/al means away from the mouth. Ab/errant (ab **er´** ənt) means wandering *_____ the normal course.

away from

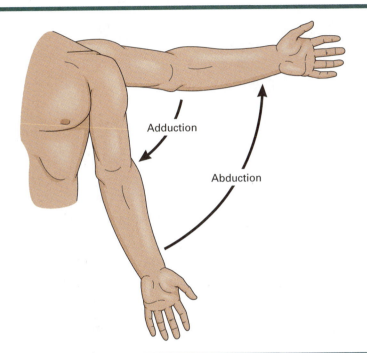

Adduction

Abduction

ANSWER COLUMN	
away from away from	**10.4** An ab/irritant is something that takes irritation *_____ the patient. Ab/lact/ation means taking the baby *_____ the breast feeding or the cessation of milk secretion.
ab/ort/ion a **bôr**′ shən	**10.5** Ab/ort was, literally, built by joining **ab-** to a word part meaning to be born (Latin: *oriri*, to be born). A naturally occurring termination of pregnancy (miscarriage) is called a spontaneous ____ /_____ /_____.
ab/ort/ed	**10.6** In an induced abortion, the products of conception are taken away from the uterus or ____ /_____ /____.
💡 *INFORMATION FRAME*	**10.7** Three types of wounds are lacerations (cuts), contusions (bruises), and abrasions (scrapes).
away from ab/rasion a **brā**′ shən	**10.8** To ab/rade (a **brād**′) the skin is to scrape some of the skin *_____ the surface of the body. A scrape type of injury is called an ____ /_____.

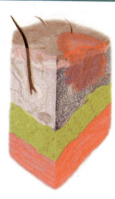

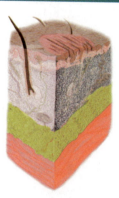

A. Bruise, also known as a contusion, results from damage to the soft tissues and blood vessels, which causes bleeding beneath the skin surface. A bruise in a light-skinned individual will change from red to purple to greenish yellow before fading. In a dark-skinned person, the bruise will first look dark red, then darker red, brown, or purple, and slowly fade.

B. Abrasion, also known as a scrape or rug burn, results when the outer layer of skin is scraped or rubbed away. Exposure of nerve endings makes this type of wound painful, and the presence of debris from the scraped surface (rug fibers, gravel, sand) makes abrasions highly susceptible to infection.

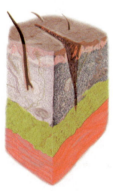

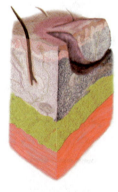

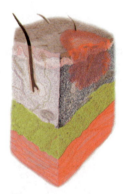

C. Laceration, cut, or incision, are caused by sharp objects such as knives or glass, or from trauma due to a strike from a blunt object that opens the skin, such as a baseball bat. If the wound is deep, the cut may bleed profusely; if nerve endings are exposed, it could also be painful.

D. Avulsion results when the skin or tissue is torn away from the body, either partially or completely. The bleeding and pain depends on the depth of tissue affected.

E. Puncture results when the skin is pierced by a sharp object such as a pencil, nail, or bullet. If a piece of the object remans in the skin, or if there is little bleeding due to the depth and location of the puncture, infection is likely.

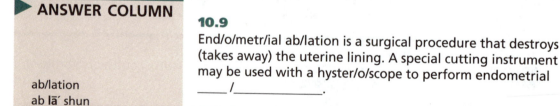

ANSWER COLUMN	
	10.9 End/o/metr/ial ab/lation is a surgical procedure that destroys (takes away) the uterine lining. A special cutting instrument may be used with a hyster/o/scope to perform endometrial
ab/lation ab lā′ shun	_____ /_____.
	10.10 These gynecologic procedures get pretty technical for the nonsurgeon, but remember, the part of the term ablation that means something is taken away is _____.
ab	

ANSWER COLUMN	
from	**10.11** de- is another prefix that means _____.
down from	**10.12** One who de/scends the stairs comes down from a higher level. A de/scend/ing nerve tract comes *_____ the brain.
de/cid/uous dē **sij**′ ōō əs	**10.13** De/ciduous leaves fall from a tree. "Baby teeth" that fall from a child's mouth are called _____ /_____ /_____ teeth.
deciduous	**10.14** There are thirty-two secondary (permanent) and twenty primary (_____) teeth.
from	**10.15** When water is taken from a substance, the substance is less than it was. De/hydr/ation takes water _____ something.
de/hydr/ation dē hī **drā**′ shən	**10.16** When water is taken from plums to make prunes, de/hydr/ation occurs. When water is taken from a cell, _____ /_____ /_____ also occurs.
de/hydr/ated dē **hī**′ drā tid	**10.17** When something is dehydrated, it has less water than it did before. When water is lost from the body due to excessive vomiting or diarrhea, the patient is _____ /_____ /_____.
dehydration	**10.18** Vomiting can cause dehydration. A high fever can also cause _____.
de/calci/fication dē kal′ si fi **kā**′ shən	**10.19** When calcium is removed from the bones, there is less calcium than before. This process is called _____ /_____ /_____.
decalcification	**10.20** De/calci/fication can occur from many causes. When a pregnant woman does not eat enough calcium for the growing baby, her own bones will be robbed of calcium, and _____ will occur.
decalcification	**10.21** Because vitamin D helps control calcium metabolism, inadequate vitamin D in the diet can account for some _____.

ANSWER COLUMN	
	10.22 Oste/o/por/osis may occur in postmenopausal women due to
decalcification	_____ of the bones.
	10.23
out from	ex- also means from, but in the sense of *_____.
	10.24
out ex/cis/ed ek **sīz′** d	To ex/cise is to cut _____ and remove a part. A diseased gallbladder may be _____ /_____ /_____.
	10.25
from	To ex/hale (ex/pire) is to breathe out waste matter _____ the body.
	10.26
ex/cretion eks **krē′** shən	Ex/cretion is the process of ex/pelling (or getting out from the body) a substance. Expelling urine is urinary _____ /_____.
	10.27
excretion excretion	Expelling carbon dioxide is respiratory _____. Expelling sweat is dermal _____.
	10.28
excretion excretion	Expelling menses is menstrual _____. Expelling fecal matter is gastrointestinal (GI) _____.
✓ SPELL CHECK	**10.29** Excretions are usually waste substances. Secretions, such as hormones, are useful substances, so, do not use them as synonyms. You may think "exit—out," "keep the secret—in."
	10.30
ex/traction eks **trak′** shən	An ex/traction is a procedure in which something is pulled out. When all of a patient's teeth have to be pulled out, it is called a full-mouth _____ /_____ (FME).
	10.31
ex/tends eks **tendz′**	Recall the word flexion, meaning to bend or shorten. The opposite of flexion is ex/tension, meaning to straighten or lengthen. Bending flexes the arm. Straightening _____ /_____ the arm.
	10.32
ex/tension eks **ten′** shun	Contracting the biceps muscle of the upper arm causes flex/ion of the arm. Relaxing this muscle causes _____ /_____.

Extension   Flexion

ANSWER COLUMN	
	10.33 Try to work this summary frame without referring to page 320. Give the prefix meaning from in the following sense:
ab- ex- de-	away from _____; out from _____; down from or from, resulting in less than _____.
	10.34 **narc/o** is the combining form for sleep. A narc/o/tic is a drug that produces sleep. Opium produces stuporous sleep. Opium is a
narc/o/tic när **kot´** ik	_____ /_____ /_____.
	10.35 A narcotic produces pain relief as well as numbness, or stuporous sleep. A narcotic should be used only when advised by a physician. Codeine produces pain relief and sleep. Codeine is a
narcotic	_____.
🏛 **WORD ORIGINS**	**10.36** Morpheus was the Greek god of dreams. Morphine is a narcotic derived from opium poppies and produces a dreamlike state as well as analgesia.
	10.37 Morphine is used as a pain reliever (analgesic) and is also a
narcotic	_____.
	10.38 Because narcotics can also cause addiction, a physician must have a narcotic license in order to dispense or write orders for _____ (plural).
narcotics	
narc/osis när **kō´** sis	**10.39** The condition induced by narcotics is called _____ /_____.

▶ **ANSWER COLUMN**

TAKE A CLOSER LOOK

10.40
Epilepsia is a Greek word meaning to seize upon. In the past epilepsy was classified by types of seizures described as petit mal and grand mal. Today epilepsy is described by the area of the brain involved and divided into two categories including partial and general. Medical and new surgical therapies are used in treatment of seizure disorders called _____.

epilepsy
ep´ i lep sē

10.41
-lepsy is used in words to mean seizure. Narc/o/lepsy means seizure or attacks of sleep. A person who is absolutely unable to stay awake suffers from _____ /_____ /_____.

narc/o/lepsy
när´ kō lep sē

10.42
Narcolepsy is a type of sleep disorder. A person may fall sound asleep standing at a bus stop. This is _____.

narcolepsy

10.43
A cerebroma, cerebral arteriosclerosis, and paresis are some causes of sleep seizures, which are called _____.

narcolepsy

10.44
You may get "tired" of hearing this, but **narc/o** any place in a word makes you think of *_____
_____.

sleep, stupor, or
stuporous sleep

10.45
iso- is used in words to mean equal or the same. Something that is iso/metr/ic is of _____ dimensions.

equal

10.46
Something that is iso/cellular is composed of cells of _____ size.

equal

10.47
An isotonic solution has the same osmotic pressure as red blood cells. Normal saline is an _____ /_____ /_____ solution.

iso/ton/ic
ī sō **ton**´ ik

10.48
Intra/ven/ous glucose is another _____ solution.

isotonic

▶ ANSWER COLUMN	**10.49** Any solution that will not destroy red blood cells because it is of equal osmotic pressure is an _____ solution.
isotonic	

higher lower same or equal	**10.50** Hyper/tonic solutions have a _____ osmotic pressure than blood cells, hypo/tonic solutions have a _____ osmotic pressure than blood cells, and iso/tonic solutions have the _____ osmotic pressure as blood cells. Good try!

℮ eee *TAKE A CLOSER LOOK*	**10.51** Many physiologic processes rely on the movement of fluids and substances in and out of the cells and bloodstream. Look up diffusion, osmosis, and filtration in your dictionary or medical text and read about how each causes movement of substances. You may think it would be nice if we could learn through osmosis just by holding this book.

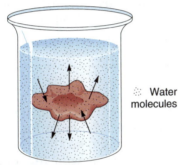 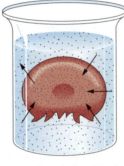 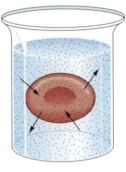

⠿ Water molecules

Hypertonic solution (sea-water) a red blood cell will shrink and wrinkle up because water molecules are moving out of the cell.

Hypotonic solution (fresh-water) a red blood cell will swell and burst because water molecules are moving into the cell.

Isotonic solution (human blood serum) a red blood cell remains unchanged, because the movement of water molecules into and out of the cell are the same.

Movement of water molecules in solutions of different osmolaties

iso/dactyl/ism
ī sō **dak**´ til izm
iso/therm/al (ic)
ī sō **thûr**´ məl (ik)
	10.52
	Build words meaning
	    fingers or toes of equal length
	    _____ /_____ /ism;
	    pertaining to equal temperature
	    _____ /_____ /____.

an/iso aniso	**10.53** iso- is a prefix for equal. an- is a prefix meaning without or lack of. Something that is without equality is unequal. The combining form for unequal is _____ /_____ or _____.

ANSWER COLUMN	
	10.54 Aniso/mastia means that a woman's breasts are of
unequal	_____ size.
	10.55 *Mastos* (or *mazos*) is the Greek word for breast. Inflammation of the breast is mast/itis. Surgical excision of part or all of the breast
mast/ectomy mast **ek**′ tōm ē	is a _____ /_____.
	10.56 Radical and simple are two main types of surgery for excising
mastectomy	diseased breast tissue or _____.
	10.57 Build a term that means a cancerous tumor of the breast:
mast/o/carcin/oma mast′ ō kär sin **ō**′ mə	_____ /____ /_____ /_____. See the case study on mastectomy at the end of this unit.
🏛 *WORD ORIGINS*	**10.58** A legendary tribe of women warriors in Asia Minor were known to have removed one breast so that they could more powerfully draw their bows. They were named the Amazons, meaning without a breast (a, *without*; mazos, *breast*). In the 1500s, a Spanish explorer named a river the Amazon after doing battle with a South American tribe that included its women in the fight.
aniso/cyt/osis an ī′ sō sī **tō**′ sis	**10.59** Aniso/cyt/osis means that cells are of unequal sizes. This word is commonly limited to red blood cells in medical usage. A word indicating a condition of inequality in cell size is _____ /_____ /_____.
anisocytosis	**10.60** Normal red blood cells are the same size (7.2 μm). An abnormal condition resulting in unequal size of red blood cells is _____.
anisocytosis	**10.61** Red blood cells are formed in the bone marrow. An unhealthy bone marrow can result in unequal red blood cells, or _____.

ANSWER COLUMN	Use the following information to work Frames 10.62–10.87. This is another group of prefixes of place.

Prefix	Meaning	Differentiation
dia-	through, complete	used with the combining forms for medical terminology
per-	through	prefix from Latin used more often in ordinary English
peri-	around	prefix from Greek used with the combining forms for medical terminology
circum-	around	Latin prefix used more often in ordinary English

---

around the tonsil

10.62
Peri/articular means around articulations or joints. Peri/tonsill/ar means *_____.
(Refer back to Frames 9.59–9.62.)

---

around the colon or pertaining to around the colon

10.63
Peri/col/ic means *_____
_____.

---

peri/chondr/al
per i **kon**´ drəl
peri/odont/al
per i ō **don**´ təl

10.64
Peri/odont/al means pertaining to diseases of the support structures around (peri-) the teeth (odont/o). A word that means around a cartilage is _____ /_____ /_____. Gum disease may require _____ /_____ /_____ surgery.

---

peri/aden/itis
per´ i ad en ī´ tis
peri/colp/itis
per´ i kol **pī**´ tis
peri/hepat/itis
per´ i hep ə **tī**´ tis
peri/cardi/ectomy
per´ i kär´dē **ek**´ tō mē

10.65
Build words meaning
  inflammation around a gland
  _____ /_____ /_____;
  inflammation around the vagina
  _____ /_____ /_____;
  inflammation around the liver
  _____ /_____ /_____;
  excision of tissue (pericardium) around the heart
  _____ /_____ /_____.

---

circum-

10.66
Another prefix that means around is _____.

ANSWER COLUMN

around

10.67
Circum/ocular means _____ the eyes.

around

10.68
Circum/or/al means _____ the mouth.

circum/scribed
sûr′ kəm skrīb′d

10.69
Circumscribed means limited in space (as though a line were drawn around it). A hive is limited in space—does not spread. A hive may be called a _____ / _____ wheal.

SURFACE LESIONS

A.
Papule:
    Solid, elevated lesion less than 0.5 cm in diameter
Example:
    Warts, elevated nevi

B.
Macule:
    Localized changes in skin color of less than 1 cm in diameter
Example:
    Freckle

C.
Wheal:
    Localized edema in the epidermis causing irregular elevation that may be red or pale
Example:
    Insect bite or a hive

D.
Crust:
    Dried serum, blood, or pus on the surface of the skin
Example:
    Impetigo

FLUID FILLED

E.
Boil (Furuncle):
    Skin infection originating in gland or hair follicle
Example:
    Furunculosis

F.
Bullae:
    Same as a vesicle only greater than 0.5 cm
Example:
    Contact dermatitis, large second-degree burns, bulbous impetigo, pemphigus

G.
Pustule:
    Vesicles or bullae that become filled with pus, usually described as less than 0.5 cm in diameter
Example:
    Acne, impetigo, furuncles, carbuncles, folliculitis

H.
Cyst:
    Encapsulated fluid-filled or a semi-solid mass in the subcutaneous tissue or dermis
Example:
    Sebaceous cyst, epidermoid cyst

Lesions

ANSWER COLUMN	
circumscribed	**10.70** A boil is also limited in the space it covers. A boil is a _____ lesion.
circumscribed	**10.71** Pimples and pustules are also _____ lesions.
circum/duction sûr kəm **duk´** shən	**10.72** Moving toward is ad/duction. Moving away is ab/duction. Moving around (circular motion) is _____ /_____.

Circumduction

to cut around (actually a surgical procedure for removing the foreskin of the penis)	**10.73** From the word parts you have already learned, think of the meaning for the following term and write it below: circum/cision *_____ _____.
circum/cision sûr´ kum si shun	**10.74** The pediatrician performed a _____ /_____ on the new baby boy soon after birth.
dia	**10.75** There are two prefixes that mean through. The one that you would expect to use more often in medical terminology is _____.
through through	**10.76** You have already learned dia/gnosis, which means knowing _____, and dia/thermy, which means heating _____.

ANSWER COLUMN	
	10.77 Build words meaning flowing through _____ /_____; pertaining to heating through _____ /_____ /_____.
dia/rrhea dia/therm/al, /ic (You pronounce)	
Thinking Frame dia/phor/esis dī ə fôr ē´ sis	**10.78** **-esis** is a suffix meaning action or process. Dia/phor/esis is an action of profuse sweating. Diaphoretic is the adjectival form. Can you think of the reason for using **dia-** as the prefix in these terms?
di/ur/esis dī yōōr ē´ sis	**10.79** Arthr/o/desis is the action of immobilizing (binding) a joint. Hemat/o/poi/esis is the process of forming blood. The process of causing urine to flow through more rapidly is ____ /____ /_____. **NOTE:** In the term diuretic the dia is shortened to di and still means through.
di/ur/etic dī yōōr ē´ tik	**10.80** A substance that causes increase in urine output (water excretion) is called a ____ /____ /_____.
nighttime bed wetting	**10.81** From what you have just learned in the past few frames decipher and recall the meaning of this condition: noct/urnal en/ur/esis * _____.
through	**10.82** Per/for/ation (noun) means puncturing _____.
through	**10.83** To per/for/ate (verb) means to puncture or make a hole _____.
per/for/ated **per´** fōr ā t'd	**10.84** The past tense of per/for/ate is per/for/ated. A _____ /_____ /_____ (past tense) ulcer is one that has eaten through the stomach.
per/for/ate **per´** fōr āt	**10.85** Ulcers can also _____ /_____ /_____ (present tense) the duodenum.

ANSWER COLUMN

per/for/ation
per fōr ā′ shən

per/cussion
per **kush**′ ən

10.86
When ulcers perforate an organ, a _____ /_____ /ation (noun) is formed.

10.87
Percussion (noun) means a striking through. Read the section on percussion in a dictionary. Analyze the word here:
_____ /_____.

NOTE: A drum is a percussion instrument.

1. stethoscope
2. penlight
3. guaiac/occult blood test developer
4. guaiac/occult blood test
5. flexible tape measure
6. urine specimen container
7. metal nasal speculum
8. tuning fork
9. percussion hammer
10. tongue depressor
11. ophthalmoscope head
12. okastic ear/nose speculum
13. otoscope head attached to base handle
14. sphygmomanometer
15. latex gloves

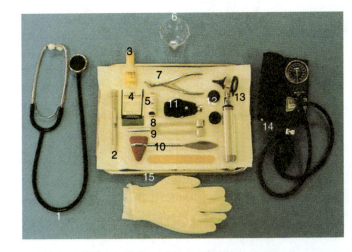

A. Instruments and supplies used in the physical examination for auscultation, percussion, inspection, and palpation

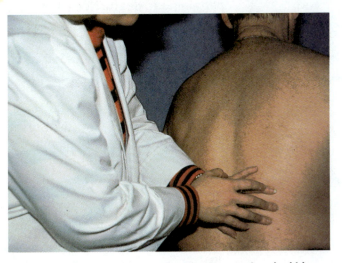

B. The examiner uses blunt percussion to examine the kidney.

ANSWER COLUMN	
	10.88 Supplying tissues with oxygen and nutrients through the blood supply or other tissue fluids is called perfusion. The passage of blood through the arteries of the heart is called coronary _____ /_____.
per/fusion per **fyoo**′ shun	
per/fuse per **fyooz**′	**10.89** A perfusate is a fluid used to _____ /_____ (verb form) tissues.
per dia circum peri	**10.90** Summarize: Two prefixes meaning through are _____ and _____. Two prefixes meaning around are _____ and _____.
through the skin across the lumen vessel repair	**10.91** Look up the following terms in your dictionary. Notice that medical specialists use the word-building system to name new procedures. Write the meaning of each term. per/cutaneous *_____; trans/luminal *_____; angi/o/plasty *_____. Abbreviation: PTA.
death	**10.92** *Necros* is a Greek word meaning corpse. **necr/o** is used in words pertaining to death. Necr/o/cyt/osis is cellular _____.
dead	**10.93** A necr/o/parasite is one that lives on _____ organic matter.
necr/osis ne **kro**′ sis	**10.94** Necr/osis refers to a condition in which dead tissue is surrounded with healthy tissue. Certain diseases can cause _____ /_____ of the bones.
necrosis	**10.95** When blood supply is cut off from an arm, gangrene sets in. This results in _____ (death) of the arm tissue.
necrosis	**10.96** When gangrene occurs anywhere in the body, _____ is seen.

ANSWER COLUMN	

10.97
Build words meaning
   excision of dead tissue
   _____ /_____;
   incision into (dissection of) a dead body
   _____ /_____ /_____;
   abnormal fear of death
   _____ /_____ /_____.

necr/ectomy
ne **krek**´ tō mē
necr/o/tomy
ne **krot**´ ō mē
necr/o/phobia
ne krō **fōb**´ ē ə

10.98
There are three ways of saying postmortem (after death) examination. One is aut/o/psy. The other is _____ /_____ /psy and another is necr/o/scopy.

necr/o/psy
nek´ rop sē

10.99
If the cause of death is unknown, an _____ /_____ /_____ may be required to examine the body.

aut/o/psy or
aw´ top sē
necropsy or
postmortem exam or
necr/o/scopy
ne **kros**´ kō pē

10.100
Cyan/o/tic is the adjectival form of cyanosis. Build the adjectival form of necrosis: _____ /_____ /_____

necr/o/tic
ne **kro**´ tik

10.101
De/bride/ment (dā brēd´ **mən**´) of dead tissue is often done for patients with severe burns. The _____ /_____ /_____ (dead) tissue is removed.

necr/o/tic
nek **rot**´ ik

INFORMATION FRAME

10.102
-philia is the opposite of -phobia. -phobia is abnormal fear of; -philia is abnormal or unusual attraction to.

10.103
Necr/o/phobia is an abnormal fear of dead bodies. Necr/o/philia is
*_____.

abnormal attraction to dead bodies

10.104
Words that can end in -phobia, can end in -philia.
Morbid fear of water is
_____ /_____.
Strong attraction to water is
_____ /_____.

hydro/phobia
(You pronounce)
hydro/philia
hī drō **fil**´ ē ə

ANSWER COLUMN

hemat/o/philia
pyr/o/philia
aer/o/philia
aut/o/philia
(You pronounce)

10.105
Think of the meaning while building words opposite to:
hemat/o/phobia _____ /_____ /_____ ;
pyr/o/phobia _____ /_____ /_____ ;
aer/o/phobia _____ /_____ /_____ ;
aut/o/phobia _____ /_____ /_____ .

attraction to, liking, loving

10.106
phil/o is the combining form that means
* _____ .

philosopher, philosophy,
Philadelphia, etc.

10.107
Can you think of a nonmedical word that involves **phil/o**? If so,
write it here: _____ .

Abbreviation	Meaning
ab I, II, III, AB	abortion (number of)
bid	twice a day
Ca	calcium
D/W	dextrose in water
Dx	diagnosis
exc	excision
FME	full-mouth extraction
hs	hour of sleep (at bedtime)
NS	normal saline (isotonic)
PTCA	percutaneous transluminal coronary angioplasty
PCA	percutaneous coronary angioplasty
q2h, q4h	every two hours, every four hours
qid	four times a day
tid	three times a day
μm	micrometer (0.000001 m)
†	death symbol

To complete your study of this unit, work the review activities on the next pages. Also, listen to the audiotapes that accompany *Medical Terminology: A Programmed Text,* 8th edition, and practice your pronunciation.

Additional practice exercises for this unit are available on the Student Practice disk found in the back of the textbook.

▶ REVIEW ACTIVITIES

Write the prefix that represents the direction, then build a word using that prefix.

Prefix   *Word*

_____ 1. away from   move away from
                               the body   _____

_____ 2. down from   part of the aorta
                               that moves down
                               from the heart   _____

_____ 3. out of   to cut out   _____

_____ 4. equal/same   equal osmotic
                               pressure (solution)   _____

_____ 5. unequal   condition of unequal
                               sized cells   _____

_____ 6. through   treatment by heating
                               through tissues   _____

_____ 7. through   to strike through
                               (part of physical
                               examination)   _____

_____ 8. around   membrane around
                               the heart   _____

_____ 9. around   circular motion   _____

_____ 10. under   below the tongue   _____

▶ REVIEW ACTIVITIES

Select and Construct
Select the correct word parts from the list below and construct medical terms that represent the given meaning.

a(b)	aden	a(n)	aniso	a/t/ion	blat	bort
brade	bras	calcific	carcin	cardium	circum	cision
coction	cre(t)	cussion	cyt	de	dia	duct
ecto	ex	fusion	hale	hepat	hydr	irritant
iso	itis	lact	lation	lepsy	mast/o	narco
oma	osis	per	peri	rade	tic	tion
tonic						

1. removal of waste from the body   _____

2. to take away the products of
    conception   _____

3. sleep attacks (seizures)   _____

4. cancer of the breast   _____

5. take away skin by scraping (verb)   _____

6. inflammation around the liver   _____

7. drug that produces sleep   _____

8. process of taking calcium from bone   _____

9. IV solutions are _____
    compared to blood cells   _____

10. process of cutting around (usually the
    foreskin for removal)   _____

11. take away tissue (i.e., endometrial
    _____)   _____

12. striking through (i.e., hammer)   _____

13. condition of cells of unequal size   _____

14. taking the baby away from the breast
    (weaning)   _____

15. condition of water taken away from
    the body   _____

16. process of supplying blood through
    tissue   _____

Now, build some other terms.

17. _____   _____
        word   meaning

18. _____   _____
        word   meaning

19. _____   _____
        word   meaning

20. _____   _____
        word   meaning

▶ **REVIEW ACTIVITIES**

Define and Dissect
Give a brief definition and dissect each term listed into its word parts in the space provided on the right. Check your answers by referring to the frame listed in parentheses and your medical dictionary. Then, listen to the audiotapes to practice pronunciation.

1. aberrant (10.3)

    _____ / _____
    pre   rt/suffix

    _____
    definition

2. ablactation (10.4)

    _____ / _____ / _____
    pre   rt   suffix

3. abrasion (10.8)

    _____ / _____
    pre   rt/suffix

4. deciduous (10.13)

    _____ / _____
    pre   rt/suffix

5. dehydrated (10.17)

    _____ / _____ / _____
    pre   rt   suffix

6. decalcification (10.19)

    _____ / _____ / _____
    pre   rt   suffix

7. excised (10.24)

    _____ / _____ / _____
    pre   rt   suffix

8. narcosis (10.39)

    _____ / _____
    rt   suffix

9. anisocytosis (10.59)

    _____ / _____ / _____
    pre   rt   suffix

10. mastectomy (10.55)

    _____ / _____
    rt   suffix

11. periodontal (10.64)

    _____ / _____ / _____
    pre   rt   suffix

12. circumscribed (10.69)

    _____ / _____
    pre   rt/suffix

▶ REVIEW ACTIVITIES

13. perforated (10.84)

_____ / _____ / _____
   pre   rt   suffix

_____

14. diaphoresis (10.78)

_____ / _____ / _____
   pre   rt   suffix

_____

15. percutaneous (10.91)

_____ / _____ / _____
   pre   rt   suffix

_____

16. necrotic (10.100)

_____ / _____ / _____
   rt   v   suffix

_____

17. necrophobia (10.97)

_____ / _____ / _____
   rt   v   suffix

_____

18. circumcision (10.73)

_____ / _____
   pre   rt/suffix

_____

19. extension (10.32)

_____ / _____
   pre   rt/suffix

_____

20. flexion (10.32)

_____ / _____
   rt   suffix

_____

21. diuresis (10.79)

_____ / _____ / _____
   pre   rt   suffix

_____

22. enuresis (10.81)

_____ / _____ / _____
   pre   rt   suffix

_____

23. percussion (10.87)

_____ / _____
   pre   rt/suffix

_____

24. pericardiectomy (10.65)

_____ / _____ / _____
   pre   rt   suffix

_____

25. ablation (10.9)

_____ / _____
   pre   rt/suffix

_____

26. perfuse (10.89)

_____ / _____
   pre   rt/suffix

_____

▶ REVIEW ACTIVITIES

Abbreviation Matching
Match the following abbreviations with their definition.

_____ 1. bid

_____ 2. q2h

_____ 3. PTA

_____ 4. exc

_____ 5. hs

_____ 6. Ca

_____ 7. tid

_____ 8. μm

a. every night
b. micrometer
c. three times a day
d. normal saline
e. parent teacher agency
f. at bedtime
g. twice a day
h. every two hours
i. excision
j. calcium
k. full-mouth extraction
l. dextrose in water
m. percutaneous transluminal angioplasty
n. millimeter

Abbreviation Fill-ins
Fill in the blank with the correct abbreviation.

9.   every four hours _____

10. dextrose in water _____

11. normal saline _____

12. four times a day _____

13. death (symbol) _____

14. diagnosis _____

▶ **CASE STUDIES**

Write the term next to its meaning given below. Then, draw slashes to analyze the word parts. Note the use of medical abbreviations. Look these up in your dictionary or find them in Appendix B. If you have any questions about the answers, refer to your medical dictionary or check with your instructor for the answers in Appendix A.

CASE STUDY 10-1
MASTECTOMY

Pt: 50-year-old female   Surgeon: Sharon Rooney-Gandy D.O.

Preoperative Dx: **Multifocal** ductal **carcinoma in situ** left breast
Postoperative Dx: Multifocal ductal carcinoma in situ left breast, pathology pending
Operation performed: Left simple **mastectomy**

Pathology: The patient was noted to have calcifications on routine **mammogram**. She does not practice breast self-exam and did not feel any lumps herself. Upon needle localization left breast **biopsy** she was found to have multifocal ductal carcinoma in situ, non-comedo type with tumor extending to margin of excision and **microcalcifications**. *Hx:* Grav 0, Para, AB 0, and is in menopause with history of ependymoma and radiation of her spine, paternal grandmother with bilateral breast cancer, paternal aunt with bilateral breast cancer. Physical examination of the right breast revealed essentially unremarkable. The left breast revealed a well healed upper medial quadrant curvilinear incision from previous biopsy. There was no **retraction**, discharge, masses, or **axillary** nodes. After biopsy she was evaluated by an oncologist for treatment of carcinoma in situ. Dr. Peter, radiation oncologist, evaluated her for radiation therapy. It was felt best that the patient undergo simple mastectomy, not so much because of previous radiation therapy, but because of the residual multicalcifications remaining in her left breast. The patient did understand this and also because of her small breasts, cosmetically we thought she would be best treated with a left simple mastectomy. The patient tolerated the procedure well and was taken to the recovery room in satisfactory condition.

Procedure: The patient was taken to the operating room, given general **anesthesia**, prepped and draped in a **sterile** manner. Elliptical incisions were made in a horizontal fashion incorporating the previous biopsy site. The skin was incised and minor bleeding controlled using Bovie cautery. The breast tissue was **dissected** down to the pectoral fascia up to the clavicle, elevating the superior skin flap. The lower skin flap was developed using Bovie cautery down to the pectoral fascia. The breast was excised using Bovie cautery, **hemostasis** secured with Bovie cautery. The incision was irrigated with saline. No other masses or axillary masses could be palpated. The skin was closed with interrupted 4-0 Vicryl followed by a continuous **subcuticular** 4-0 Prolene. Prior to closing the skin a JP drain was placed through a separate stab incision. Steri-strips were applied and the drain was sutured in place. A sterile pressure dressing was applied. Postoperative condition was stable. The case was clean and elective.

1. pertaining to below the epidermis   _____
2. condition creating no sensation   _____
3. having more than one focus (location)   _____
4. type of cancer in one location   _____
5. was cut apart   _____
6. area under the arm   _____
7. control of blood flow   _____
8. excision of the breast   _____
9. breast x-ray   _____
10. absence of organisms   _____
11. pulling and holding back   _____
12. small calcium deposits   _____
13. examination of living tissue   _____

► CROSSWORD PUZZLE

Check your answers by going back through the frames or checking the solutions in Appendix C.

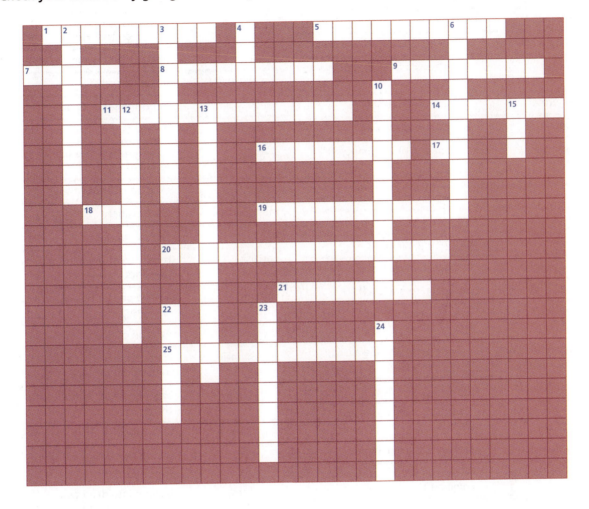

Across

1. make a hole in (verb)
5. seizures of sleep
7. combining form for dead
8. teeth that fall out (primary)
9. agent that causes diuresis
11. encircled
14. synonym for necropsy
16. seizure disorder
17. hour of sleep, at bedtime (abbreviation)
18. excision (abbreviation)
19. water loss (noun)
20. excision of the pericardium
21. wandering from the norm
25. loves blood

Down

2. waste removal
3. movement away from the midline
4. twice a day (abbreviation)
6. striking to examine
10. different size breasts
12. same size digits
13. breast cancer
15. percutaneous transluminal angioplasty (abbreviation)
22. breathe out
23. termination of pregnancy
24. sleeping drug

► GLOSSARY

abduction	movement away from the midline
aberrant	wandering away from the norm
ablactation	weaning a baby from the breast
ablation	takes away a layer or destroys a tissue layer
abnormal	unusual (not normal)
aboral	away from the mouth
abortion	termination of pregnancy
abrasion	scraping
adduction	movement toward the midline
aerophilia	attraction to air
anisocytosis	cells of unequal sizes
anisomastia	breasts of unequal size
autophilia	attraction to one's self
autopsy	necropsy, postmortem examination
circumduction	moving as to describe a circle with a body part
circumocular	encircling the eye
circumscribed	encircling or in the shape of a circle
decalcification	calcium loss (from bone)
deciduous	falls down (primary teeth that come out)
dehydration	water loss
descending	moving downward
diaphoresis	profuse sweating
diuresis	increase in urine output
diuretic	agent that causes diuresis
epilepsy	disorder characterized by seizures
excision	removing a body part
excretion	removal of waste (urination, defecation)
exhale	breathe out (expire)
extension	to straighten or lengthen a body part
extraction	removal or pulling out of a body part
flexion	to shorten or bend a body part
hematophilia	attraction to blood
hydrophilia	attraction to water
hydrophobia	fear of water (symptom of rabies)
isocellular	equal size cells
isodactylism	digits the same length
isometric	measures the same on all sides
isotonic	osmotic pressure equal to the inside of a cell
mastectomy	excision of breast tissue
mastocarcinoma	breast cancer
narcolepsy	seizures of sleep
narcosis	condition of sleep induced by narcotics
narcotic	a sleep producing agent (also an analgesic)
necrectomy	excision of dead tissue
necrocytosis	condition of cell death or decomposition
necroparasite	organism that lives off dead tissue
necrophobia	abnormal fear of dead bodies
necrotic	pertaining to necrosis (condition of dead tissue)
necrotomy	incision into dead tissue
nocturnal enuresis	bedwetting
percussion	striking or tapping
percutaneous	through the skin
perforation	puncturing
periarticular	area surrounding a joint
pericardiectomy	excision of the membrane around the heart
perihepatitis	inflammation around the liver
pericolic	area surrounding the colon
peritonsillar	area surrounding the tonsils
pyrophilia	attraction to fire
transluminal	across the lumen

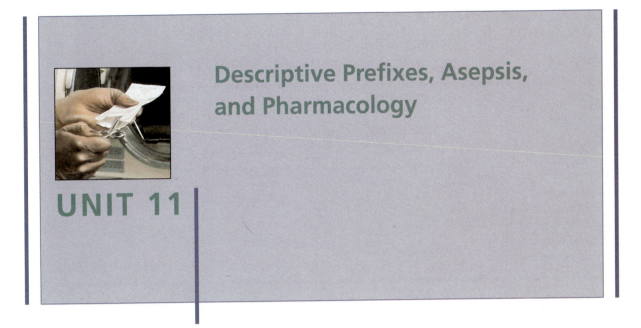

Descriptive Prefixes, Asepsis, and Pharmacology

UNIT 11

ANSWER COLUMN	
same gland	**11.1** homo- means same. Homo/genized milk has the same amount of cream throughout. Homo/gland/ular means pertaining to the *_____.
same	**11.2** Homo/therm/al means having the _____ body temperature all the time (i.e., 98.6°F).
same	**11.3** Homo/later/al means pertaining to the _____ side.
homo/sex/ual hō′ mō **sek**′ shōō əl	**11.4** Homo/sex/ual means being attracted to the same sex. When men are attracted to men much more than to women, they are said to be _____ /_____ /_____.
homosexual	**11.5** When women are attracted to women rather than to men, they too are called _____.
different different	**11.6** hetero- is the opposite of homo-. hetero- means _____. Heter/opia (het ûr ō′ pē ə) means _____ vision in each eye.

ANSWER COLUMN	
different	**11.7** Hetero/sex/ual means being attracted to a _____ sex.

homo/gen/eous
hō′ mō **jē**′ nē us
pertaining to the same
  throughout
hetero/gen/eous
het′ ûr ō **jē**′ nē us
pertaining to different
  throughout
	11.8
	Look up the meanings of homogeneous and heterogeneous. Draw the slashes and write the definitions below:
	
	* _____ ,
	   _____ ;
	* _____ ,
	   _____ .

hetero/gen/esis
het′ ûr ō **jen**′ ə sis
hetero/sex/ual
het′ ûr ō **seks**′ ū əl
	11.9
	Open your dictionary and look up these terms while you think of their meanings. Form *opposites* of the following:
	      homo/gen/esis
	
	      _____ / _____ / _____ ;
	      homo/sex/ual
	
	      _____ / _____ / _____ .

anterior
iso
hyper
adduction
	11.10
	Think of their meanings while you recall these or other opposites:
	      posterior _____ ;
	      aniso- (prefix) _____ ;
	      hypo- (prefix) _____ ;
	      abduction _____ .

together or joined	**11.11** Good. Now you'll study syn- and sym-. They are different forms of the same prefix. syn- and sym- mean * _____ .
	11.12 Review: You have already learned syn- in the words syndactylism, synergetic, synarthrosis, and syndrome. (Review Frames 4.131–4.141.)
sym-	**11.13** syn- is the form of the prefix that is used to mean fixed or joined, except when it is followed by the sound of "b," "m," "f," "ph," or "p." Then, _____ is used. **EXAMPLES:** symbol, symphony, sympathy.

> **ANSWER COLUMN**

11.14
Sym/pathy is an ordinary word that has a special medical meaning. From either a medical or regular English dictionary, find what it takes to fill this blank: **sym-** + **path/os**, the Greek word for
_____.

suffering (medical) or
  feeling (standard)

11.15
blephar/o means eyelid. A sym/physis is a growing together of parts. Sym/blepharon means *_____
_____.

eyelids have grown
  together, or adhesions
  of the eyelids

11.16
pod/o is one combining form for foot. Build words meaning
lower extremities are grown together (united)
    _____ /pod/ia;
excision of a sympathetic nerve
    _____ /path/_____;
tumor of a sympathetic nerve
    _____ /_____ /_____.

sym/podia
sim **pō´** dē ə
sym/path/ectomy
sim pa **thek´** tō mē
sym/path/oma
sim path **ō´** mə

11.17
Find a fairly common word in your medical dictionary in which **sym-** is followed by m. (There are only two or three to choose from.) One is _____.

symmetry, symmetric, or
  symmetrical

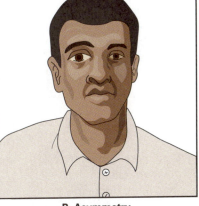

A. Symmetry   **B. Asymmetry**

► **ANSWER COLUMN**

11.18
Find a common word in your medical dictionary that is used in ordinary English in which sym- is followed by b:
*_____.

symbol or symbolism

11.19
syn- and sym- both mean together. sym- is used when followed by the sound of the letters _____, _____, _____, _____, and _____. syn- is used in other medical words.

b
m
p
f
ph

TAKE A CLOSER LOOK

11.20
super- and supra- are both prefixes that mean above or beyond. Analyze the following words in which super- and supra- are used. Write the meaning of the word as you analyze it. If necessary, consult a dictionary.

11.21
Draw the slashes as you write the following:

super/fici/al
super/cili/ary
super/infect/ion
super/ior/ity
super/leth/al
super/numer/ary

superficial _____;
superciliary _____;
superinfection _____;
superiority _____;
superlethal _____;
supernumerary _____.
Look up their meanings in your dictionary.

11.22
Draw the slashes as you write the following:

supra/lumb/ar
supra/pub/ic
supra/mammary
supra/ren/al
supra/inguin/al
supra/ren/o/pathy

supralumbar _____;
suprapubic _____;
supramammary _____;
suprarenal _____;
suprainguinal _____;
suprarenopathy _____.
Look up their meanings.

11.23
Draw a conclusion about super- and supra- from your answer in the last two frames:
super- is *_____
_____.

supra- is *_____
_____.

used more frequently in modern English
used more frequently in straight medical words

a- and **an-** are prefixes that mean without or lack of. Examine the following list of words:

an/al/ges/ia	a/bi/o/tic
ana/phy/lax/is	a/blast/emic
an/emia	a/chol/ia
an/encephal/us	a/derm/a
an/esthesi/a	a/febrile
an/iso/cyt/osis	a/galact/ia
an/hidr/osis	a/kinesi/a
an/irid/ia	a/men/o/rrhea
an/onych/ia	a/phasia
an/orex/ia	a/pnea
an/ur/ia	a/seps/is
an/ur/esis	a/symmetry

11.24
Draw a conclusion.
Use **a-** if it is followed by a (choose one) _____ (vowel/consonant).

consonant

Use **an-** if it is followed by a (choose one) _____ (vowel/consonant).

vowel

More prefixes! Use this table to work Frames 11.25–11.61.

Prefix	Meaning	Special Comment
epi-	over, upon	epicenter of an earthquake
extra-	outside of, beyond, in addition to	extracurricular activities
infra-	below, under	almost always below a part of the body; almost always adjectival in form; there are fewer words beginning with infra- than with sub-
sub-	under, below	Many words of all kinds begin with sub-
meta-	beyond, after, occurring later in a series	also used with chemical names

Directional prefixes

ANSWER COLUMN	
	11.25
	epi- means upon or over. The epi/gastr/ic region is the region
over the stomach	*_____.
	11.26
	Epi/splen/itis means inflammation of the tissue
over the spleen	*_____.
	11.27
	Build words meaning
	inflammation of the area over the bladder
epi/cyst/itis	_____ / _____ / _____;
ep´ i sis **tī´** tis	inflammation (of the tissue) upon the kidney
epi/nephr/itis	_____ / _____ / _____.
ep´ i nef **rī´** tis	
	11.28
	Build words meaning
	excision of the tissue upon the kidney
epi/nephr/ectomy	_____ / _____ / _____;
ep´ i nef **rek´** tə mē	suture of the region over the stomach
epi/gastr/o/rrhaphy	_____ / _____ / ____ / _____.
ep´ i gas **trôr´** ə fē	
	11.29
	Build words meaning pertaining to
	(the tissue) upon the skin (outer most layer)
epi/derm/al	_____ / _____ / ____;
	(the tissue) covering the cranium
epi/crani/al	_____ / _____ / ____;
	the area above the stern/um
epi/stern/al	_____ / _____ / ____;
	the tissues upon the heart
epi/card/ium	_____ / _____ / _____.
(You pronounce)	

► ANSWER COLUMN

INFORMATION
FRAME

11.30
Didymos is another Greek word for testis. The epi/didymis is a small oblong body resting upon the testicle, containing convoluted tubules. The epididymis is involved in sperm production and transportation.

epi/didym/itis
ep´ i did i mī´ tis
epi/didym/ectomy
ep´ i did i mek´ tōm ē

11.31
Build words that mean
    inflammation of the epididymis
    _____ /_____ /_____;
    excision of the epididymis
    _____ /_____ /_____.

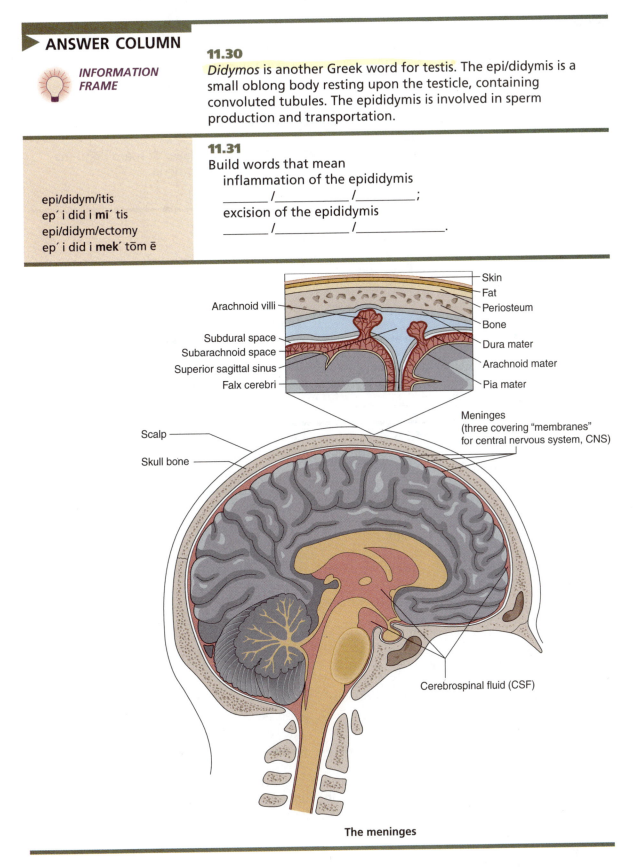

Skin
Fat
Periosteum
Bone
Dura mater
Arachnoid mater
Pia mater

Arachnoid villi

Subdural space
Subarachnoid space
Superior sagittal sinus
Falx cerebri

Meninges
(three covering "membranes"
for central nervous system, CNS)

Scalp

Skull bone

Cerebrospinal fluid (CSF)

The meninges

ANSWER COLUMN	
upon	**11.32** Recall your previous study of the meninges, the membranes that surround the brain and spinal cord. The dura (**dur**) mater is a layer of the meninges. The epi/dur/al layer is located _____ the dura.
epi/dur/al ep´ i **dur**´ əl	**11.33** Anesthetic can be administered in the layer or space upon the dura. This is _____ /_____ /_____ anesthesia.

sub/dur/al
sub **dur**´ əl
epi/dur/al
ep´ i **dur**´ əl
	11.34
	Using dur/al build words meaning
	  below the dura mater
	  _____ /_____ /_____ ;
	  upon the dura mater
	  _____ /_____ /_____ .

outside of or beyond	**11.35** **extra-** means outside or beyond. Think of extraterrestrial. Extra/nuclear (eks tra nōō´ klē är) means * _____ the nucleus of a cell.
outside of or beyond	**11.36** Extra/uterine is an adjective meaning * _____ the uterus.

extra-/articul/ar
eks´ trə är **tik**´ yə lər
extra/cyst/ic
eks´ trə **sis**´ tik
extra/dur/al
eks´ trə **dōōr**´ əl
extra/genit/al
eks´ trə **jen**´ i təl
extra/hepat/ic
eks´ trə hep **at**´ ik
extra/cerebr/al
eks´ trə ser **ē**´ brəl
	11.37
	Build words meaning outside of the
	  joint
	  _____ /_____ /____ ;
	  urinary bladder
	  _____ /_____ /____ ;
	  dura mater (meninges)
	  _____ /_____ /____ ;
	  genitals
	  _____ /_____ /____ ;
	  liver
	  _____ /_____ /____ ;
	  cerebrum
	  _____ /_____ /____ .

adjectives	**11.38** Look at the words in the last frame. Draw a conclusion. **extra-** is used as a prefix in words that are usually (choose one) _____ (nouns/adjectives).

▶ ANSWER COLUMN	
mamm/o/graphy mam **og**´ raf ē	**11.39** Recall that **mamm/o** is one combining form for breast. An x-ray picture of the breast is a mammogram. The process of taking this x-ray is called _____ /____ /_____.
both sides both breasts	**11.40** **bi-** means both or two. Whenever a procedure is performed on both sides, it is said to be bilateral. A bilateral hernia repair is on * _____. A bilateral mammogram is a radiograph of * _____.

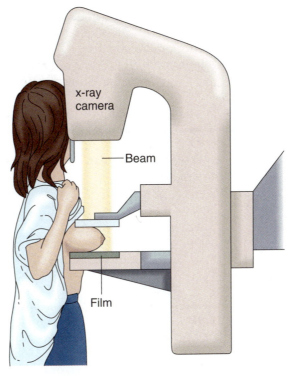

x-ray camera

Beam

Film

During a mammomgraphy, the breast is gently flattened and then radiographed.

| bi/later/al
bī **lat**´ er əl | **11.41**
In humans, since most body parts are in pairs, the opposite of unilateral is ____ /_____ /____. |
| below or under | **11.42**
infra- means below or under. Infra/mammary means
* _____ the mammary gland. |

ANSWER COLUMN	
below or under	**11.43** Infra/patell/ar means *_____ the patella (kneecap).
sub	**11.44** Below the tongue is _____ /lingual.
under or below under	**11.45** sub- is a prefix that means *_____. A sub/dural hematoma is a mass of clotted blood _____ the dura mater.
under below below	**11.46** Sub/abdominal means _____ the abdomen. **aur** from the Latin word *auris* is one word root for ear. Sub/aur/al means _____ the ear. Sub/cutaneous means _____ the skin.
sub/dur/al sub/aur/al sub/cutan/eous (You pronounce)	**11.47** Build words that mean below or under the dura mater _____ /_____ /_____; ear _____ /_____ /_____; skin _____ /_____ /_____.
under below	**11.48** The prefixes infra- and sub- are sometimes confusing in word building. For that reason, you will build words that can take either prefix. When you see sub- or infra-, you will think of _____ or _____.
infra/stern/al inˊ fra **stûrˊ** nəl sub/stern/al subˊ **stûrˊ** nəl supra/stern/al sooˊ pra **stûrˊ** nəl	**11.49** Using **stern/o**, build two words meaning below the sternum: _____ /_____ /al; _____ /_____ /_____. A word meaning above the sternum is supra/_____ /_____.

ANSWER COLUMN	

11.50
Using **cost/o**, build two words meaning under the ribs:

infra/cost/al
sub/cost/al
supra/cost/al
inter/cost/al
(You pronounce)

_____ /_____ /____ ;
_____ /_____ /____ .
A word meaning above the ribs is _____ /_____ /____ .
The _____ /_____ /____ muscles are between the ribs.

11.51
Using **pub/o**, build two words meaning under the pubis:

infra/pub/ic
sub/pub/ic
supra/pub/ic
(You pronounce)

_____ /_____ /____ ;
_____ /_____ /____ .
A word meaning above the pubis is _____ /_____ /____ .

INFORMATION FRAME

11.52
meta- is a prefix used in many ways. Look at the table on page 349 to discover its meanings.

11.53
Analyze the term metaphysics. It is the study of things

beyond the physical or
of the spirit

*_____ .

11.54
The bones of the hand that are beyond the carpals (wrist) are the

meta/carpals
me´ tə **kar´** palz

_____ /_____ .

11.55
The bones of the foot that are beyond the tarsals (ankle) are the

meta/tarsals
me´ tə **tar´** salz

_____ /_____ .

11.56
A meta/stasis occurs when a disease spreads beyond its point of origin. A meta/static (adjective) tumor is a secondary growth from a malignant tumor. This secondary growth is a

meta/stasis
me **tas´** tə sis
meta/stases
me **tas´** tə sēs

_____ /_____ (singular noun). The plural form of this word is _____ /_____ .

11.57
The area of the origin of cancer or the first discovered site in a patient is said to be the primary site. If a secondary site is found,

metastasis

it is a _____ .

▶ **ANSWER COLUMN**

ultra/violet ul′ tra **vi**′ ō let	**11.58** ultra- is a prefix meaning beyond or in excess. Light waves that are beyond the violet frequency are _____ /_____ (UV).
ultra/son/o/graphy ul′ tra son **og**′ raf ē	**11.59** Sound waves that are beyond the audible frequency are ultra/son/ic. The process of making an image using ultrasound (US) is called _____ /_____ /___ /_____ or sonography. See the case study at the end of this unit.
ultrasonography ultrasonography	**11.60** Ultra/sound may be used for therapy or for diagnostic testing. To detect gallstones in a diseased gallbladder, the sonographer uses diagnostic _____. To treat a patient with kidney stones, the sonographer uses therapeutic _____.
Do it	**11.61** You have now learned many prefixes of location. Review them by making a list, with their meaning plus anything special about them.

Professional Profiles ◀◀◀◀◀◀◀◀◀◀◀◀◀◀◀◀◀◀◀◀◀◀◀◀◀◀◀◀◀◀◀◀◀

Registered Diagnostic Medical Sonographers (RDMSs) are highly skilled allied health professionals who use ultrasound (high-frequency sound) to create images of organs and tissues that are displayed on a computerized monitor in real time and on still films (sonograms). Knowledge of sectional anatomy, pathology, computer technology, and medical ethics is essential. The American Registry of Diagnostic Medical Sonographers (ARDMS) determines educational requirements and criteria for registration of diagnostic medical sonographers.

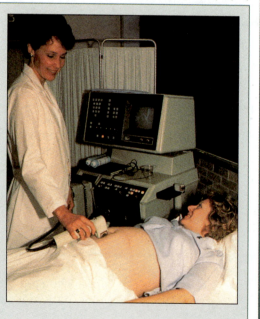

Sonographer performing fetal ultrasound (Courtesy of Jackson Community College, Jackson, MI)

02-FEB-90
02:23:28PM
L382| 28HZ
DEPTH= 100
OB

PWR =| -3dB
50dB |1/3/2
GAIN=| -6dB

HEAD   ←CHIN

EYE

17 WEEK FETUS

Fetal ultrasound (Prepared by Lynne Schreiber, BS, RDMS, RT[R])

ANSWER COLUMN

11.62
Recall that path/o/genic refers to disease production. Sepsis is a noun meaning a poisoned state or infection caused by absorption of pathogenic bacteria and their products into the bloodstream. A noun meaning a state without or lack of sepsis is

_____ /_____.

a/sepsis
ə **sep**′ sis, ā **sep**′ sis

11.63
Sept/ic is the adjectival form of sepsis. The adjectival form for the word meaning free from infection is _____ /_____ /_____.

a/sept/ic
ə **sep**′ tik, ā **sep**′ tik

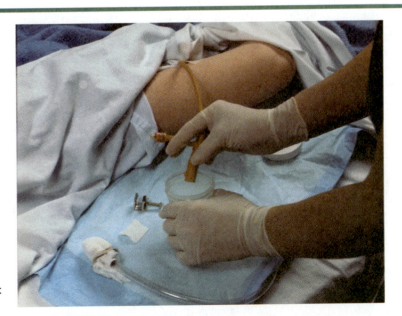

Catheterization requires strict asepsis

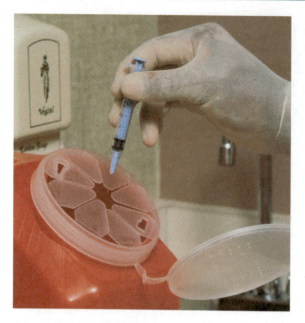

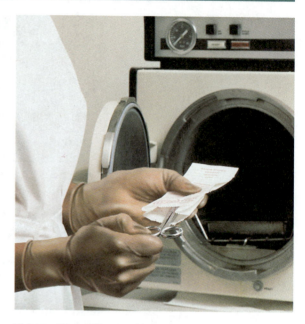

Proper disposal of contaminated needles and syringes in biohazard containers prevents accidental exposure to potentially infectious fluids

This medical assistant places an instrument into an envelope package for autoclaving

ANSWER COLUMN	
	11.64 Sept/i/cemia is an infection (poisoned state) in the bloodstream. Sept/o/py/emia means *_____ _____.
infection with pus in the bloodstream	
	11.65 Study the last two frames. A combining form for infection is _____ /____.
sept/o (used most) or seps/o	
	11.66 Review the material from Frames 11.62–11.65. Give words that mean noun for infection _____ /____; adjective for infected _____ /____; noun for state free from infection ____ /_____ /____; adjective for free from infection ____ /_____ /____.
seps/is sept/ic a/seps/is ā **sep´** sis a/sept/ic ā **sep´** tik	
	11.67 anti- is a prefix meaning against. An anti/pyretic is an agent that works _____ a fever. An anti/toxin is an agent that works _____ a toxin. A pyr/o/toxin is a _____ produced by fever (heat). **NOTE:** A toxin is a poisonous substance produced by an organism.
against against toxin	

ANSWER COLUMN

The following is a table listing categories of drugs that work against something:

Drug Category	Works Against
anti/arrhythmic	irregular heartbeats
anti/arthritic	arthritis
anti/biotic	bacteria
anti/cholinergic	parasympathetic impulses
anti/convulsive	seizures
anti/depressant	depression
anti/diarrheal	diarrhea
anti/emetic	vomiting
anti/fungal	fungi
anti/histamine	histamine (allergic reactions)
anti/hypertensive	high blood pressure
anti-/inflammatory	inflammation
anti/narcotic	narcotics
anti/neoplastic	tumors
anti/pruritic	dry skin (itching)
anti/septic	infective agents
anti/spasmodic	muscle spasms
anti/toxin	poisons (toxins)

against

11.68
An anti/narcotic is an agent that works ______________ narcotics.

against

11.69
An anti/biotic is an agent that works ______________ living bacterial infections.

anti/biotic
an´ ti bī **ot´** ik

11.70
Erythromycin is one type of ________/____________.

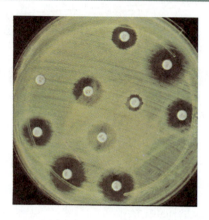

Antibiotic susceptibility test (C&S) plate

▶ **ANSWER COLUMN**

Confused about agents that fight pathogenic organisms? Study the following table:

AGENTS THAT FIGHT PATHOGENIC ORGANISMS

Antiseptics are agents that prevent sepsis by inhibiting growth of causative organisms. They may be inorganic, such as mercury and iodine preparations, or organic, such as carbolic acid (phenol) and alcohol.

Antibiotics are mostly prescription drugs that inhibit growth or destroy microorganisms, especially bacteria. Antibiotics can be used topically or taken internally for a systemic effect. Examples: penicillin, Keflex, erythromycin. Antibiotics can be bacteriocidal (kill bacteria) or bacteriostatic (inhibit growth, keep the numbers down).

Disinfectants are chemical or physical agents that prevent infection by killing microorganisms. They are used to clean equipment or surfaces rather than in or upon the body (i.e., Virex, bleach).

Sterilization is a process that kills organisms of all sorts. An autoclave uses pressure and steam and is the most effective form of sterilization. Chemical sterilization using disinfectants like bleach kills most organisms but not the ones that form spores.

11.71

Now, build words describing the agents that work against
   rheumatic disease

anti/rheumatic
an´ ti rōō ma´ tik

_____ /_____;

spastic muscle

anti/spasmodic
an´ ti spaz **mod**´ ik

_____ /_____;

toxins

anti/toxin
an´ ti **toks**´ in

_____ /_____.

11.72
Build adjectives describing the agents that work against
   convulsive states

anti/convulsive
an´ ti kon **vul**´ siv
_____ /_____;

arthritic diseases

anti/arthritic
an´ ti ar **thri**´ tik
_____ /_____;

toxic states

anti/toxic
an´ ti **toks**´ ik
_____ /_____;

sepsis

anti/septic
an´ ti **sep**´ tik
_____ /_____.

11.73
contra- is a prefix that means against. contra- is usually used with
modern English words. To contra/dict someone is to speak

against
_____ what the person is saying.

11.74
Contra/ry things are _____ each other. A contra/ry

against
against
person is one who is _____ your wishes.

11.75
In medical terminology, contra- is mainly confined in use to four
words. However, in these four words contra- still means

against
_____.

11.76
Analyze these three words:
   contraindication

contra/indication
kon´ tra in di **kā**´ shun
_____ /_____;

contraceptive

contra/ceptive
kon´ tra **sep**´ tiv
_____ /_____;

contralateral

contra/later/al
kon´ tra **lat**´ ur əl
_____ /_____ /_____.

11.77
Using the words in Frame 11.76, fill the following blanks with a
word whose literal meaning is:

contraindication
contraceptive
contralateral
   against indication   _____;
   against conception   _____;
   opposite (against) side   _____.

11.78
Using the noun contra/indication, build other parts of the same
word:

contra/indicate
contra/indicated
(You pronounce)
_____ /_____ (present tense verb);
_____ /_____ (past tense verb).

ANSWER COLUMN	
	11.79 Before beginning a drug therapy of any kind on a pregnant woman, a physician will consult a drug reference guide to see if the medication is safe to use during pregnancy. If it is not, the guide will say the medication is contra/indicated during pregnancy. Narcotic medications are not advisable during pregnancy;
contra/indicated kon′ tra **in**′ di kā ted	therefore, they are _____ /_____.
across or over	**11.80** trans- is a Latin prefix meaning across or over. To trans/port a cargo is to carry it *_____ the ocean or land.
across or over	**11.81** Trans/position means literally position *_____.
trans/position trans′ pə **zish**′ ən	**11.82** When an organ is placed across to the other side of the body from where it is normally found (e.g., liver on the left side), _____ /_____ occurs.
transposition	**11.83** Cardi/ac transposition means that the heart is on the right side of the body. If the stomach is on the right side of the body, the condition is gastr/ic _____.
across or over	**11.84** When a trans/fusion is given, blood is passed *_____ from one person to another.
trans-	**11.85** Recall that the procedure performed across the lumen of an artery of the heart is percutaneous _____ /luminal angioplasty (PTA).
trans/sex/ual trans/illumin/ation trans/vagin/al trans/thorac/ic trans/urethr/al trans/fusion (You pronounce)	**11.86** Analyze the following by drawing the slashes and writing the meaning: transsexual _____, _____ meaning transillumination _____, _____ meaning transvaginal _____, _____ meaning transthoracic _____, _____ meaning transurethral _____, _____ meaning transfusion _____, _____ meaning

▶ **ANSWER COLUMN**

💡 **INFORMATION FRAME**

11.87
A catheter (**kath´ e ter**) is a flexible tube. When a sterile urine specimen is needed, the urologist may introduce a catheter through the urethra into the bladder to obtain the specimen.

💡 **INFORMATION FRAME**

11.88
A procedure for enlarging heart vessels is called trans/catheter therapy or angioplasty. It is possible to introduce an intravascular occlusion balloon "through" a catheter. Look up these terms in your dictionary and note the use of the prefix trans-.

catheterization

11.89
Inserting a catheter for urine collection is called

_____ / _____.

heart

11.90
Cardiac catheterization allows the physician to view the inside of the vessels of the _____.

▶▶▶▶◀◀◀◀

Abbreviation	Meaning
A, B, O, AB	blood types
AAMA	American Association of Medical Assistants
ARDMS	American Registry of Diagnostic Medical Sonographers
c̄	with
cath	catheter
cm	centimeter
CMA	certified medical assistant
C&S	culture and sensitivity (antibiotic)
inf	infusion
met., metas., mets.	metastasis
RDMS	registered diagnostic medical sonographer
s̄	without
trans	transverse
US	ultrasound
UV	ultraviolet
XM	cross match (as in blood type and cross match)

To complete your study of this unit, work the review activities on the next pages. Also, listen to the audiotapes that accompany *Medical Terminology: A Programmed Text,* 8th edition, and practice your pronunciation.

Additional practice exercises for this unit are available on the Student Practice disk found in the back of the textbook.

► **REVIEW ACTIVITIES**

Select and Construct
Select the correct word parts from the list below and construct medical terms that represent the given meaning.

a(an)	algesia	aniso	anti	bi
ceptive	contra	cyst/o(ic)	cyt(o)(ic)	derm/o(al)
didym/o(is)	dur/a(al)	ectomy	epi	extra
gastr/o	genit/o(al)	graph/o(y)(er)	hetero	homo
infra	iso	itis	later/o(al)	lumb/ar
mamm/o	meta	oma	osis	otic
path(o)(y)	pod/o(ia)	ren/o(al)	rrhaphy	sept/o(ic)
sex(ual)	son/o	stasis	stern/o(al)	sub
sym	syn	tox/o(in)(ic)	tri	ultra

1. agent that works against infection _____

2. agent that works against fertilization of an ovum _____

3. attracted to the same sex _____

4. cells of different sizes _____

5. feet joined (grown) together _____

6. below the sternum _____

7. breast x-ray procedure _____

8. one who uses reflected sound to make images _____

9. upon the dura mater _____

10. outside of the urinary bladder _____

11. three sides _____

12. disease that goes beyond its original growth _____

▶ REVIEW ACTIVITIES

Write the prefix that represents the direction. Then, build a word using that prefix.

Prefix   *Word*

_____   1. same   attracted to the same sex   _____

_____   2. different   made of different substances   _____

_____   3. join   feet grown together
                                     (followed by b, m, f, ph, p)   _____

_____   4. above   above the surface   _____

_____   5. above   above the kidneys   _____

_____   6. without   absence of menstruation   _____

_____   7. without   without feeling or sensation   _____

_____   8. upon/over   upon the stomach (adjective)   _____

_____   9. outside of   outside of the cell (adjective)   _____

_____   10. below/under   below the sternum (adjective)   _____

_____   11. beyond   bones beyond the carpals   _____

_____   12. beyond   beyond audible sound waves   _____

_____   13. both   including both sides (adjective)   _____

_____   14. against   against arthritis (adjective)   _____

_____   15. against   against indications
                                     (not indicated)   _____

_____   16. across   across the urethra (adjective)   _____

▶ REVIEW ACTIVITIES

Define and Dissect

Give a brief definition and dissect each term listed into its word parts in the space provided on the right. Check your answers by referring to the frame listed in parentheses and your medical dictionary. Then, listen to the audiotapes to practice pronunciation.

1. homolateral (11.3)

_____ / _____ / ____
pre   rt   suffix

_____
definition

2. heterosexual (11.9)

_____ / _____ / ____
pre   rt   suffix

3. sympathectomy (11.16)

_____ / _____ / _____
pre   rt   suffix

4. symmetrical (11.17)

_____ / _____ / _____
pre   rt   suffix

5. superinfection (11.21)

_____ / _____ / _____
pre   rt   suffix

6. suprarenopathy (11.22)

_____ / ____ / ___ / _____
pre   rt   v   suffix

7. analgesia (table)

____ / _____
pre   rt/suffix

8. asepsis (11.62)

____ / _____
pre   rt/suffix

9. episplenitis (11.26)

_____ / _____ / _____
pre   rt   suffix

10. extra-articular (11.37)

_____ / _____ / ____
pre   rt   suffix

11. extracerebral (11.37)

_____ / _____ / ____
pre   rt   suffix

12. inframammary (11.42)

_____ / _____
pre   rt/suffix

13. mammography (11.39)

_____ / ____ / _____
rt   v   suffix

14. metastasis (11.56)

_____ / _____
pre   rt/suffix

15. ultrasonography (11.59)

_____ / _____ / ____ / _____
pre   rt   v   suffix

16. anti-inflammatory (table)

_____ / _____ / _____ / _____
pre   pre   rt   suffix

17. contraceptive (11.76)

_____ / _____
pre   rt/suffix

18. transcatheter (11.88)

_____ / _____
pre   rt/suffix

19. homogeneous (11.8)

_____ / _____ / ____
pre   rt   suffix

20. antiseptic (11.72)

_____ / _____ / ____
pre   rt   suffix

21. antibiotic (11.70)

_____ / _____ / ____
pre   rt   suffix

22. bacteriostatic (table)

_____ / ____ / _____ / ____
rt   v   rt   suffix

23. epididymitis (11.31)

_____ / _____ / _____
pre   rt   suffix

24. epidural (11.33)

_____ / _____ / ____
pre   rt   suffix

25. contraindication (11.76)

_____ / _____ / _____
pre   rt   suffix

▶ REVIEW ACTIVITIES

Abbreviation Matching
Match the following abbreviations with their definition.

_____	1. c̄
_____	2. trans
_____	3. C&S
_____	4. CMA
_____	5. UV
_____	6. mets.
_____	7. RDMS
_____	8. A, B, O, AB

a. ultraviolet
b. transurethral
c. blood group types
d. catheter
e. fractured metatarsals
f. transverse
g. with
h. certified medical assistant
i. culture and sensitivity
j. metastasis
k. registered dietitian
l. registered diagnostic medical sonographer
m. without
n. infrared
o. certified physician's assistant

Abbreviation Fill-ins
Fill in the blank with the correct abbreviation.

9. American Association of Medical Assistants _____

10. without _____

11. infusion _____

12. cross match _____

▶ CASE STUDIES

Write the term next to its meaning given below. Then, draw slashes to analyze the word parts. Note the use of medical abbreviations. Look these up in your dictionary or find them in Appendix B. If you have any questions about the answers, refer to your medical dictionary or check with your instructor for the answers in Appendix A.

CASE STUDY 11-1
NEUROLOGY OPERATIVE REPORT

Pt: male, age 46

Preoperative diagnosis: Left **hemiparesis** with right **subdural** hygroma (Postoperative Dx: same)

Procedure: Burr hole with evacuation of subdural fluid

Anesthesia: 1% Xylocaine with standby—**Anesthesiologist**

Having shaved his head and properly positioned him the patient was turned slightly to the left. IV Valium was given by the anesthetist who was monitoring his vital signs, including oxygenation.

The right **temporoparietal** region was prepared and draped in the usual fashion. Xylocaine 1% was administered locally and thereafter a scalp **incision** was carried out which was deepened down through the **subcutaneous** tissue. The galea was incised. **Hemostasis** was achieved. The muscle fascia and muscle fibers were incised and thereafter the wound was **retracted** and the **pericranium** was thus opened and incised. Using McKenzie's **perforator**, a burr hole was made which was widened and thereafter the **dura mater** was thus exposed. **Cauterization** was carried out. Bone wax was applied to the scalp margin and thereafter a **cruciate** incision was carried out. Clean Fluid with pressure was obtained, however, there was no evidence of any blood. The fluid was allowed to seep out, was suctioned out, and a small amount of dura was removed, using Kerrison rongeur. I did not feel that a drain would be necessary in the absence of blood and so having done this, the wound was closed in layers, closing the **temporalis** muscle fascia, the galea and skin. Steri-strips were applied and the patient was **transferred** to his room.

1. below the dura mater _____
2. physician specializing in painless surgery _____
3. making a cut into (noun) _____
4. controlling blood flow _____
5. below the skin _____
6. membrane surrounding the skull _____
7. pulled back _____
8. instrument used to make a hole _____
9. outermost layer of the meninges _____
10. placed in another location _____
11. half (partially) paralyzed _____

▶ CROSSWORD PUZZLE

Check your answers by going back through the frames or checking the solutions in Appendix C.

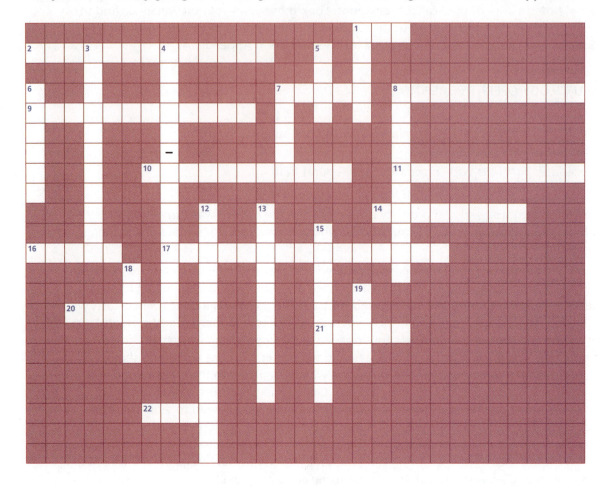

Across

1. synonym for syn-
2. prevents pregnancy
7. prefix meaning between
8. toxins in the blood from infection
9. inflammation upon the kidney
10. x-ray of the breast (process)
11. agent that fights bacteria
14. below the dura mater
16. prefix meaning across
17. used to obtain a sterile urine specimen
20. prefix meaning against
21. prefix meaning outside
22. prefix meaning same

Down

1. prefix meaning above
3. Donors give blood for _____.
4. outside of a joint
5. prefix meaning against
6. prefix meaning different
7. prefix meaning within
8. above the pubic bone
12. made of different substances or tissues
13. cleans the skin before surgery
15. both sides
18. prefix meaning beyond
19. prefix meaning beyond

▶ **GLOSSARY**

antiarthritic	agent that works against arthritis
antibiotic	agent that works against organisms, especially bacteria
anticonvulsive	agent that prevents seizures
antinarcotic	agent that works against the effects of narcotics
antipyretic	agent that works against fever
antirheumatic	agent that works against rheumatic disease
antiseptic	agent that protects against infection (external cleaner)
antispasmodic	agent that prevents muscle spasms
antitoxin	agent that works to destroy toxins
asepsis	without poisons or infection
bilateral	including both sides (adjective)
catheterization	using a tube (catheter) inserted into the bladder or vessels to obtain specimens, to look, or to keep the vessel open
contraceptive	agent that prevents conception
contraindicated	not recommended in these circumstances
contravolitional	against one's will
disinfectants	chemical or physical agents that kill organisms; not used on the body
epicystitis	inflammation upon the urinary bladder
epidural	pertaining to the layer upon the dura mater (adjective)
epigastric	upon the stomach
epigastrorrhaphy	suturing of tissue in the region upon the stomach
epinephrectomy	excision of tissue upon the kidney
epinephritis	inflammation upon the kidney
episplenitis	inflammation upon the spleen
extra-articular	outside of a joint (adjective)
extracerebral	outside of the cerebrum (adjective)
extracystic	outside of the bladder (adjective)
extradural	outside of the dura mater (adjective)
extragenital	outside of the genital area (adjective)
extranuclear	outside of the nucleus (adjective)
heterogeneous	different throughout (adjective)
heteropia	different vision in each eye
heterosexual	attracted to the opposite sex (adjective)
homogeneous	the same throughout (adjective)
homoglandular	same gland (adjective)
homosexual	attracted to the same sex (adjective)

► GLOSSARY

infracostal	below the ribs (adjective)
inframammary	below the breast (adjective)
infrapatellar	below the patella (adjective)
infrapubic	below the pubic bone (adjective)
mammogram	breast x-ray film or x-ray picture
mammography	process of taking a breast x-ray
metacarpals	bones of the hand beyond the wrist bones (carpals)
metastasis	disease that spreads beyond its origin
metatarsals	bones of the foot beyond the ankle (tarsals)
pyrotoxin	toxin produced by fever or heat
septicemia	infection in the blood
septopyemia	infection and pus in the blood
sterilization	process that kills all organisms
subdural	below the dura mater (adjective)
superciliary	pertaining to the eyebrow
superficial	on the surface (adjective)
superinfection	an infection on top of another infection
supracostal	above the ribs (adjective)
suprainguinal	above the groin
supralumbar	above the lumbar spine (adjective)
suprapubic	above the pubic bone (adjective)
suprarenal	above the kidney
suprarenopathy	disease of the suprarenal glands (adrenals)
symmetry	the same size and shape all around or on both sides
sympathetic	suffering along with, functional part of the autonomic nervous system
sympathoma	tumor of a sympathetic nerve
transcatheter	across a catheter
transfusion	transferring blood from one person to another
transillumination	use of light across a tube to view organs
transluminal	across the lumen of a vessel
transposition	placement of an organ on the opposite side
transsexual	a person who has changed sexes
transurethral	across the urethra
transvaginal	across the vagina
ultrasonography	use of ultrasound to make images from sound reflected through the body and computerized
ultrasound	high frequency sound beyond audible frequency
ultraviolet	light beyond the violet light frequency

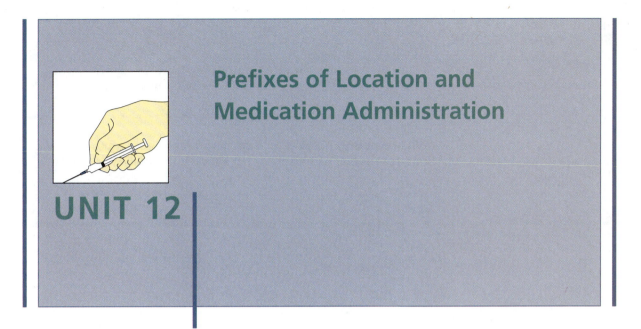

UNIT 12

Prefixes of Location and Medication Administration

ANSWER COLUMN	
	12.1 *Spirare* is a Latin word meaning to breathe. Breathing is respiration. Breathing consists of the following two processes: expiration and inspiration. Think of the meaning as you analyze:
ex/pir/ation in/spir/ation ex/cise in/cise	expiration _____ /_____ /_____; inspiration _____ /_____ /_____; excise _____ /_____; incise _____ /_____. **NOTE:** The s is dropped from spire when preceded by ex.
	12.2 Look at the words in Frame 12.1. The word that means breathing
inspiration	in is _____.
	12.3 in- is a prefix that means in, into, or not. In/compatible drugs are
not	drugs that do _____ mix with each other.
	12.4 In/compet/ency occurs in an organ when it is _____ able to
not	perform its function.
	12.5 Incompetence is a noun. When the ile/o/cec/al valve cannot perform its function, the result is ileocecal valve
in/compet/ence in **kom**′ pə təns	_____ /_____ /_____.

► ANSWER COLUMN	
incompetence	**12.6** When blood seeps back through the aortic valves, aortic _____ or insufficiency occurs.
incompetence incompetent	**12.7** When a person is not able to think rationally enough to care for himself or herself, you may call it ment/al _____. You may even say the person is mentally _____ (adjective).
in/continence in **kon**´ ti nəns	**12.8** Continence is the ability to control defecation and urination. Lack of control of waste removal is called _____ /_____.

in/sane
in/somnia
in/coherent
	12.9
	Build words meanings
	   not sane _____ /sane;
	   inability to sleep _____ /somnia;
	   not coherent _____ /coherent.

in/cision in **sizh**´ ən	**12.10** in- also means into. To in/cise is to cut into. This is a verb. The noun from in/cise is _____ /_____.
ex/cise ek´ **sīz**´	**12.11** To cut into is to incise. To cut out (remove) is to _____ /_____.
in/flammation in flə **mā**´ shən	**12.12** Look up the meaning of in/flammation. **-itis** is the suffix for _____ /_____. Think of the meaning of in as a prefix in this word.
verb form of inject one who (thing which) injects procedure of injecting	**12.13** In/ject means to introduce a substance into the body (usually through a needle). Define the following: inject, injected *_____; injector *_____; injection *_____.

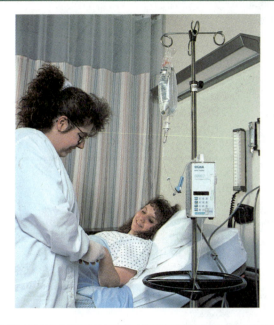

Intravenous infusion (IV) using an infusion pump
(Photo by Marcia Butterfield, Courtesy of Jackson Community College, Jackson, MI)

ANSWER COLUMN	
in/fusion in **fyoo**′ shən	**12.14** Fluids such as normal (isotonic) saline with 5 percent dextrose may be introduced into a vein. This is an IV _____ /_____.
infusion	**12.15** The pump used to regulate the speed of flow of an IV is called an _____ pump.
in/stillation in stil **ā**′ shən	**12.16** In Latin *stillare* means to drip. In/stillation is putting medicated drops into an eye or body cavity. Medication (otic solution) dropped into an ear is an _____ /_____.
in/semin/ation in sem i **nā**′ shun	**12.17** Recall that semen is a fluid substance that contains sperm. **SEMIN/O** is the combining form. Artificial in/semin/ation is a process of placing semen into the opening of the cervix using either husband (AIH) or donor (AID) sperm. Couples having difficulty with conception may be successful using artificial _____ /_____ /_____.
insemination	**12.18** Use of a husband's sperm to fertilize an egg is called artificial _____ by husband (AIH).

▶ **ANSWER COLUMN**

12.19
Now, see how many new vocabulary word you have just learned.
Build words that mean

ex/pire or ex/hale
ex/cision
in/spiration
in/cise

to breath out (verb) _____ /_____;
cutting out (noun) _____ /_____;
breathing in (noun) _____ /_____;
to cut into (verb) _____ /_____.

12.20
Build words that mean

in/compentency
in/compatible
in/coherent
in/fusion
in/stillation

not competent (noun) _____ /_____;
not compatible _____ /_____;
not able to be understood _____ /_____;
solution introduced into a vein _____ /_____;
medication administration by drops _____ /_____.

12.21

in, not, into

Remember that **in-** means _____, _____, or _____.

12.22

**TAKE A
CLOSER LOOK**

Use your dictionary to
find the answer

Analyze the following **in-** words by writing their meaning and
indicating the part of speech:

	meaning	part of speech
injected	_____	(_____)
incision	_____	(_____)
inflamed	_____	(_____)
infusion	_____	(_____)
infested	_____	(_____)

12.23

bad

mal- is a French word that means bad. **mal-** is also a prefix that
means bad or poor. Mal/odor/ous means having a _____ odor.

12.24

poorly formed or
poor formation

Mal/aise (ma **lāz´**) means a general feeling of illness or feeling
poorly. Mal/formation means *_____
_____.

12.25

poor nutrition

poor absorption
(as of nutrients)

Good nutrition is essential for good health. Mal/nutrition means
*_____.

Mal/absorption means
*_____.

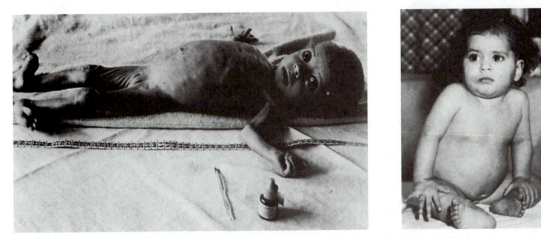

A. **B.**
a. A four-month-old baby suffering from severe malnutrition b. The same child at the age of ten months after having been properly fed (Courtesy of the Food and Agriculture Organization of the United Nations)

ANSWER COLUMN	
	12.26 Build a "bad" word that means feeling bad
mal/aise ma lāz´ mal/nutrition mal nōō **tri**´ shun mal/absorbtion mal ab **sorb**´ shun mal/formation mal fôr **mā**´ shun	_____ /_____; bad (poor) nutrition _____ /_____; bad (poor) absorption _____ /_____; bad (poor) formation _____ /_____. Good!
malari/o	**12.27** Look at the words in the next two frames. Now find the combining form for the disease malaria: _____ /_____.
malari/a mə **lair**´ ē ə	**12.28** Before people knew that mosquitoes carry the malaria parasite (*Plasmodium vivax*), they thought this disease was caused by "bad" night air. Analyze malaria (means bad air): _____ /_____.
malari/al malari/ous malari/o/logy malari/o/therapy (You pronounce)	**12.29** Analyze these words involving the disease malaria by drawing the diagonals and giving the part of speech: *part of speech* malarial _____ (_____) malarious _____ (_____) malariology _____ (_____) malariotherapy _____ (_____)

page 378 Unit 12

▶ **ANSWER COLUMN**

three three three	**12.30** uni- means one. bi- means two. tri- means three. The tri/ceps muscle has _____ heads. A tri/cuspid valve has _____ cusps. The tri/gemin/al nerve has _____ branches. Look back to the numerical prefix table on page 304 to review Latin and Greek word parts.
tri/ceps **trī´** seps	**12.31** The three-bellied muscle in the posterior upper arm is the _____ /_____.
tri/plets **trip´** letz	**12.32** Quintuplets are five infants born at the same time. Giving birth to three infants during the same pregnancy is having _____ /_____.
tri/gemin/al trī **jem´** i nəl	**12.33** The three-branched cranial nerve is the _____ /_____ /_____ nerve.
bi/furc/ates **bī´** fər kāts	**12.34** bi- means two. furco- means branching or dividing. To bi/furc/ate is to divide into two branches. When an artery divides into two, it _____ /_____ /_____ (verb) (e.g., carotid artery; see the illustration).
bi/furc/ation bī fer **kā´** shən	**12.35** Bi/furcate is a verb. The noun is bi/furc/ation. When a nerve divides into two branches, a _____ /_____ /_____ (noun) is formed.
bifurcations	**12.36** Various ducts in the body also form _____ (plural).

Bifurcation of the carotid artery

Blood vessels of the head and neck

ANSWER COLUMN	

> ◣ **ANSWER COLUMN**

12.37
The bi/ceps is a muscle with _____ bellies.
A bi/cusp/id is a tooth with _____ cusps.
Bi/foc/al glasses have _____ foci in one lens.
A bi/furc/ation has _____ branches.

two
two
two
two

12.38
Build words that mean
   a tooth with two cusps
   _____ /_____;
   lenses with two areas of focus
   _____ /_____;
   one who is sexually attracted to both males and females
   _____ /_____;
   the part of a structure that divides into two branches
   _____ /_____;
   a muscle with two bellies (b. brachii)
   _____ /_____.

bi/cuspid
bī **kus´** pid
bi/focals
bī´ fō kəlz
bi/sexual
bī **sex´** yoo̅ əl
bi/furcation
bī fer **kā´** shun
bi/ceps
bī´ seps

12.39
uni- means one. A uni/corn has _____ horn. Uni/ovular pertains
to twins who develop from _____ ovum. Uni/vers/al means
combined into _____ whole.

one
one
one

12.40
Later/al means pertaining to the side. Build words meaning
pertaining to
   one side
   _____ /_____ /_____;
   two sides
   _____ /_____ /_____;
   three sides
   _____ /_____ /_____.

uni/later/al
yoo̅ ni **lat´** er əl
bi/later/al
bī´ lat er əl
tri/later/al
trī´ lat er əl

12.41
multi- means many. Multi/cell/ular means made of many cells.
Build words meaning
   made of two cells
   _____ /_____ /_____;
   made of one cell only
   _____ /_____ /_____.

bi/cell/ular
bī **sel´** yoo̅ lar
uni/cell/ular or
yoo̅´ nē **sel´** yoo̅ lar
mono/cell/ular
mon ō **sel´** yoo̅ lar

► **ANSWER COLUMN**

12.42

Some cells are multi/nucle/ar in nature. Build words meaning
 having one nucle/us (adjective)

uni/nucle/ar or
yōō ni **nōō**´ klē ar
mono/nucle/ar
mon ō **nōō**´ klē ar
bi/nucle/ar
bī´ nōō klē ar

_____ / _____ / _____;
 having two nucle/i
 _____ / _____ / _____.

NOTE: Nucleus is singular, nuclei is plural, and nuclear is the
adjectival form.

12.43

Bi/sexual has two meanings. It can indicate a person with physical
characteristics of both males and females (hermaphrodite) or a
person attracted to both males and females. A person with both
male and female genitals may be said to be _____ / _____
or a _____ / _____.

bi/sexual
bī **seks**´ yōō əl
herm/aphrodite
herm **af**´ rō dīt

🏛 **WORD ORIGIN**

12.44

Hermaphrodites was the child of the god Hermes and the goddess
Aphrodite. S/he exhibited characteristics of both the father and
mother, male and female genders.

12.45

Affective disorders are disturbances in emotional mood or mental
state. Some people experience severe mood swings from a manic
(excited) to a depressive state. This experience of two polar
extremes is called _____ / _____ affective disorder

bi/polar
bī **pōl**´ ar

12.46

Build words that mean
 sexually attracted to both sexes

bi/sexual
bi/polar

 _____ / _____;
 having two poles
 _____ / _____.

12.47

Review:

one
two
three
many

uni-   means _____;
bi-   means _____;
tri-   means _____;
multi- means _____.

▶ **ANSWER COLUMN**

12.48
Give the meaning of the following terms:
bifurcation
* _____ ;
bisexual
* _____ ;
bilateral
* _____ ;
uninuclear
* _____ ;
hermaphrodite
* _____ .

dividing into two
  branches
attracted to both males
  and females
pertaining to both sides

pertaining to having one
  nucleus
individual possessing both
  male and female genitals

PREFIX	MEANING	EXPLANATION
semi-	half	used with modern English words or words closer to modern English
hemi-	half	used more with straight medical words

semi-
hemi-

12.49
There are two prefixes that mean half. They are _____ and
_____.

semi/circle
semi/conscious
semi/private

12.50
Form words that mean
  half circle   _____ / _____ ;
  half conscious   _____ / _____ ;
  half private (hospital room) _____ / _____ .

hemi/cardi/a
hem ē **kär′** dē ə
hemi/gastr/ectomy
hem ē gast **rek′** tom ē
hemi/plegia or
hem ē **plē′** jē ə
hemi/paralys/is
hem ē par **al′** ə sis

12.51
Build words meaning
  presence of only half a heart (noun)
  _____ / _____ / _____ ;
  removal of half the stomach
  _____ / _____ / _____ ;
  paralysis of half the body (on one side)
  _____ / _____ .

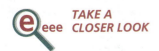
*TAKE A
CLOSER LOOK*

12.52
Note the difference between these two words: hemiplegia—
paralysis of one side of the body; paraplegia—paralysis of the
lower half of the body. Look up paraplegia, hemiplegia, and
quadriplegia in your dictionary and read about these conditions.

► **ANSWER COLUMN**

semi/circul/ar
semi/norm/al
semi/coma/tose
(You pronounce)
	12.53
	Build words meaning
	    half circular _____ /_____ /____ ;
	    half normal _____ /_____ /____ ;
	    half comatose _____ /_____ /_____ .

hemi/plegia
hem´ ē **plē**´ jē ə
hemi/sphere
hem´ i sfēr
hemi/an/esthesi/a
hem´ ē an es **thēs**´ ē ə
	12.54
	Build words with the literal meaning of
	    paralysis of half (one side) of the body
	    _____ /_____ ;
	    half of a sphere (e.g., cerebral)
	    _____ /_____ ;
	    anesthesia of half the body
	    _____ /____ /_____ /____ .

💡 *INFORMATION FRAME*	**12.55** **genit/o** comes from the Greek word *genesis*, meaning the beginning or formation. The reproductive system structures are called genit/als.
genit/al **jen**´ i təl	**12.56** A herpes simplex II infection in the area around the external genitalia is called _____ /_____ herpes.
with	**12.57** con- is a prefix that means with. Con/genit/al means born _____ .
born with	**12.58** A child with con/genit/al cataracts is *_____ cataracts.
con/genit/al kon **jen**´ i təl	**12.59** There are many con/genit/al deformities. A child born with a lateral curvature of the spine has _____ /_____ /____ scoliosis.
congenital	**12.60** Another way of saying a deformity that one is born with is to say congenital anomaly. A child born with kyphosis (posterior curvature of the spine) has a _____ anomaly (abnormality).
congenital	**12.61** A child born with hydr/ophthalm/os has _____ glaucoma (increased fluid pressure condition of the eye).
congenital	**12.62** A child born with syphilis has _____ syphilis.

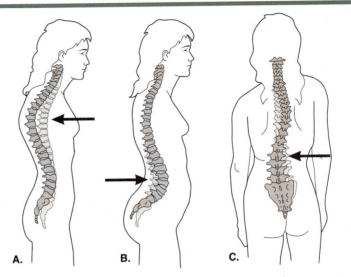

Abnormal curvatures of the spine: a. kyphosis, b. lordosis, c. scoliosis

ANSWER COLUMN	
	12.63 **con-** prefix—with **sanguin/o** combining form—blood **-ity** noun suffix—quality Using what you need of the above word parts, build a word meaning literally with blood or, in usage, blood relationship: _____ /_____ /_____.
con/sanguin/ity kon´ sang **gwin**´ i tē	
	12.64 Con/sanguin/ity is a relationship by descent from a common ancestor. The noun that expresses the relationship of cousins is _____.
consanguinity	
	12.65 **sanguin/o** means bloody. Build a word meaning pertaining to bloody draining on a dressing: _____ /_____.
sanguin/eous or sang **gwin**´ ē us sanguin/ous **sang**´ gwin us	

	12.66
	Build words meaning
	   having blood relationship _____ /_____ /_____;
	   bloody _____ /_____;
	   born with _____ /_____ /____.

con/sanguin/ity san/guin/ous or san/guin/eous con/genit/al	
	12.67 **dis-** is a prefix that means to free of, to separate, or to undo. Dis/ease means, literally, *_____.
free of ease	

> **ANSWER COLUMN**

12.68
To dis/sect is to cut a tissue or to undo it (into parts) for purposes of study. Write the following forms of the word dissect below:

dis/sect
dis **sekt´**
dis/section
dis **sek´** shən
dis/sected
dis **sek´** td

verb

_____ /_____;

noun

_____ /_____;

past tense verb

_____ /_____.

12.69
To dis/infect is to free of infective agents. Analyze the following terms and check definitions:

dis/infect
dis/infect/ant
dis/infect/ion
dis/infect/ed

disinfect _____ /_____;
disinfectant _____ /_____ /_____;
disinfection _____ /_____ /_____;
disinfected _____ /_____ /____.

12.70
People with multiple personality disorder (MPD) dis/associate and experience various personas. Analyze and check definitions:

dis/associate
dis/sociate
dis/sociated
dis/sociation

disassociate _____ /_____;
dissociate _____ /_____;
dissociated _____ /_____;
dissociation _____ /_____.

12.71
Recall that **dys-** means difficult or painful.

to free of, to undo
with

dis- is a prefix that means *_____.
con- is a prefix that means _____.

Use the following table to work Frames 12.71–12.77.

Prefix	Meaning	Look Up Meanings
post-	behind after	postnasal postmastectomy
ante-	before forward	antecubital anteverted
pre-	before in front of	premolar pretibial

ANSWER COLUMN	
	12.72
	post- means after.
after	Post/prandial (pp) means _____ meals.
after	Post/cibal (pc) means _____ meals.
after	Post/glucose (pg) means _____ ingesting glucose.
behind	Post/esophageal means _____ the esophagus.
after	Post/menopausal means _____ menopause.

	12.73
	pre- means before or in front of.
before	Pre/an/esthetic means _____ anesthesia.
in front of	Pre/hyoid means *_____ the hyoid bone.

	12.74
	ante- means before or forward.
before	Ante/pyretic means _____ the fever.
forward	Ante/flexion means _____ bending.

	12.75
	Peri/natal concerns events that are around birth. Nat/al means birth. Think of the meaning while you analyze:
	postnatal
post/nat/al	_____ /_____ /____;
pōst **nā**′ təl	prenatal
pre/nat/al	_____ /_____ /____;
prē **nā**′ təl	antenatal
ante/nat/al	_____ /_____ /____.
an tē **nā**′ təl	

	12.76
	Febris in Latin means fever. Febr/ile means pertaining to fever. Build words meaning
	pertaining to after a fever
post/febr/ile	_____ /_____ /_____;
pōst′ **fē**′ brəl	pertaining to before a fever
ante/febr/ile	_____ /_____ /_____.
an′ tē **fē**′ brəl	

	12.77
	Build words meaning pertaining to:
	after an operation
post/operative	_____ /_____ (po);
pōst **op**′ er a tiv	after coitus (intercourse)
post/coit/al	_____ /_____ /____;
pōst **kō**′ it əl	after delivery (refers to the mother)
post/part/um	_____ /_____ /____;
pōst **par**′ tum	after delivery or birth (refers to the baby)
post/nat/al	_____ /_____ /____.
pōst **nāt**′ al	**NOTE:** Notice that most of the terms you are learning here start with prefixes and are adjectives.

> ▶ **ANSWER COLUMN**

12.78

pre- means before. Build a word (adjective) that means:
before an operation _____ /_____ ;
before maturity (readiness) _____ /_____ ;
write before you can take (Rx) _____ /_____ ;
before cancer develops _____ /_____ /_____ .

pre/operative
pre/mature
pre/scribe
pre/cancer/ous
(You pronounce)

NOTE: Natal refers to birth and terms related to the newborn baby. **Partum** refers to delivery and terms related to the mother.

✔️ **SPELL CHECK**

12.79

A precription is written before a medication may be dispensed. It is prescribed (Rx).

12.80

Build terms that begin with ante-:
turning forward
_____ /_____ ;
before delivery
_____ /_____ /_____ ;
position in front
_____ /_____ .

ante/version
an´ tē ver shən
ante/part/um
an tē **par´** tum
ante/position
an tē pos **i´** shən

12.81

Mortem means death (think of mortal). What do these terms mean?
postmortem *_____ ;
antemortem *_____ .

after death
before death

NOTE: A.M. means ante- meridiem—before noon.
P.M. means post- meridiem—after noon.

12.82

In medicine mort/ality refers to the death rate and morbid/ity refers to the rate of occurrence of disease. Statistics giving the ratio of deaths in a given population is the _____ /_____ rate. The ratio of disease in a given population is the _____ /_____ rate.

mort/ality
mor **tal´** it ē
morbid/ity
mor **bid´** it ē

12.83

Recall that inter- means between. intra- means within. Intra-abdominal means *_____ .

within the abdomen

12.84

Intra/cellular means *_____ .
Intra/uterine means *_____ .

within a cell
within the uterus

Professional Profiles ◀◀◀◀◀◀◀◀◀◀◀◀◀◀◀◀◀◀◀◀◀◀◀◀◀◀◀◀◀

A **nurse** is a health care professional who provides a wide variety of services including the most simple patient care tasks, sophisticated lifesaving procedures, management of health care teams, education, and research. The level of responsibility of each nurse is related to education, licensure, and experience. The following are descriptions of various levels and credentials:

Licensed practical nurse (LPN), a graduate of a practical nursing program who has passed a state practical nursing licensing exam; most programs grant a certificate of completion.

Registered nurse (RN), a graduate of a state board-approved school of nursing who has passed a state registered nurse exam; he or she may earn an associate degree, diploma, or bachelor's degree.

Nurse practitioner (NP), an RN with advanced preparation for practice including clinical experience in diagnosis and treatment of illnesses. NPs may be allowed to practice independently depending upon state laws; this is a master's degree level.

Certified registered nurse anesthetist (CRNA), an RN who administers anesthesia under the supervision of an anesthesiologist and receives specialized training and certification recognized by the American Association of Nurse Anesthetists.

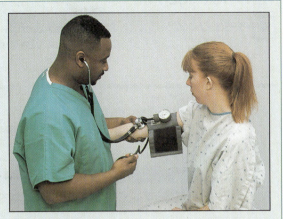

This nurse is assessing a young adult's blood pressure as part of a health program to enhance patient wellness

Clinical nurse specialist, an RN with a master's degree with a special competence in an area such as obstetrics, cardiology, or intensive care nursing.

Masters of Science in Nursing (MSN), completion of a board-approved MSN program including clinical practicum and research. MSNs may work directly with patients, manage teams, or serve as administrators and educators in nursing programs.

RNs with Doctorate Degrees in Nursing (PhDs) work as educators and researchers in colleges and universities, or may serve as hospital administrators.

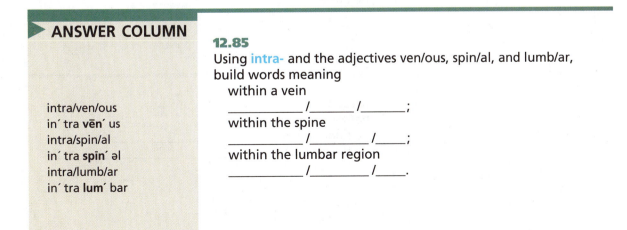

▶ **ANSWER COLUMN**

intra/ven/ous
in´ tra **vēn**´ us
intra/spin/al
in´ tra **spīn**´ əl
intra/lumb/ar
in´ tra **lum**´ bar

12.85

Using intra- and the adjectives ven/ous, spin/al, and lumb/ar, build words meaning

within a vein

_____ /_____ /_____;

within the spine

_____ /_____ /_____;

within the lumbar region

_____ /_____ /_____.

▶ **ANSWER COLUMN**

☑ *SPELL CHECK*

12.86
Intravenous ends in -ous, not -eous. Watch the pronunciation, too.
It is in´ tra **vēn**´ us.

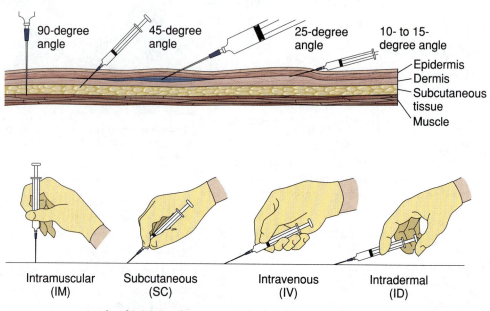

90-degree angle   45-degree angle   25-degree angle   10- to 15-degree angle
— Epidermis
— Dermis
— Subcutaneous tissue
— Muscle

Intramuscular (IM)   Subcutaneous (SC)   Intravenous (IV)   Intradermal (ID)

Angle of injection for parenteral administration of medications

12.87
Using **intra-** build adjectives meaning
    within an artery
    _____ /_____ /____;
    within the cranium
    _____ /_____ /____;
    within the bladder
    _____ /_____ /____;
    within the aorta
    _____ /_____ /____.

intra-/arteri/al
in´ tra är **tēr**´ ē əl
intra/crani/al
in´ tra **krā**´ nē əl
intra/cyst/ic
in´ tra **sis**´ tik
intra-/aort/ic
in´ tra ā **ôr**´ tik

12.88
Build adjectives meaning
    within the skin _____ /_____ /____;
    within the duodenum _____ /_____ /____;
    within the thoracic cavity _____ /_____ /____.

intra/derm/al
intra/duoden/al
intra/thorac/ic
(You pronounce)

Abbreviation	Meaning
ac	before meals (ante cibum)
AID	artificial insemination by donor's sperm
AIH	artificial insemination by husband's sperm
am	ante meridiem (morning)
CRNA	certified registered nurse anesthetist
exc	excision
GNID	gram-negative intracellular diplococcus
I&O	intake and output
IABP	intra-aortic balloon pump
ID	intradermal, identification
IM	intramuscular
inf	infusion
instill	instillation
IU	international units
IUD	intrauterine device
IV	intravenous
IVP	intravenous pyelogram
LPN	licensed practical nurse
MSN	Masters of Science in Nursing
NP	nurse practitioner
pc	after meals (post cibum)
pm	post meridiem (after noon)
PO	postoperative, by mouth (per os)
RN	registered nurse
sc, subcu, sq, subq	subcutaneous
ī, īi, īii, īv, v̄	one, two, three, four, five (apothecary numbers)
†	death

To complete your study of this unit, work the review activities on the next pages. Also, listen to the audiotapes that accompany *Medical Terminology: A Programmed Text,* 8th edition, and practice your pronunciation.

Additional practice exercises for this unit are available on the Student Practice disk found in the back of the textbook.

▶ REVIEW ACTIVITIES

Write the prefix that represents the direction. Then, build a word using that prefix.

Prefix   *Word*

_____	1. out	breathe out (verb)	_____
_____	2. in	cut into (verb)	_____
_____	3. not	not competent	_____
_____	4. bad/poor	poor nutrition	_____
_____	5. three	three branched nerve	_____
_____	6. two	two foci in one lens	_____
_____	7. one	one sided	_____
_____	8. half	half conscious	_____
_____	9. half	atrophy of half the body	_____
_____	10. with	born with	_____
_____	11. to free of	substance used to free of infective agents	_____
_____	12. after	after mastectomy	_____
_____	13. before	before surgery	_____
_____	14. in front of	in front of the frontal lobe	_____
_____	15. behind	behind the esophagus	_____
_____	16. before	before a fever	_____
_____	17. within	within the dermis	_____
_____	18. between	between the cells (review)	_____
_____	19. below	below the cutaneous (dermis) layer (review)	_____

▶ REVIEW ACTIVITIES

Select and Construct

Select the correct word parts from the list below and construct medical terms that represent the given meaning.

ante	aria(l)	bi	cancer/ous	card/ia(o)	cell/ular
cibal	coit(us)(al)	comatose	con	continence(y)	febrile
fest(ed)(ing)	formation	fus(ed)(ion)	glucose	hemi	in
intra	ject(ion)(ed)	mal	natal	nuclear(us)	partum
plegia	post	pre	sane	semi	tri
uni					

1. before birth   _____
2. after delivery   _____
3. half of a heart   _____
4. partially (half) in a coma   _____
5. pertaining to one cell   _____
6. having one nucleus   _____
7. before the development of cancer   _____
8. put in using a needle (verb)   _____
9. not able to control urination   _____
10. not sane   _____
11. poor growth   _____
12. parasitic disease caused by Plasmodium vivax   _____

Now use the word parts above to build other medical terms.

13. _____ (word)   _____ (meaning)
14. _____ (word)   _____ (meaning)
15. _____ (word)   _____ (meaning)
16. _____ (word)   _____ (meaning)
17. _____ (word)   _____ (meaning)
18. _____ (word)   _____ (meaning)

► **REVIEW ACTIVITIES**

Define and Dissect
Give a brief definition and dissect each term listed into its word parts in the space provided on the right. Check your answers by referring to the frame listed in parentheses and your medical dictionary. Then, listen to the audiotapes to practice pronunciation.

1. expiration (12.1)

    _____ / _____ / _____
    pre   rt   suffix

    _____
              definition

2. incompetency (12.4)

    _____ / _____ / _____
    pre   rt   suffix

3. inflammation (12.12)

    _____ / _____
    pre   rt/suffix

4. malaise (12.24)

    _____ / _____
    pre   rt/suffix

5. infusion (12.14)

    _____ / _____
    pre   rt/suffix

6. malariology (12.29)

    _____ / ___ / _____
    rt   v   suffix

7. bicuspid (12.37)

    _____ / _____ / _____
    pre   rt   suffix

8. uniovular (12.39)

    _____ / _____ / _____
    pre   rt   suffix

9. bifurcation (12.35)

    _____ / _____ / _____
    pre   rt   suffix

10. semicomatose (12.53)

    _____ / _____ / _____
    pre   rt   suffix

11. hemigastrectomy (12.51)

    _____ / _____ / _____
    pre   rt   suffix

12. consanguinity (12.63)

    _____ / _____ / _____
    pre   rt   suffix

13. dissection (12.68)   _____ / _____
                                          pre   rt/suffix

14. postfebrile (12.76)   _____ / _____ / _____
                                          pre   rt   suffix

15. precancerous (12.78)   _____ / _____ / _____
                                          pre   rt   suffix

16. anteversion (12.80)   _____ / _____
                                          pre   rt/suffix

17. intravenous (12.85)   _____ / _____ / _____
                                          pre   rt   suffix

18. incontinence (12.8)   _____ / _____ / _____
                                          pre   rt   suffix

19. insemination (12.17)   _____ / _____ / _____
                                          pre   rt   suffix

20. bisexual (12.43)   _____ / _____ / _____
                                          pre   rt   suffix

21. triplets (12.32)   _____ / _____
                                          pre   rt/suffix

22. hemiplegia (12.51)   _____ / _____
                                          pre   suffix

23. disassociate (12.70)   _____ / _____
                                          pre   rt/suffix

24. perinatal (12.75)   _____ / _____ / _____
                                          pre   rt   suffix

25. intradermal (12.88)   _____ / _____ / _____
                                          pre   rt   suffix

► REVIEW ACTIVITIES

Abbreviation Matching
Match the following abbreviations with their definition.

_____ 1. IUD
_____ 2. IM
_____ 3. PO
_____ 4. IV
_____ 5. ac
_____ 6. IVP
_____ 7. pc
_____ 8. IU

a. drops
b. international units
c. intravenous
d. subcutaneous
e. intake and output
f. intramuscular
g. intrauterine device
h. before meals
i. postoperative
j. intradermal
k. intravenous pyelogram
l. after meals
m. infusion
n. input and outtake
o. postprandial

Abbreviation Fill-ins
Fill in the blanks with the correct abbreviation.

9. excision _____

10. artificial insemination (husband) _____

11. intradermal _____

12. apothecary number three _____

13. before noon _____

14. infusion _____

▶ CASE STUDIES

Write the term next to its meaning given below. Then, draw slashes to analyze the word parts. Note the use of medical abbreviations. Look these up in your dictionary or find them in Appendix B. If you have any questions about the answers, refer to your medical dictionary or check with your instructor for the answers in Appendix A.

CASE STUDY 12-1
OPERATIVE REPORT

Preoperative diagnosis: **bilateral** adnexal masses, probable pelvic endometriosis and **endometriomata**

Postoperative diagnosis: bilateral adnexal masses, probable pelvic endometriosis and endometriomata

Procedure: Total abdominal hysterectomy, bilateral **salpingo-oophorectomy**, lysis of **adhesions**, incidental **appendectomy**

Technique and findings: Under adequate general anesthesia the patient was prepped and draped in the supine position with an **intracystic** Foley catheter. A lower abdominal midline **incision** was made and the abdominal wall opened in the usual fashion. Upon entering the abdominal cavity no unusual peritoneal fluid was noted. The upper abdomen was explored and found to be within normal limits. There were noted bilateral large ovarian endometriomata. The anterior cul-de-sac was free of adhesions, but the lower part of the sigmoid colon was adhered to the **posterior** wall of the cul-de-sac. The sigmoid adhesion was taken off the posterior wall of the uterus by sharp and blunt **dissection**, down past the uterosacral ligaments and freeing the cul-de-sac area. The bilateral endometriomata were ruptured, freeing the ovaries from the lateral pelvic walls. The round ligaments were bilaterally clamped, cut, and ligated with #1 chromic sutures. The **visceroperitoneum** between the round ligaments was **transversely incised** and the bladder bluntly **dissected** off the lower uterine segment of the cervix.

1. both sides _____
2. tumors of the endometrium _____
3. cut into (verb) _____
4. across (adverb) _____
5. the membrane on the abdominal organs _____
6. before surgery _____
7. cut apart (verb) _____
8. back _____
9. within the urinary bladder _____
10. excision of the appendix _____
11. excision of the ovaries and uterine tubes _____
12. tissues grown together _____
13. after surgery _____
14. cutting apart (noun) _____

► CROSSWORD PUZZLE

Check your answers by going back through the frames or checking the solutions in Appendix C.

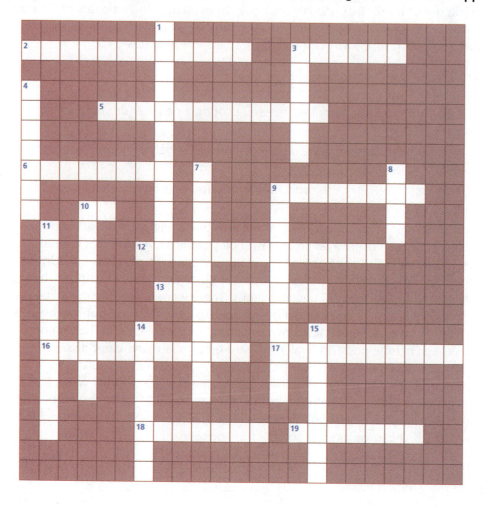

Across

2. subcu. means _____
3. two bellied muscle
5. poor nutritional status
6. a cut made into the body
9. synonym for antenatal
10. after meals (abbreviation)
12. partially conscious
13. involving both sides
16. medicines to fight bacteria (plural)
17. born with
18. three bellied muscle
19. to cut apart

Down

1. unable to control urination or defecation
3. sanguinous means _____
4. general poor feeling
7. process of administering medication using drops
8. hemiplegia is paralysis of _____ the body
9. before surgery
10. after delivery (the mother)
11. branched in two (noun)
14. at the site
15. introducing a substance into the body, such as IV

▶ GLOSSARY

antefebrile	before a fever
anteflexion	bending forward
antemortem	before death
antenatal	before birth (prenatal)
antepartum	before delivery (mother)
anteposition	in front of
antepyretic	before a fever
anteversion	turning toward
anteversion	turning forward
bicellular	made of two cells
biceps	a two-bellied muscle (i.e., b. femoris, b. brachii)
bifocal	lens having two focus strengths
binuclear	having two nuclei
bipolar	having two poles
bisexual	attracted to two sexes
congenital	born with
consanguinity	with blood relationship
disassociate	to break apart
disinfect	to rid of infectious agents
dissect	to cut apart
excise	to take out
exhale	to breathe out
expire	breathing out
genitals	reproductive system structures
hemianesthesia	anesthesia involving half the body
hemicardia	half a heart
hemigastrectomy	excision of half the stomach
hemiplegia	paralysis of one side of the body (right or left) (hemiparalysis)
incise	to cut into
incoherent	unable to be understood (speech)
incompatible	not compatible, does not associate well with
incompetency	not able to function properly
incontinence	inability to control urination or defecation
infested	organisms living within or on another organism
inflammation	condition with such symptoms as a red, swollen, and warm area
infusion	introducing a substance into a vein through a needle
inhale	to breathe in
injection	procedure of introducing a substance into the body through a needle
insane	not sane
insemination	process of introducing semen into the uterus or tubes
insomnia	unable to fall asleep
inspiration	breathing in

▶ GLOSSARY

instillation	applying drops
intercellular	between the cells
intra-abdominal	within the abdomen
intra-aortic	within the aorta
intra-arterial	within the artery
intracranial	within the cranium
intracystic	within the urinary bladder
intradermal	within the dermis layer
intraduodenal	within the duodenum
intrathoracic	within the chest (thoracic cavity)
malaise	generally poor feeling, not feeling well
malformation	poor formation
malnutrition	poor nutrition, missing essential nutrients
malodorous	smelling bad
morbidity	related to illness
mortality	related to death
postcibal	after meals
postcoital	after intercourse
postesophageal	in back of the esophagus
postfebrile	after a fever
postglucose	after glucose is administered
postmastectomy	after mastectomy surgery

postmenopausal	after menopause is complete
postmortem	after death
postnatal	after birth (baby)
postoperative	after surgery
postpartum	after delivery (mother)
postprandial	after meals
preanesthetic	before anesthesia
precancerous	condition that may lead to cancer
prefrontal	in front of the frontal bone
preoperative	before surgery
prescribe	write an order for before it can be done
sanguineous	bloody (also, sanguinous)
semicircle	half of a circle
semicomatose	partially in a coma
semiconscious	partially conscious (half)
semiprivate	situation in which half a room is shared
subcutaneous	the layer below the dermis of the skin
triceps	a three-bellied muscle (i.e., t. femoris, t. brachii)
unicellular	of one cell (also, monocellular)
unilateral	one sided
uninuclear	having one nucleus (also, mononuclear)

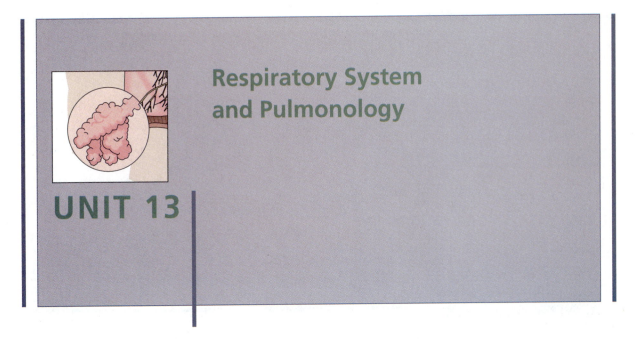

Respiratory System and Pulmonology

UNIT 13

Notice how these word roots were built from each other.

Combining Form	Meaning	Medical Term
pne/o (pnea, suffix)	breathing	tachy/**pne**a
pneum/o	air (lung)	**pne**um/o/thorax
pneumon/o	lung	**pne**umon/ectomy

13.1

pne/o refers to breathing. The lungs are the organs of the body that take in air (breathe). **Pneumon/o** is used in medical words concerning lungs.

excision of part or all of a lung
pneumon/o/tomy
no͞o´ mə **nôt´** ə mē

Pneumon/ectomy means *_____.
Incision of a lung is a
_____ /_____ /_____.

13.2

any disease of the lungs

pneumon/o/rrhagia
no͞o´ mə nō **rā´** jē ə

Pneumon/o/pathy means *_____.
Form a word meaning hemorrhage of a lung:
_____ /_____ /_____.

399

X-ray of lung with pneumonia

▶ **ANSWER COLUMN**

INFORMATION FRAME

13.3
Pneumonia is an acute inflammation of the lungs caused by a variety of organisms and viruses. Often, antibiotics are used to treat pneumonia. Another word for pneumonia is pneumonitis.

---

pneumon/o/centesis
noo′ mə nō sen tē′ sis
pneum/o/centesis
noo′ mō sen tē′ sis

13.4
Form a word meaning surgical puncture of a lung to remove fluid:
_____ /_____ /_____ or
_____ /_____ /_____.

---

pneumon/ia
noo **mōn**′ yə
pneumon/itis
noo′ mə **ni**′ tis

13.5
There are two words meaning inflammation of the lungs:
_____ /_____ and
_____ /_____.

---

lungs

13.6
Pneumocystis carinii pneumonia is an infection caused by a protozoan-like organism. People debilitated by immunodeficiency disease such as AIDS are particularly susceptible to this disease, which affects the _____.

✓ **SPELL CHECK**

13.7
Think of the "pn" rule for pronunciation when saying words like pneumonia. The "p" is silent when "pn" begins the word. Also, remember "eu" makes the "ū" sound. The "e" is written in front of the "u."

ANSWER COLUMN	
	13.8 Lung tissue can be surgically attached (fixated) by a procedure called _____ /_____ /_____.
pneumon/o/pexy noo′ mə no pek′ sē	
	13.9 Recall that **melan/o** means black. Pneumon/o/melan/osis is a lung disease in which lung tissue becomes black due to breathing black dust. The word root for black is _____.
melan	
	13.10 Pneumon/o/melan/osis literally means a condition of black lungs. Analyze this word: _____ /_____ combining form for lung _____ word root for black _____ suffix—condition
pneumon/o melan osis	
	13.11 Construct a word meaning condition of lung blackness: _____ /_____ /_____ /_____.
pneumon/o/melan/osis noo′ mə no mel′ ə **no**′ sis	
	13.12 The inhalation (breathing) of black dust results in _____. The inhalation of much soot or black smoke can also cause _____.
pneumonomelanosis pneumonomelanosis	
	13.13 Pneumon/o/myc/osis means a fungus disease of the lungs. The word root that means fungus is _____.
myc	
	13.14 **myc/o** seen any place in a word should make you think of _____. *myces* is a Greek word meaning mushroom.
fungus (singular) or **fung**′ gəs fungi (plural) **fun**′ jī, **fung**′ gī	
	13.15 In high school biology, you read or even learned the words mycelium and mycelial. **myc** refers to *_____.
fungi or fungus	

ANSWER COLUMN	
	13.16 A myc/osis is any condition caused by a fungus. A condition of lung fungus is _____ /_____ /_____ /_____.
pneumon/o/myc/osis no͞o **mon′** ō mī kō′ sis	

	13.17
	Build words meaning
	   resembling fungi
	   _____ /_____;
	   science and study of fungi
	   _____ /_____ /_____.

myc/oid **mī′** koid myc/o/logy mī **kol′** ə jē	

	13.18
	Build words meaning
	   fungal disease (condition) of the pharynx (throat)
	   pharyng/o/_____ /_____;
	   fungal disease (condition) of the nose
	   _____ /_____ /_____ /_____;
	   fungal disease of the skin
	   _____ /_____ /_____ /_____;
	   inflammation of the skin caused by a fungus
	   _____ /_____ /_____ /_____.

pharyng/o/myc/osis rhin/o/myc/osis dermat/o/myc/osis myc/o/dermat/itis (You pronounce)	
INFORMATION FRAME	**13.19** **pneum/o** and **pneumon/o** can both refer to the lung. **pneum/o** is derived from the Greek word *pneuma* (for wind or breath). **pneum/o** is used in words to mean air.
	13.20 **pneumon/o** comes from the Greek word *pneumon* (lung). **pneumon/o** is used in words that refer to the
lung or lungs	*_____. The lungs are shown on page 405.
	13.21 **pneum/o** is used in most words to mean _____, as in pneumatic drill, but it can also be used to mean lung.
air	
	13.22 **thorax** is a noun and suffix for chest cavity. Your use of **pneum/o** will be in words about air. Pneum/o/derm/a means a collection of air under the skin. A collection of air in the chest cavity (thorax) is a _____ /_____ /_____.
pneum/o/thorax no͞o′ mō **thôr′** aks	

ANSWER COLUMN	
thorac/o pneum/o/thorac/ic (You pronounce)	**13.23** The combining form for thorax (chest cavity) is _____ /_____. The adjective that pertains to a collection of air in the chest cavity is _____ /_____ /_____ /_____.
pneum/o/therapy noō′ mō **ther′** ə pē	**13.24** Hydrotherapy means treatment with water. Treatment with compressed air is called _____ /_____ /_____.
pneum/o/meter noō **mom′** ə tər	**13.25** A tacho/meter in cars measures the number of revolutions per minute of the drive shaft. An instrument that measures air volume in respiration is a _____ /_____ /_____.
pneum/o/py/o/thorax pneum/o/hem/o/thorax (You pronounce)	**13.26** A collection of air and serum (**ser/o**) in the chest cavity is pneum/o/ser/o/thorax. A collection of air and pus in the thoracic cavity is a _____ /_____ /_____ /_____ /_____, while a collection of air and blood in this same cavity is a _____ /_____ /_____ /_____ /_____.
pulmon/ary **pul′** mon air ē	**13.27** Pulmonary and pulmonic are both used as adjectives meaning pertaining to the lungs. **pulmon/o** is another combining form for lung used only in a few words. The heart valve through which blood travels to the lungs is the _____ /_____ valve.
pulmon/ary or pulmon/ic pul **mon′** ik	**13.28** Blood flows from the heart to the lungs via the _____ /_____ artery.
pulmonary embolus **pul′** mon air ē **em′** bol us	**13.29** Look up embolus in your dictionary. An embolus is a thrombus (clot) that moves. A blood clot moving to the lung is called a *_____.

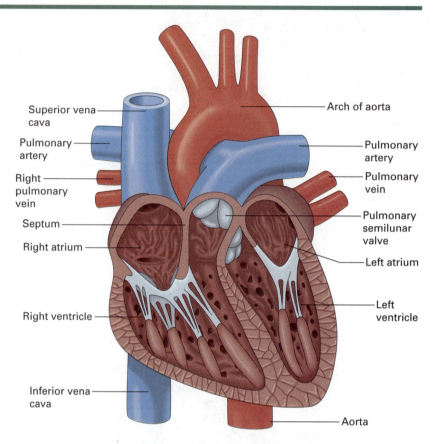

Heart—pulmonary arteries and veins

Study the following table of respiratory symptoms:

Term	Symptom
a/pnea	absence of breathing
dys/pnea	difficult breathing
hyper/pnea	increased rate and depth of breathing
tachy/pnea	rapid breathing
brady/pnea	slow breathing
ortho/pnea	able to breathe only when sitting or standing
hem/o/pty/sis	expectoration (coughing up) blood
hyper/ventil/ation	excessive movement of air in and out of lungs, sighing respirations
hyp/oxia	low oxygen in organs and tissues
cyan/osis	bluish color due to hypoxia

ANSWER COLUMN

a/pnea
ap´ nē ə
brady/pnea
brad ip **nē´** ə
orth/o/pnea
ôr **thop´** nē ə
hem/o/pty/sis
hēm **op´** tə sis

13.30
Build breathing words that mean
absence of breathing
_____ /_____;
slow breathing
_____ /_____;
able to breathe only when sitting up
_____ /_____ /_____;
coughing up blood
_____ /_____ /_____ /_____.

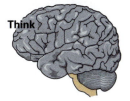
Think

Use the following information to work Frames 13.31–13.57. If you have forgotten a word part, remember, you may look back. The respiratory system is illustrated in the figure below. Seeing the parts as you work will make your work more interesting.

Air
    enters the nose and nasal cavity—**nas/o** (Remember **rhin/o**? Use **nas/o** in this work.)
    goes to the pharynx—**pharyng/o**
    to the larynx—**laryng/o**
    to the trachea—**trache/o**
    to the bronchi (us)—**bronch/o**
    to the alveoli (us)—**alveol/o** (part of the lung where it enters the bloodstream).
The lungs
    are covered by the pleura—**pleur/o**.
The diaphragm
    (**phren/o**) is a muscle that assists with inhalation and exhalation. The phrenic nerve innervates the diaphragm.

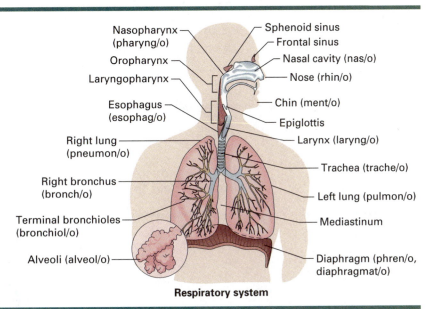

Nasopharynx (pharyng/o)
Oropharynx
Laryngopharynx
Esophagus (esophag/o)
Right lung (pneumon/o)
Right bronchus (bronch/o)
Terminal bronchioles (bronchiol/o)
Alveoli (alveol/o)
Sphenoid sinus
Frontal sinus
Nasal cavity (nas/o)
Nose (rhin/o)
Chin (ment/o)
Epiglottis
Larynx (laryng/o)
Trachea (trache/o)
Left lung (pulmon/o)
Mediastinum
Diaphragm (phren/o, diaphragmat/o)

Respiratory system

ANSWER COLUMN	
nasal cavity	**13.31** **nas/o** is used in words about the nasal cavity. Nas/o/antr/itis means inflammation of the antrum (maxillary sinus) and the *_____.
chin	**13.32** Taken from the Latin *mentum*, **ment/o** is the combining form for chin. Nas/o/ment/al means pertaining to the nasal cavity and _____.

nas/al
nā´ zəl
nas/itis
nā **zi´** tis
nas/o/scope
nā´ zō skōp
	13.33
	Build words meaning
	   pertaining to the nose (cavity)
	   _____ /____;
	   inflammation of the nose (cavity)
	   _____ /_____;
	   instrument to examine the nose (cavity)
	   _____ /____ /_____.

nas/o/pharyng/itis
nās´ ō far in **ji´** tis
nas/o/front/al
nās´ ō **front´** əl
nas/o/lacrim/al
nās´ ō **lak´** rim əl
	13.34
	Build words (you may use your dictionary if necessary) meaning
	   inflammation of nose and pharynx
	   _____ /____ /_____ /_____;
	   pertaining to the nasal and frontal bone
	   _____ /____ /_____ /____;
	   pertaining to the nose and lacrimal duct
	   _____ /____ /_____ /____.

nose and pharynx (throat)	**13.35** Nas/o/pharyng/eal means pertaining to the *_____.
pharynx **far´** inks	**13.36** A pharyng/o/lith (far **ing´** ō lith) is a calculus in the wall of the _____. **NOTE:** Pronounced like "fair" and "inks." Larynx is pronounced like "lair" and "inks."
pharynx (work on the pronunciation)	**13.37** A pharyng/o/myc/osis (far ing´ ō mī **kō´** sis) is a fungus disease of the _____.

▶ **ANSWER COLUMN**

13.38
Build words meaning
    inflammation of the pharynx

pharyng/itis
far´ in **ji**´ tis
    _____ /_____;
pharyng/o/cele
fə **ring**´ gō sēl
    herniation of the pharynx
pharyng/o/tomy
far´ ing **got**´ ə mē
    _____ /____ /_____;
    incision of the pharynx
    _____ /____ /_____.

13.39
The pharynx is the throat. Build words meaning (you put in slashes):
    disease of the pharynx

pharyng/o/pathy
    _____;
    surgical repair of the pharynx

pharyng/o/plasty
    _____;
    instrument to examine the pharynx

pharyng/o/scope
(You pronounce)
    _____.

13.40
laryng/o is used to build words that refer to the larynx. The larynx contains the vocal cords. When referring to the organ of sound, use _____ /____.

laryng/o
(You pronounce)

NOTE: laryng/o is also used to indicate "throat," as in otorhinolaryngologist (ENT).

13.41
Form a word that means inflammation of the larynx:

laryng/itis
lar´ in **ji**´ tis
_____ /_____.

13.42
After a bad cold, a patient may have laryngitis with accompanying pain. Pain in the larynx is called _____ /_____.

laryng/algia
lar´ in **gal**´ jē ə

13.43
Anything that obstructs the flow of air from the nose to the larynx may call for creating a new opening, or a
_____ /____ /_____.

laryng/o/stomy

13.44
When a temporary opening is wanted into the larynx, the surgical procedure is a laryng/o/tomy. An incision into the larynx is called a
_____ /____ /_____.
Remember the "g" rule for pronunciation in Frames 5.81–5.89.

laryng/o/tomy
lar´ ing **got**´ ə mē

ANSWER COLUMN	
	13.45
herniation of the larynx	A laryng/o/cele is a *_____.
	13.46
	Build words meaning
	any disease of the larynx
laryng/o/pathy	_____ /_____ /_____;
	instrument used to examine the larynx
laryng/o/scope	_____ /_____ /_____;
	spasm of the larynx
laryng/o/spasm	_____ /_____ /_____.
(You pronounce)	
	13.47
	The trachea (**trache/o**) is the windpipe. Trache/o/py/osis means
a condition of the trachea	*_____
with pus formation	_____.
	13.48
	Trache/o/rrhagia means
hemorrhage from the	*_____
trachea	_____.
	13.49
	Build words meaning
	pain in the trachea
trache/algia	_____ /_____;
trā′ kē **al**′ jē ə	incision into the trachea
trache/o/tomy	_____ /_____ /_____;
trā′ kē **ot**′ ə mē	herniation of the trachea
trache/o/cele	_____ /_____ /_____.
trā′ kē ō sēl	
	13.50
	Build words meaning
	examination of the trachea
trache/o/scopy	_____ /_____ /_____ ;
trā′ kē **os**′ kō pē	pertaining to the trachea
trache/al	_____ /_____;
trā′ kē əl	incision of trachea and larynx
trache/o/laryng/o/tomy	_____ /_____ /_____ /_____ /_____;
trā′ kē ō lär′ in **go**′ tō mē	surgical creation of a new opening in the trachea
trache/ostomy	_____ /_____;
trā′ kē **os**′ tō mē	within the trachea
endo/trache/al	_____ /_____ /____.
en′dō **trā**′ kē əl	

► **ANSWER COLUMN**

inflammation of the
  bronchi
an instrument to
  examine the bronchi
use of a flexible
  bronchofiberscope to
  examine the
  tracheobronchial tree

13.51
Bronch/itis means *_____
_____.
A bronch/o/scope is *_____
_____.
Bronch/o/fiber/o/scopy is *_____
_____.

bronch/o/lith
bron´ kō lith
bronch/o/scopy
bron **kos´** kə pē
bronch/o/rrhagia
bron´ kô **rā´** jē ə

13.52
Build words meaning
  calculus in a bronchus
  _____ /_____ /_____;
  examination of a bronchus (with instrument)
  _____ /_____ /_____;
  bronchial hemorrhage
  _____ /_____ /_____.

bronch/o/stomy

bronch/o/spasm

bronch/o/rrhaphy
(You pronounce)

13.53
Build words meaning
  formation of a new opening into a bronchus
  _____ /_____ /_____;
  spasm of a bronchus
  _____ /_____ /_____;
  suturing of a bronchus
  _____ /_____ /_____.

pertaining to the pleura
inflammation of the
  pleura

13.54
Pleur/al means *_____.
Pleur/itis means *_____
_____.

pleur/algia
plōō **ral´** jē ə
pleur/o/dynia
plōōr´ ō **din´** ē ə
pleur/o/centesis
plōōr´ ō sen **tē´** sis

13.55
Build words meaning
  pain in the pleura _____ /_____
  or
  _____ /_____ /_____;
  surgical puncturing of the pleura
  _____ /_____ /_____.

ANSWER COLUMN

viscer/o/pleural

pleur/o/lith

pleur/ectomy
(You pronounce)

13.56
Build words meaning
pertaining to the membrane attached to the lung
_____ /_____ /_____;
calculus in the pleura
_____ /_____ /_____;
excision of part of the pleura
_____ /_____.

TAKE A CLOSER LOOK

13.57
Look up the word pleurisy. Read all your dictionary has to say about this disease. Its synonym is pleuritis. Write the treatment described here:

_____

_____

_____

pleur/isy
plōō′ ri sē

13.58
Inflammation of the pleura is pleuritis, or
_____ /_____.

phren/o/plegia
fren ō **plē′** jē ə

13.59
The phrenic nerve controls the diaphragm. The combining form for diaphragm is **phren/o**. -plegia is the suffix for paralysis. Paralysis of the diaphragm is _____ /_____ /_____.

Professional Profiles ◄◄◄◄◄◄◄◄◄◄◄◄◄◄◄◄◄◄◄◄◄◄◄◄◄◄◄◄◄◄

Respiratory therapists (RRTs or CRTs) perform physiologic (i.e., arterial blood gases) and pulmonary (i.e., breathing) tests to determine respiratory health or impairment. They administer breathing treatment and other respiratory procedures to maintain or improve ventilatory function to patients in hospital and ambulatory care settings. It is also possible for the respiratory therapist to specialize in pulmonary function testing or to be cross-trained to perform cardiopulmonary testing such as stress tests. The National Board for Respiratory Care (NBRC) sets standards for education and credentialing of registered respiratory therapists (minimum two years) and certified respiratory therapists (minimum one year).

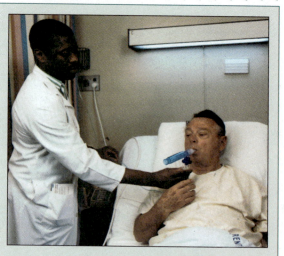

Respiratory therapist (RT) administering nebulizing mist treatment (NMT)

► **ANSWER COLUMN**

✔ *SPELL CHECK*

13.60
Watch your spelling of the word diaphragm. It has a silent "g."

---

phren/ectomy
fren **ek´** tō mē
phren/ic/ectomy
fren i **sek´** tō mē

13.61
Removal of a portion of the phrenic nerve is a
_____ /_____
or
_____ /_____ /_____.

---

left

13.62
In medicine you go back to the original meaning of sinister to find the combining form **sinistr/o**, which means _____.

---

left

13.63
ad- as a prefix or **-ad** as a suffix means toward. Sinistr/ad means toward the _____.

---

sinistr/al
sin´ is trəl
sinistr/o/cardi/a
sin´ is trō **kär´** dē ə
sinistr/o/cerebr/al
sin´ is trō **ser´** ə brəl

13.64
Using **sinistr/o**, build words meaning
    pertaining to the left
    _____ /_____;
    displacement of the heart to the left
    _____ /_____ /_____ /_____;
    pertaining to the left half of the cerebrum
    _____ /_____ /_____ /_____.

---

sinistr/o/man/ual

sinistr/o/ped/al
(You pronounce)

13.65
Using manual (hand) and pedal (foot), build words meaning
    left-handed
    _____ /_____ /_____ /_____;
    left-footed
    _____ /_____ /_____ /_____.

---

right

13.66
The opposite of **sinistr/o** is **dextr/o**. **dextr/o** means _____.

---

right

13.67
Dextr/ad means toward the _____.

► **ANSWER COLUMN**

13.68
Build words meaning
   pertaining to the right
   _____ /____;
   displacement of the heart to the right
   _____ /____ /_____ /____;
   displacement of the stomach to the right
   _____ /____ /_____ /____.

dextr/al
dek´ strəl
dextr/o/cardi/a
dek´ strō **kär´** dē ə
dextr/o/gastr/ia
dek´ strō **gas´** trē ə

13.69
Refer to Frame 13.65 if necessary and build words meaning
   right-handed _____ /____ /_____ /____;
   right-footed _____ /____ /_____ /____.

dextr/o/man/ual
dextr/o/ped/al
(You pronounce)

13.70
pod/o (Greek) and **ped/i** (Latin) are both combining forms for foot. Two terms for foot pain are _____ /____ /_____
and _____ /_____.

ped/i/algia
ped ē **al´** jē ə
pod/algia
pod **al´** jē ə

13.71
The two combining forms for foot are _____ /____ and
_____ /____.

ped/i
pod/o

13.72
Suffixes **-iatrist** (noun) and **-iatric** (adjective) are used to indicate medical professionals or physicians. A health professional responsible for care of conditions of the feet is a _____ /_____ (DPM). The specialty is called podiatry.

pod/iatrist
pō **dī´** ə trist

13.73
A hammertoe operation is a type of _____ /_____ (adjective) treatment.

pod/iatric
pō dē a´ trik

13.74
Cheir is a Greek word for hand. Look up chir/o/spasm; it means
*_____.
The combining form for hand is _____ /____.

spasm of the hand
chir/o

13.75
Chir/o/practors (DC—doctor of chiropractic) use their hands to manipulate the body for therapy. In the adjective chir/o/practic, the word root **chir/o** means _____.

hands

13.76
Spinal manipulation is a form of _____ /____ /_____ (adjective) treatment.

chir/o/practic
kī´ rō **prak´** tik

ANSWER COLUMN

chir/o/plasty
kī´ rō plas tē

13.77
Surgical repair of the hand is called
_____ /_____ /_____.

pedi/a/trician
pē´ dē a **tri´** shən

13.78
pedi/a is a combining form that comes from the Greek word
pedias, meaning child. A physician specialist who treats children is
a _____ /_____ /_____.

pedi/a/trics
pē´ dē a´ triks

13.79
Recall -iatric is a suffix meaning medical or physician. The
medical specialty for treatment of diseases of children is
_____ /_____ /_____.

-iatrist

13.80
A psych/iatrist is a medical doctor who specializes in the study
of diagnosing and treating mental disorders. _____
is the suffix used to indicate a medical professional.

psych/i/atric
sī´ kē a´ trik

13.81
A psychiatrist provides _____ /_____ /_____ treatment.

Professional Profiles ◀◀◀◀◀◀◀◀◀◀◀◀◀◀◀◀◀◀◀◀◀◀◀◀◀◀◀◀◀◀◀◀◀◀

**Registered Health Information Administrators
(RHIAs)** manage medical record departments in
hospitals to ensure accurate, complete, orderly,
and timely record keeping. They help plan
hospital systems for better patient care and
provide statistics for research, accreditation, and
assistance with financial management.

**Registered Health Information Technicians
(RHITs)** complete, index, code, file, and abstract
statistical information and prepare medical
records for release. In many institutions they also
perform management functions. The American
Health Information Management Association
(AHIMA) sets standards for education programs
(ranging from correspondence courses to
bachelor's degrees), registration, and accreditation of medical records professionals.

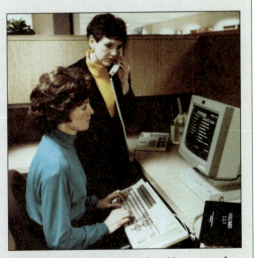

Health Information technician (Courtesy of
Hinsdale Hospital, Hinsdale, IL)

▶ **ANSWER COLUMN**

13.82

ger/i means old age. Ger/ont/o/logy is the study of treatment of aging and the elderly. The medical specialty involving treating diseases related to old age is _____/_____/_____.
The study of aging is _____/_____/_____/_____.

ger/i/atrics
jer´ ē a´ triks
ger/ont/o/logy
jer´ on **tol**´ ō jē

Abbreviation	Meaning	Abbreviation	Meaning
ABG	arterial blood gases	NBRC	National Board for Respiratory Care
AD	right ear (auris dexter)	NMT	nebulizing mist treatment
AHIMA	American Health Information Management Association	O_2	oxygen
		PD	pulmonary disease
RHIT	registered health information	PE	pulmonary edema, physical exam, pulmonary embolism
AS	left ear (auris sinister)	Peds	pediatrics
CO_2	carbon dioxide	PFT	pulmonary function test
COLD	chronic obstructive lung disease	PND	paroxysmal nocturnal dyspnea, postnasal drip
COPD	chronic obstructive pulmonary disease	R	respiration (rate)
CRT	certified respiratory therapist	RHIA	registered health information administrator
DC	doctor of chiro-practic medicine	RRT	registered respiratory therapist
DPM	doctor of podiatric medicine	RT	respiratory therapist
		TB	tuberculosis
ICU	intensive care unit	TC & DB	turn, cough, and deep breathe
IS	incentive spirometer	URI	upper respiratory infection

To complete your study of this unit, work the review activities on the next pages. Also, listen to the audiotapes that accompany *Medical Terminology: A Programmed Text,* 8th edition, and practice your pronunciation.

Additional practice exercises for this unit are available on the Student Practice disk found in the back of the textbook.

▶ REVIEW ACTIVITIES

Circle and Correct

Circle the correct answer for each question. Then, check your answers in Appendix A.

1. Word root for lung:
   a. pnea   b. pneumonia
   c. pneumon   d. pulmonary

2. Combining form for fungus:
   a. monilo   b. myo
   c. myco   d. mycelio

3. Noun for throat:
   a. pharynx   b. trachea
   c. esophagus   d. phalanx

4. Adjective for kidney:
   a. nephriac   b. nephroc
   c. cystic   d. renal

5. Which of the following does *not* refer to the lung?
   a. thoraco   b. pulmonary
   c. pneumono   d. pneumo

6. Combining form for air:
   a. pneumono   b. pneumo
   c. pnea   d. pulmono

7. Combining form for nasal cavity:
   a. rhin   b. mento
   c. naso   d. antro

8. Singular of pharynges:
   a. pharynx   b. pharyngos
   c. pharyno   d. pharynge

9. Sound made by the "g" in laryngocele:
   a. s   b. k
   c. j as in job   d. g as in goat

10. Combining form for right:
    a. dextro   b. dextrose
    c. dextrous   d. dexter

11. Combining form for the windpipe:
    a. esphago   b. laryngo
    c. pharyngo   d. tracheo

► **REVIEW ACTIVITIES**

Select and Construct
Select the correct word parts from the list below and construct medical terms that represent the given meaning.

al	algia	ary	atrician	blast	bronch(o)(i)
centesis	chir(o)	constriction	dermat/o	dextr(o)	dilatation
dilation	dynia	ectasis	ectomy	embol	fungi
hist(o)	iatrist	ic	ism	itis	laryn(x)(g)(o)
lith	(o)logy	lysis	manual	melan(o)	mental
myc(o)	nas(o)	oma	osis	pathy	pedal
pedi	pharynx(go)	phren(o)	plegia	pleur(o)(a)	pneumon/o
practor	psych	pulmon/o	rrhagia	scope (y)	sinistr/o
stomy	thorac/o	trache(o)	us		

1. adjective for lung

2. black lung disease

3. fungus infection of the skin

4. moving blood clot

5. the study of fungi

6. pertaining to the nose and chin

7. instrument used to look at the throat

8. surgical puncture of the membrane around the lung

9. right-footed

10. left-handed

11. physician specialist for children

12. destruction of tissue

13. inflammation of the bronchi

14. pain in the voice box

15. paralysis of the diaphragm

16. dilatation of the bronchi

17. physician specialist in mental disorders

18. making a new opening in the trachea

19. doctor using hands to manipulate the spine

> ## ▶ REVIEW ACTIVITIES

Define and Dissect

Give a brief definition and dissect each term listed into its word parts in the space provided on the right. Check your answers by referring to the frame listed in parentheses and your medical dictionary. Then, listen to the audiotapes to practice pronunciation.

1. pneumonocentesis (13.4)

    _____/____/_____
           rt   v   suffix

    _____
                definition

2. pneumonomelanosis (13.11)

    _____/____/_____/_____
           rt   v   rt   suffix

3. pharyngomycosis (13.18)

    _____/____/_____/_____
           rt   v   rt   suffix

4. pneumothorax (13.22)

    _____/____/_____
           rt   v   rt

5. pulmonic (13.28)

    _____/_____
           rt   suffix

6. pneumopyothorax (13.26)

    _____/____/____/____/_____
           rt   v   rt   v   rt

7. pneumohemothorax (13.26)

    _____/____/____/____/_____
           rt   v   rt   v   rt

8. pulmonary (13.27)

    _____/_____
           rt   suffix

9. embolus (13.29)

    _____/_____
           rt   suffix

10. pneumonia (13.5)

    _____/_____
           rt   suffix

11. mycology (13.17)

    _____/____/_____
           rt   v   suffix

12. dermatomycosis (13.18)

    _____/____/_____/_____
           rt   v   rt   suffix

13. nasitis (13.33)

    _____/_____
           rt   suffix

14. pharyngomycosis (13.37)

    _____/____/_____/_____
           rt   v   rt   suffix

418   Unit 13

▶ **REVIEW ACTIVITIES**

15. nasoantritis (13.31)

_____ / _____ / _____ / _____
rt   v   rt   suffix

16. nasopharyngitis (13.34)

_____ / _____ / _____ / _____
rt   v   rt   suffix

17. tracheolaryngotomy (13.50)

_____ / _____ / _____ / _____ / _____
rt   v   rt   v   suffix

18. pleurisy (13.58)

_____ / _____
rt   suffix

19. bronchorrhaphy (13.53)

_____ / _____ / _____
rt   v   suffix

20. phrenectomy (13.61)

_____ / _____
rt   suffix

21. sinistrocardia (13.64)

_____ / _____ / _____ / _____
rt   v   rt   suffix

22. dextromanual (13.69)

_____ / _____ / _____ / _____
rt   v   rt   suffix

23. podiatric (13.73)

_____ / _____
rt   suffix

24. pediatrician (13.78)

_____ / _____ / _____
rt   v   suffix

25. chiropractor (13.75)

_____ / _____ / _____
rt   v   rt/suffix

26. laryngotomy (13.44)

_____ / _____ / _____
rt   v   suffix

27. bronchoscopy (13.52)

_____ / _____ / _____
rt   v   suffix

28. pleurocentesis (13.55)

_____ / _____ / _____
rt   v   suffix

29. psychiatrist (13.80)

_____ / _____
rt   suffix

30. gerontology (13.82)

_____ / _____ / _____ / _____
rt   rt   v   suffix

▶ REVIEW ACTIVITIES

Abbreviation Matching
Match the following abbreviations with their definition.

_____ 1. PND	a. intensive care unit
_____ 2. RT	b. partial pressure of oxygen
	c. registered respiratory therapist
_____ 3. ICU	d. tuberculosis
_____ 4. AS	e. North American Breathing Corporation
	f. postnasal drip
_____ 5. URI	g. urinary tract infection
_____ 6. ABG	h. doctor of chiropractic
	i. right ear
_____ 7. DC	j. nebulizing mist treatment
_____ 8. NMT	k. arterial blood gases
	l. left ear
_____ 9. RRT	m. upper respiratory infection
_____ 10. NBRC	n. respiratory therapy (department)
	o. arteriobiogram
	p. National Board of Respiratory Care
	q. dentist

Abbreviation Fill-ins
Fill in the blanks with the correct abbreviation.

11. pulmonary edema _____

12. pulmonary function test _____

13. carbon dioxide _____

14. respiration (rate) _____

15. chronic obstructive pulmonary disease _____

16. registered records administrator _____

Matching
Match the breathing term on the left with its desctription on the right.

_____ 1. apnea	a. difficult (painful) breathing
_____ 2. hemoptysis	b. fast breathing
_____ 3. dyspnea	c. slow breathing
_____ 4. orthopnea	d. bloody sputum
_____ 5. bradypnea	e. absence of breathing
_____ 6. tachypnea	f. best breathing when sitting up

▶ CASE STUDIES

Write the term next to its meaning given below. Then, draw slashes to analyze the word parts. Note the use of medical abbreviations. Look these up in your dictionary or find them in Appendix B. If you have any questions about the answers, refer to your medical dictionary or check with your instructor for the answers in Appendix A.

CASE STUDY 13-1
CONSULTATION NOTE

Pt: male, age 11

Dx: 1. status asthmaticus

    2. probable viral syndrome

Peter Puffer is an eleven-year-old boy with no known previous history of asthma, although he does have a history of bronchitis during which he has had episodes of wheezing. Master Puffer has had respiratory symptoms and fever since Monday morning and now has increasing respiratory distress on the day of admission. He was seen in the office of Dr. Neumo who reported tightness in the chest. Pulse oximetry revealed an O_2 saturation of 83%. Peter Puffer was therefore sent to the hospital, treated overnight with oxygen, intravenous Aminophylline and Bronkosol, as well as IV Zinacef. He appears to be more comfortable at this point with less tachypnea and better oxygen saturation.

1. inflammation of the bronchi   _____

2. heart rate   _____

3. fast breathing   _____

4. within a vein   _____

5. measurement of oxygen   _____

6. oxygen symbol   _____

7. percent symbol   _____

8. pertaining to breathing   _____

9. spasms of the bronchi   _____

10. pertaining to a virus   _____

▶ CROSSWORD PUZZLE

Check your answers by going back through the frames or checking the solutions in Appendix C.

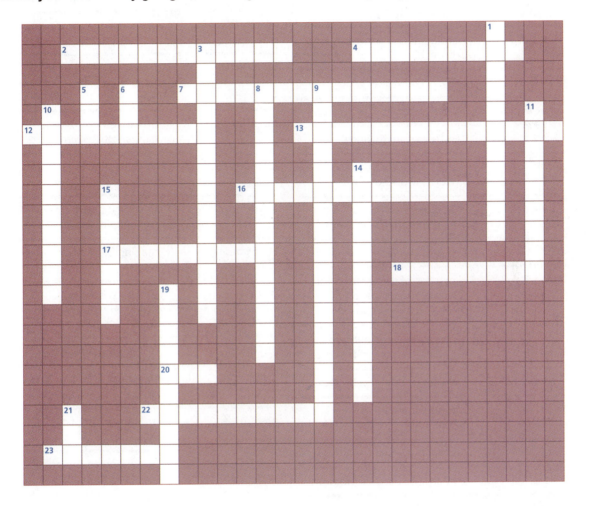

Across

2. instrument to look at the voice box
4. sit up straight to breath
7. cancer-fighting drugs
12. synonym for gerontology
13. condition known as athlete's foot
16. DC
17. pertaining to lung
18. synonym for pleuritis
20. arterial blood gases (abbreviation)
22. inflamed bronchi
23. moving clot

Down

1. right-footed
3. left-handed
5. upper respiratory infection
6. pulmonary function test (abbreviation)
8. back of the throat up near the nose (adj.)
9. black lung disease
10. coughing up blood (bloody sputum)
11. study of tissues
14. new permanent opening in the windpipe
15. difficulty breathing
19. foot doctor
21. podiatrist (abbreviation)

GLOSSARY

apnea	absence of breathing
bradypnea	slow breathing
bronchitis	inflammation of the bronchi
broncholith	bronchial stone
bronchorrhagia	hemorrhage of the bronchi
bronchorrhaphy	suture of the bronchi
bronchoscopy	examination of the bronchi with a bronchoscope
bronchospasm	uncontrolled contraction of the bronchial muscles
chiroplasty	surgical repair of the hand
chiropractic	practice of using hands for therapeutic spinal and skull manipulation, a philosophy of medicine based on musculoskeletal alignment and holistic health practices
chiropractor	doctor of chiropractic (DC)
dermatomycosis	fungal infection of the skin (mycodermatitis)
dextral	pertaining to the right
dextrocardia	heart displaced to the right
dextrogastria	stomach displaced to the right
dyspnea	difficulty (painful) breathing
embolus	moving blood clot (embolism)
endotracheal	inside the trachea
fungi	plural of fungus
geriatrics	medical specialty studying aging and related diseases (gerontology)

hyperpnea	increase in depth and rate of breathing
laryngalgia	larynx pain (laryngodynia)
laryngitis	inflammation of the voice box (larynx)
laryngocele	herniation of the larynx
laryngopathy	any disease of the larynx
laryngoscope	an instrument used to examine the larynx
laryngospasm	uncontrolled contraction of the vocal cords
laryngostomy	making a new permanent opening in the larynx
laryngotomy	making an incision into the larynx
larynx	the voice box
manual	pertaining to the hands
mycoid	resembling a fungus
mycology	the science and study of fungi
nasoantritis	inflammation of the nose and antrum
nasofrontal	pertaining to the nasal and frontal bones
nasolacrimal	pertaining to the nose and lacrimal ducts
nasomental	pertaining to the nose and chin
nasopharyngeal	pertaining to the nasopharynx (nose and pharynx)
nasophryngitis	inflammation of the nose and throat
nasoscope	instrument used to examine the nose
orthopnea	dyspnea when lying down (straight) or any position other than sitting or standing

▶ GLOSSARY

otorhino-laryngologist	physician specialist in diseases of the ear, nose, and throat
pedal	pertaining to the foot
pedialgia	foot pain (podalgia)
pediatrician	physician specialist in children's diseases and development
pharyngocele	herniation (weakening of the wall) of the throat
pharyngomycosis	fungal infection of the throat
pharyngoplasty	surgical repair of the throat
pharyngoscope	instrument used to examine the throat
pharynx	throat
phrenectomy	excision of part of the phrenic nerve (phrenicectomy)
phrenoplegia	paralysis of the diaphragm
pleural	pertaining to the pleura
pleuralgia	pleural membrane pain (pleurodynia)
pleurectomy	excision of part of the pleura
pleurisy	inflammation of the pleura (pleuritis)
pleurocentesis	surgical puncture of the pleura to remove fluid
pleurolith	stone in the pleural cavity
pneumohemothorax	air and blood in the thoracic cavity
pneumometer	instrument for measuring air volume
pneumonectomy	excision of the lung
pneumonia	inflammation of the lung
pneumonocentesis	surgical puncture of the lung to remove fluid (pneumocentesis)
pneumonomelanosis	black lung disease
pneumonomycosis	fungus infection of the lung
pneumonopathy	any lung disease
pneumonopexy	surgical fixation of a prolapsed lung (pneumonoplasty)
pneumonorrhagia	hemorrhage of the lung
pneumonotomy	incision into the lung
pneumotherapy	treatment using air
pneumothorax	air in the thoracic cavity
podiatrist	specialist in care of conditions of the feet; may also perform surgery of the foot
psychiatrist	physician specialist in mental disorders
pulmonary	pertaining to the lung (pulmonic)
rhinomycosis	fungal infection in the nose
sinistral	pertaining to the left
tachypnea	fast breathing
trachea	windpipe
trachealgia	tracheal pain
tracheocele	herniation of the tracheal wall
tracheopyosis	condition of pus in the trachea
tracheorrhagia	hemorrhage of the trachea
tracheoscopy	process of inspecting the trachea
tracheostomy	surgical creation of an opening in the trachea
tracheotomy	incision into the trachea

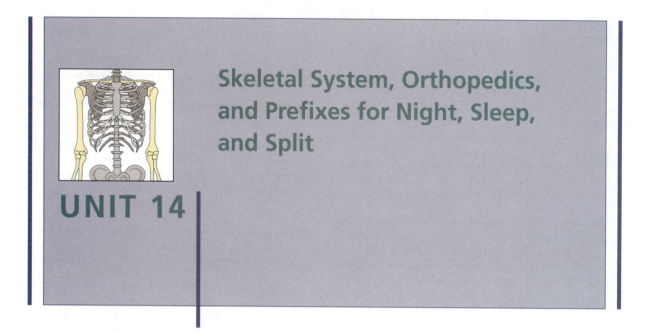

UNIT 14

Skeletal System, Orthopedics, and Prefixes for Night, Sleep, and Split

night	**14.1** There are two combining forms that mean night. One is Latin, **noct/i**, the other is Greek, **nyct/o**. Noct/i/luca are microscopic marine animals that make the ocean glow during the _____.
night	**14.2** Those of you who have studied music know that a noct/urne is dreamy music, sometimes called _____ music.
🏛 WORD ORIGIN	**14.3** In Greek mythology sleep and death were related to night. Somnus (Sleep) and Thanatos (Death) were the sons of Nox (Night).
able to walk a vehicle for transporting the sick (who can't walk)	**14.4** **ambul**, from the Latin *ambulare*, is a word root meaning walk. Look up the meaning of these terms about walking: ambul/atory *_____; ambul/ance *_____.
noct/ambul/ism nok **tam**´ byōō lizm	**14.5** **ambul** is the word root for walk. Noct/ambul/ism literally means walking at night. Sleepwalking is what you mean when you use the word _____ /_____ /_____.

424

ANSWER COLUMN

somn/ambul/ism som **nam´** by$\overline{oo}$ lizm	**14.6** **somn** is the word root for sleep. A more common term for sleepwalking is _____ /_____ /_____.
somnambulism	**14.7** Sleepwalking can occur at any age, but childhood is the most common age for _____.
somnambulism	**14.8** People are not really asleep when they sleepwalk. They appear to be asleep but are really suppressing the memory of what they do. They are indulging in _____.
night	**14.9** **nyct/o** is another combining form for night. It comes from the Greek word *nyx*. Nyct/algia means pain during the _____.
night	**14.10** Nyct/albumin/uria means the presence of albumin in the urine only during the _____.
nyct/al/opia nik´ tə **lō´** pē ə	**14.11** Nyct/al/opia means night blindness or difficulty in seeing at night. Vitamin A is associated with night vision. Lack of vitamin A in the diet is one cause of _____ /_____ /_____. **NOTE: al** comes from the Greek *alaos*, meaning blind. Nyctalopia literally means night blind vision.
nyctalopia	**14.12** Nyct/al/opia has several causes. Retinal fatigue from exposure to very bright light is a cause of _____.
nyctalopia	**14.13** Retinitis pigmentosa is another cause of _____.

nyct/o/phobia
nik´ tō **fō´** bē ə
noct/i/phobia
nok´ ti **fō´** bē ə
nyct/o/philia
nik´ tō **fil´** ē ə
noct/i/philia
nok´ ti **fil´** ē ə
	14.14
	Using **nyct/o** and **noct/i** build two words that mean
	   abnormal fear of night
	   _____ /_____ /_____
	   _____ /_____ /_____;
	   unusual attraction to the night
	   _____ /_____ /_____
	   _____ /_____ /_____.

ANSWER COLUMN	
nyct/uria nik **tyoor**′ ē ə	**14.15** Noct/uria means excessive urination during the night. Another word that means the same thing is _____ /_____.
nyct/uria noct/uria	**14.16** Two words that mean excessive urination during the night are _____ /_____ and _____ /_____.
immovable eyelids	**14.17** **ankyl/o** means immovable or fixed. Ankylosed means stiffened. Ankyl/o/blephar/on means adhesions resulting in *_____.
immobility	**14.18** Ankyl/osis, such as in ankylosing spondylitis, is a condition of _____ of the spine.

Use the following table to build words for Frames 14.19–14.21.

Combining Form	Noun
aden/o (gland)	aden/ia
cardi/o (heart)	cardi/a
cheil/o (lips)	cheil/ia
dactyl/o (digits)	dactyl/ia
dent/o (teeth)	dent/ia
derm/o (skin)	derm/a
	derm/ia
gastr/o (stomach)	gastr/ia
gloss/o (tongue)	gloss/ia
onych/o (nails)[a]	onych/ia
ophthalm/o (eyes)[a]	ophthalm/ia
ot/o (ears)	ot/ia
phag/o (eat)	phag/ia
pneumon/o (lung)	pneumon/ia
proct/o (anus + rectum)	proct/ia
urethr/o (urethra)	urethr/a
[a]new in Unit 15	

NOTE: The **-ia** suffix means condition.

▶ **ANSWER COLUMN**

14.19
Ankyl/o/stoma means lockjaw (stiff mouth). Build words meaning
(remember, you may look back)
   adhesions of lips (immovable lips)

ankyl/o/cheilia
ang´ ki lō **kī**´ lē ə
ankyl/o/proctia
ang´ ki lō **prok**´ shē ə
ankyl/o/phobia
ang´ ki lō **fō**´ bē ə

     _____ /____ /_____ ;
   closure (immobility) of the anus and rectum
     _____ /____ /_____ ;
   abnormal fear of ankylosis
     _____ /____ /_____ .

14.20
Build words meaning
   tongue tied (stiff tongue)

ankyl/o/glossia
ang´ ki lō **glos**´ ē ə
ankyl/o/dactylia
ang´ ki lō dak **til**´ ē ə

     _____ /____ /_____ ;
   adhesions of fingers (immovable fingers) or toes
     _____ /____ /_____ .

noun
condition

14.21
-ia is a (choose one) _____ (noun/adjective/verb) suffix
meaning _____ .

14.22
-stasis is used as a suffix and means stopping or controlling.
To say that you control an organ or what that organ
produces, use the combining form for the organ
or product (**viscer/o**) plus the word _____

stasis
viscer/o/stasis
vi´ ser **os**´ tə sis

to form _____ /____ /_____ .

stopped or controlled

14.23
Fung/i/stasis is a condition in which the growth of fungi is
*_____ .

control or stopping of
   bile flow

14.24
Chol/e/stasis means
*_____ .

14.25
Read Frame 14.22 again. Build words meaning
   controlling the small intestine

enter/o/stasis
en´ tə **ros**´ tə sis
py/o/stasis
pī **os**´ tə sis

     _____ /____ /_____ ;
   stopping the formation of pus
     ____ /____ /_____ .

ANSWER COLUMN

hem/o/stasis
hē **mos**′ tə sis
phleb/o/stasis or
fleb **os**′ tə sis
ven/o/stasis
vēn **os**′ tə sis
arteri/o/stasis
är tir′ ē **os**′ tə sis
	14.26
	Build words meaning
	  controlling the flow of blood
	  _____ /_____ /_____ ;
	  checking flow in the veins
	  _____ /_____ /_____ ;
	  checking flow in the arteries
	  _____ /_____ /_____ .

schizo/phas/ia
skit′ zō **fā**′ sē ə
schiz/onych/ia
skit′ zō **nik**′ ē ə
	14.27
	schizo- (prefix), schisto- (prefix), and -schisis (suffix) have a
	complicated evolution from Greek. They mean split, cleft, or
	fissure. Build words meaning split
	  speech (incomprehensible speech)
	  _____ /_____ /_____ ;
	  nails (**onych/o**)—condition
	  _____ /_____ /_____ .
	NOTE: schizo- and schisto- are combining forms used as prefixes.

schizo/phren/ia skit′ zō **fre**′ nē ə	**14.28** Schiz/o/phren/ia literally means split mind. It is really a group of severe mental disorders in which thinking, emotions, and behavior are disturbed. A person with delusions of persecution, jealousy, and hallucinations may suffer from paranoid _____ /_____ /_____ .
schizophrenia	**14.29** Anti/psych/otic medications and psych/o/therapy are treatments used for those with _____ .

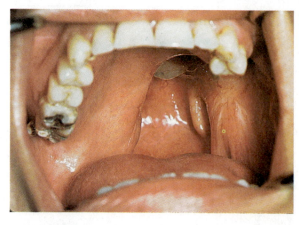

Cleft palate (Courtesy of Dr. Joseph Konzelman, School of Dentistry, Medical College of Georgia)

► **ANSWER COLUMN**

14.30
A fissure is a troughlike cleft in a structure.
Build words using schisto-:
  split tongue
  _____ /_____ /____;
  split cell (cell with a fissure)
  _____ /____ /_____;
  split chest (fissure)
  _____ /____ /_____.

schisto/gloss/ia
shis′ tō **glos**′ ē ə
schist/o/cyte
shis′ tō sīt
schist/o/thorax
shis′ tō **thôr**′ aks

14.31
Build words using -schisis as a suffix:
  cleft palate (**palat/o**)
  _____ /____ /_____;
  cleft palate (**uran/o**)
  _____ /____ /_____;
  split spine (**rach/i**)
  _____ /____ /_____.

palat/o/schisis
pal ə **tos**′ ki sis
uran/o/schisis
yōōr ə **nos**′ ki sis
rach/i/schisis
rā **kis**′ ki sis

eeee *TAKE A CLOSER LOOK*

14.32
Look up spina bifida in your dictionary. This condition is synonymous with rachischisis. Read about the two types and write notes here:
_____
_____

14.33
In your dictionary, read about the disease schistosomiasis and Schistosoma. Schistosomiasis is a very important disease in terms lof world health. Because of increased worldwide travel, all people should be concerned with the disease
_____ /_____ /_____.

schisto/som/iasis
shis′ tō sō **mī**′ ə sis

14.34
Learn the words involving the combining forms used as prefixes and suffixes for "split" that you need to know. Surely schizophrenia will be one of them. schizo-, schisto-, and -schisis mean _____.

split

14.35
Carpos is a Greek word meaning wrist. Locate the carpus. The plural of carpus is _____.

carpi
kär′ pī

14.36
From carpus and carpi, derive a word root that refers to the wrist. It is _____.

carp

430   Unit 14

ANSWER COLUMN	
carp/al kär′ pəl	**14.37** Carpal tunnel syndrome is an occupational hazard to court reporters and others who do a lot of typing. The adjectival form for carpus is _____ /____.
carp/o	**14.38** Look at the words (in your medical dictionary) that begin with **carp**. The combining form that is used in words about the wrist is _____ /____.

carp/al
kär′ pəl
carp/o/meta/carp/al
kär′ pō **met**′ ə kär pəl
carp/ectomy
kär **pek**′ tə mē
	14.39
	Close your dictionary. Build words meaning
	    pertaining to the wrist (adjective)
	    _____ /____;
	    pertaining to the wrist and metacarpals
	    _____ /____ /_____ /_____ /____;
	    excision of all or part of the wrist
	    _____ /_____.

wrist	**14.40** **carp/o** in a word refers to the _____.

Bones of the left hand

▶ **ANSWER COLUMN**

meta/carp/als met´ ə **kär**´ palz	**14.41** Recall that meta- means beyond. The bones in the hand "beyond" the carpals are called the _____ /_____ /_____.
meta/tarsals met´ ə **tar**´ salz	**14.42** Refer to the illustration of the foot on page 432. **tars/o** is the combining form for the tarsal bones. From what you already know about the prefix meta-, name the bones that are located beyond the tarsals: _____ /_____.
wrist ankle	**14.43** Locate the following bones: carpals _____; tarsals _____.

TAKE A CLOSER LOOK

14.44
The bones that protrude from the ankles on the inside and out are really parts of two bones. Look at the illustration of the bones of the foot. The lateral maleolus is a protrusion on the fibula bone. The medial maleolus is a protrusion on the distal end of the tibia.

Professional Profiles ◀◀◀◀◀◀◀◀◀◀◀◀◀◀◀◀◀◀◀◀◀◀◀◀◀◀◀◀◀◀◀◀

Registered occupational therapists (OTRs)— The American Occupational Therapy Association (AOTA) information brochure defines occupational therapy as "the use of purposeful activity with individuals who are limited by physical injury or illness, psychosocial dysfunction, developmental or learning disabilities, poverty and cultural differences, or the aging process to maximize independence, prevent disability, and maintain health. The practice encompasses evaluation, treatment, and consultation." Preparation for this profession requires completion of a baccalaureate degree from an approved college including an internship experience. An occupational therapist may specialize in a particular area of expertise such as hand therapy or substance abuse rehabilitation.

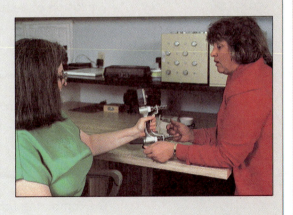

Occupational therapist assisting patient with grip strength test (Photo by Marcia Butterfield, courtesy of Foote Memorial Hospital, Jackson, MI)

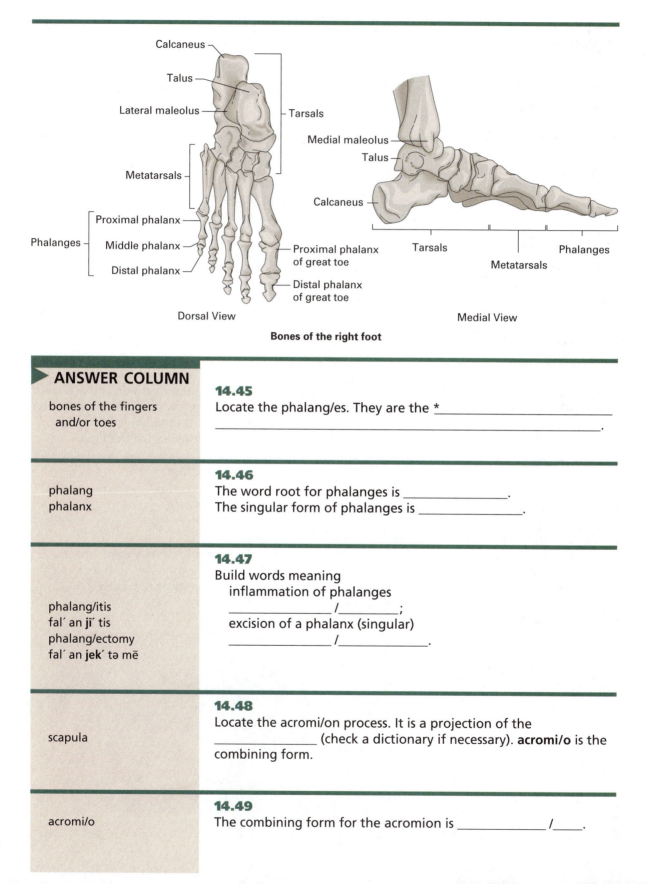

Bones of the right foot

ANSWER COLUMN	
bones of the fingers and/or toes	**14.45** Locate the phalang/es. They are the *_____ _____.
phalang phalanx	**14.46** The word root for phalanges is _____. The singular form of phalanges is _____.

phalang/itis
fal´ an **jī**´ tis
phalang/ectomy
fal´ an **jek**´ tə mē
	14.47
	Build words meaning
	   inflammation of phalanges
	   _____ /_____;
	   excision of a phalanx (singular)
	   _____ /_____.

scapula	**14.48** Locate the acromi/on process. It is a projection of the _____ (check a dictionary if necessary). **acromi/o** is the combining form.
acromi/o	**14.49** The combining form for the acromion is _____ /____.

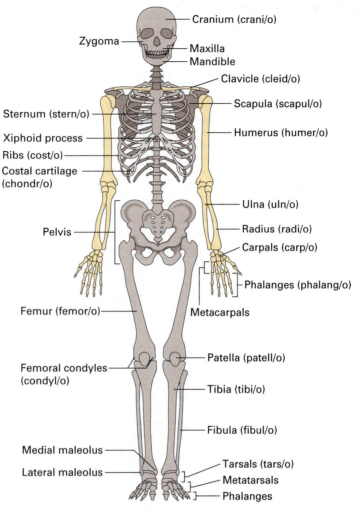

Skeletal system

ANSWER COLUMN

14.50
Find words in your dictionary meaning
    pertaining to the acromion
acromi/al
    _____ /____;
ə **krō**´ mē əl
    pertaining to the acromion and humerus
acromi/o/humer/al
    _____ /____ /humer/al;
ə krō´ mē ō **hyōō**´ mər əl
    pertaining to the acromion and the clavicle
acromi/o/clavicul/ar
    _____ /____ /clavicul/ar.
ə krō´ mē ō kla **vik**´ yōō lar

14.51
Look at Frame 14.50. Can it start you looking for another
combining form? Try. It is _____ /____.

humer/o

ANSWER COLUMN	**14.52** **humer/o** is used in words to refer to the bone of the upper arm, which is named the _____.
humerus	
(pick three out of four) humeral humeroradial humeroscapular humeroulnar	**14.53** Find three words in your dictionary that begin with **humer** or **humer/o**. They are _____ ; _____ ; _____ .
TAKE A CLOSER LOOK	**14.54** Look up the term fracture in your medical dictionary. You should find at least ten different types of fractures described. Read about them and study the illustration of fractures. Notice that some are closed, some open, some complete, incomplete, displaced, and some not. Write the terms of interest in your notebook and then take a "break."

Normal   Greenstick (incomplete)   Closed (simple, complete)   Open (compound)   Comminuted

Proximal portion of bone · Middle (medial) portion of bone · Distal portion of bone · Transverse · Oblique · Displaced · Linear

Types of bone fractures

radi/o/ulnar rā´ dē ō ul´ nar	**14.55** The radius (**radi/o**) and ulna (**uln/o**) are located in the forearm. If both are fractured, it would be described as a _____ / ____ / _____ fracture. (Abbreviation: FxBB, fracture of both bones.)
condyl	**14.56** Refer back to the drawing of the skeleton. Locate a condyle. A condyle is a rounded process that occurs on many bones. The word root for condyle is _____.

► **ANSWER COLUMN**

 INFORMATION FRAME

14.57
Falls, bumps, crashes, and disease that put stress on bones often cause cracks and breaks called fractures. Study the following table to learn about how these fractures are described; then, compare them to your notebook dictionary research and the illustration on page 434.

Fracture Facts	
Complete	through the width of the bone
Incomplete	not through the width of the bone
Closed	also called simple (skin is not broken)
Open	also called compound (bone ends protrude through the skin)
Pathologic	diseased area that weakens the bone
Fracture reduction and fixation:	
Closed manipulation	movement of body part to cause bone ends to align without surgery
Internal fixation	screws or nails in bone under the skin (ORIF)
External fixation	screws attached to an external bar (ORIF)

condyles
kon´ dīlz

14.58
Two rounded processes at the medial and lateral distal ends of the femur are the femoral _____.

femur
fē´ mer
femor/al
fem´ er əl

14.59
In Latin *femur* means thigh. **femor/o** is the combining form for the longest bone in the body, the femur (thigh bone—notice the spelling). Look at the illustration of the skeleton. The proximal end of the _____ is part of the hip joint. The artery that supplies blood to the leg is called the _____ /_____ artery.

✔ *SPELL CHECK*

14.60
Watch the spelling of femur as it changes to femor/o to make the combining form.

ANSWER COLUMN	

	14.61
	A rounded bony process on the femur is a condyle.
	Build words meaning
	  excision of a condyle
	  _____ /_____;
	  resembling a condyle
	  _____ /_____;
	  upon a condyle
	  _____ /_____.

ANSWER COLUMN

14.61
A rounded bony process on the femur is a condyle.
Build words meaning
  excision of a condyle
  _____ /_____;
  resembling a condyle
  _____ /_____;
  upon a condyle
  _____ /_____.

condyl/ectomy
kon´ di **lek**´ tə mē
condyl/oid
kon´ di loid
epi/condyle
ep i **kon**´ dil

14.62
Condyl/ar is an adjective meaning pertaining to a
_____.

condyle

14.63
Locate the calcaneus bone (also: calcaneum). The plural of
calcaneus is _____.

calcanea
kal **kā**´ nē ə

14.64
From calcaneus and calcanea, derive the word root for the heel:
_____.

calcane

14.65
In your medical dictionary, look at the words beginning with
calcane. Derive the combining form that is used in words that
refer to the heel: _____ /_____.

calcane/o

14.66
Close your dictionary. Now build words meaning
  pertaining to the heel
  _____ /_____;
  pain in the heel
  _____ /_____ /_____
  or
  _____ /_____.

calcane/al
kal **kā**´ nē əl
calcane/o/dynia
kal kā´ nē ō **din**´ ē ə
calcane/algia
kal kā nē **al**´ jē ə

14.67
The bones of the pelvis include the ischium, ilium, and pubis.
Locate them and their combining forms in the illustration on
page 437. Write the combining forms below:
  ischium _____ /_____;
  ilium _____ /_____;
  pubis _____ /_____.

ischi/o
ili/o
pub/o

The pelvis—anterior view

Sacrum (sacr/o)
Sacroiliac joint
Iliac crest (ili/o)
Ilium (ili/o)
Anterior superior iliac spine
Coccyx (coccyg/o)
Acetabulum
Ischial spine (ischi/o)
Obturator foramen
Ischium (ischi/o)
Symphysis pubis (pub/o)

ANSWER COLUMN

✓ *SPELL CHECK*

14.68
It is easy to confuse ilium with ileum because they are pronounced the same and differ by only one letter in spelling. Remember i-l-e-um because it is part of the small intestine of the digestive system and the "e" reminds us of "eat." The combining forms are also spelled differently, ile/o for ileum (small intestine) and il*i*/o for ilium (pelvic bone).

14.69
From what you have just learned, try this question. In which body system would you find the ile/i/cecal valve?

digestive system

_____

In which body system would you find the il*i*ac crest?

skeletal system

_____

Good try!

CONGRATULATIONS!

14.70
You are now finding your own combining forms. Feels good, doesn't it? Let's do some more.

---

ischia
is´ kē ə

14.71
Locate the ischium. The plural of ischium is _____.
Refer to the illustration above.

---

ischi
ischi/o

14.72
From ischium and ischia, derive a word root that refers to the part of the hip bone on which the body rests when sitting. The word root is _____; the combining form is _____ /____.

► **ANSWER COLUMN**

	14.73
	In your dictionary, find words meaning
	pertaining to ischium and rectum
ischi/o/rect/al	_____ /____ /_____ /____;
is´ kē ō **rek**´ təl	neuralgic pain in the hip (synonym is sciatica)
ischi/o/neuralgia	_____ /____ /_____;
is´ kē ō nōō **ral**´ jē ə	pertaining to the ischium and pubis
ischi/o/pub/ic	_____ /____ /_____ /____.
is´ kē ō **pyōō**´ bik	

	14.74
	Close your dictionary. Build words meaning
	pertaining to the ischium
ischi/al	_____ /____;
is´ kē əl	herniation through the ischium
ischi/o/cele	_____ /____ /_____.
is´ kē ō sēl	

	14.75
	ischi/o in a word refers to the part of the hip bone known as the
ischium	_____.
is´ kē əm	

	14.76
	Locate the pubis in the illustration on page 437. The plural of
pubes	pubis is _____. The combining form is _____ /____.
pyōō´ bēz	
pub/o	

	14.77
	Close your dictionary. Recall that **femor/o** is the combining
	form for femur. Using **pub/o** and **femor/o**, build a word
	meaning pertaining to the pubis and femur:
pub/o/femor/al	_____ /____ /_____ /____.
pyōō bō **fem**´ ər əl	

	14.78
	Use the diagram on page 433 to locate the sternum. The
stern/o	combining form for sternum is _____ /____.

	14.79
	With your dictionary open, find words meaning
	pertaining to the sternum and pericardium
stern/o/peri/cardi/al	_____ /____ /_____ /_____ /____;
stûr´ nō per i **kärd**´ ē əl	pertaining to the sternum and ribs
stern/o/cost/al	_____ /____ /_____ /____.
stûr´ nō **kos**´ təl	

ANSWER COLUMN	

stern/al
stern/algia
stern/o/dynia
(You pronounce)
	14.80
	Close the dictionary. Build words meaning
	    pertaining to the sternum _____ /____;
	    pain in the sternum _____ /_____ or
	    _____ /____ /_____.

sternum breastbone	**14.81** **stern/o** in a word makes you think of the _____, which is the _____.
xiph/o/cost/al zi′ fō kos′ təl	**14.82** Recall **cost/o** refers to ribs. The xiphoid (from the Greek *xiphos*, meaning sword) process is the projection at the inferior end of the sternum. **xiph/o** is the combining form. A word meaning pertaining to the xiphoid process and the ribs is _____/____/_____/____.
gangli/o	**14.83** The plural of gangli/on is gangli/a. A gangli/on is a collection of nerve cell bodies. Now that you have a system, form the word root/combining form for ganglion: _____ /____.
ganglia	**14.84** The main cerebral nerve centers are called the cerebral _____.
gangli/on gangli/a	**14.85** Any one of three neural masses found in the cervical region is called a cervical _____ /____, whereas all three are referred to as the cervical _____ /____.
backbone	**14.86** You are now ready to find word roots and their combining forms by another method. Look up the word spine in your dictionary. A synonym for spine is _____.
spine	**14.87** Look in your dictionary for words beginning with **rach**. **rach** is the word root for _____.
rach/itis or rə **kī**′ tis spondyl/itis spon di **lī**′ tis	**14.88** There are two word roots that mean spine. One is **rach** (**rachi/o**), the other is **spondyl** (**spondyl/o**). Build a word that means inflammation of the spine: _____ /_____.

spine

14.89
Words beginning with the combining forms **rachi/o** or **spondyl/o**
refer to the _____.

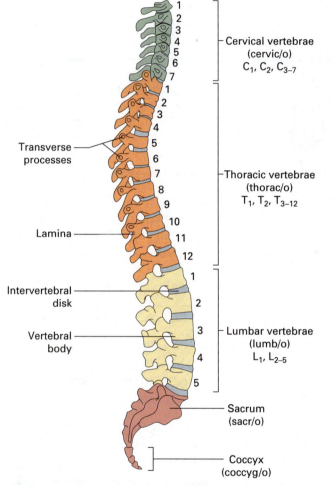

Cervical vertebrae
(cervic/o)
C_1, C_2, C_{3-7}

Thoracic vertebrae
(thorac/o)
T_1, T_2, T_{3-12}

Transverse
processes

Lamina

Intervertebral
disk

Vertebral
body

Lumbar vertebrae
(lumb/o)
L_1, L_{2-5}

Sacrum
(sacr/o)

Coccyx
(coccyg/o)

Spinal column

14.90
Using **rachi/o**, build words meaning
  spine pain
  _____ /_____;
  incision into the spine
  _____ /_____ /_____.

rachi/algia
rā´ kē **al**´ jē ə
rachi/o/tomy
rā´ kē **ot**´ ō mē

ANSWER COLUMN	

14.91
Using **rachi/o**, build words meaning
   a synonym for rachialgia
   _____ /_____ /_____;
   instrument to measure spinal curvature
   _____ /_____ /_____;
   spinal paralysis
   _____ /_____ /_____.

rachi/o/dynia
rā´ kē ō **din´** ē ə
rachi/o/meter
rā´ kē **om´** ə tər
rachi/o/plegia
rā´ kē ō **plē´** jē ə

14.92
In the same manner, using **rach/i**, build words meaning
   fissure of the spine (split spine)
   _____ /_____;
   inflammation of the spine
   _____ /_____.

rachi/schisis
rā **kis´** kis is
rach/itis
rā **kī´** tis

14.93

Ⓔ eee *TAKE A CLOSER LOOK*

There are basically three types of spinal curvature, including kyphosis (posterior curvature), lordosis (anterior curvature), and scoliosis (lateral curvature). Refer back to the illustration in Unit 12, page 383.

The following word parts refer to regions of the spine.

Combining Form	Adjective
cervic/o	cervical
thorac/o	thoracic
lumb/o	lumbar
sacr/o	sacral
coccyg/o	coccygeal

14.94
A device used to immobilize the neck is a _____ collar.

cervical

14.95
Cervic/al traction is applied as a treatment for an injured _____.

neck

14.96
Recall that the cervix is the neck of the uterus. The plural of cervix is _____.

cervices

> ANSWER COLUMN

14.97
Build a combining form for cervix. The combining form takes **o**.
The combining form is _____ /_____.

cervic/o
sûr′ vi kō

14.98
Build words meaning
   excision of the cervix
   _____ /_____;
   inflammation of the cervix
   _____ /_____;
   pertaining to the cervix
   _____ /_____.

cervic/ectomy
sûr′ vi **sek′** tō mē
cervic/itis
sûr′ vi **sī′** tis
cervic/al
sûr′ vi kəl

INFORMATION
FRAME

14.99
cervic/o can mean the neck as well as the neck of the uterus. In usage you are not likely to confuse them. The next frame will make the point. Refer to the illustration of the spinal column on page 440.

14.100
Cervic/o/faci/al means pertaining to the face and _____.
Cervic/o/brachi/al means pertaining to the arm and _____.
Cervic/o/vesic/al means pertaining to the bladder and
*_____.

neck
neck

the neck of the uterus

14.101
brachi/o is the combining form for arm. It is used to describe bones and blood vessels in the arm. The biceps brachii is a muscle in the _____. The brachial artery is an artery in the_____.

arm
arm

14.102
The muscle that extends from the upper arm to the radius bone is the _____ /_____ /_____ /_____ muscle.

brachi/o/radi/alis
brā′ kē ō rā dē **al′** is

14.103
Build words that mean pertaining to the
   artery of the arm
   _____ /_____;
   arm and radius muscle
   _____ /_____ /_____ /_____;
   arm and head
   _____ /_____ /_____ /_____.

brachi/al
brā′ kē əl
brachi/o/radi/alis
brā′ kē ō rā dē **al′** is
brachi/o/cephal/ic
brā′ kē ō se **fal′** ik

▶ **ANSWER COLUMN**

sacr/o/ili/ac
sak rō **il′** ē ak

14.104
The joint between the sacrum and the ilium is the
_____ /____ /_____ /____ joint.

---

thorac/o/lumbar
thôr′ ə kō **lum′** bär
sacr/o/sciat/ic
sak′ rō sī **a′** tik
coccyg/ectomy
kok′ si **jek′** tō mē

14.105
Build terms meaning
   pertaining to the thorax and lumbar spines
   _____ /____ /_____;
   pertaining to the sacrum and the sciatic nerve
   _____ /____ /_____ /____;
   removal of the coccyx
   _____ /_____.

---

cervic/al
thorac/ic
sacr/al
coccyg/eal

14.106
Provide the adjectival forms for
   cervix _____ /____;
   thorax _____ /____;
   sacrum _____ /____;
   coccyx _____ /_____.

---

lamin/ectomy
lam′ in **ek′** tō mē

14.107
A lamina (**lamin/o**) is a thin, flat sheet, plate, or membrane. A
lamin/ectomy is the removal of the lamina of the vertebral
posterior arch that has been ruptured (ruptured disk). One
treatment to repair an intervertebral disk herniation may be
_____ /_____.

---

disk/ectomy
dis **kek′** tō mē
myel/o/gram
mī′ el ō gram

14.108
disk is the word root for intervertebral disk. A myel/o/gram (spinal
x-ray) is used to diagnose disk herniation. Removal of a herniated
disk is called a _____ /_____. Then, spinal fusion may
be performed. The x-ray that can be used to view the spine is a
_____ /____ /_____.

Abbreviation	Meaning
AMB	ambulate, ambulatory
AOTA	American Occupational Therapy Association
C_1, C_2, C_{3-7}	cervical vertebrae 1–7
DPM	podiatrist (doctor of podiatric medicine)
Fx	fracture
FxBB	fracture both bones
hs	hour of sleep (*hora somni*), at bedtime
L_1, L_2, L_{3-5}	lumbar vertebrae 1–5
LP	lumbar puncture
lt, L	left
OREF	open reduction with external fixation
ORIF	open reduction with internal fixation
ORTH	orthopedist, orthopedics
OTR	registered occupational therapist
qn	every night
rt, R	right
T_1, T_2, T_{3-12}	thoracic vertebrae 1–12
y/o, yrs	years old (years)

To complete your study of this unit, work the review activities on the next pages. Also, listen to the audiotapes that accompany *Medical Terminology: A Programmed Text,* 8th edition, and practice your pronunciation.

Additional practice exercises for this unit are available on the Student Practice disk found in the back of the textbook.

▶ REVIEW ACTIVITIES

Circle and Correct
Circle the correct answer for each question. Then, check your answers in Appendix A.

1. Combining form for night:
    a. narco   b. necro
    c. nycto   d. noct

2. Suffix meaning in the urine:
    a. -uro   b. -uremia
    c. -urine   d. -uria

3. Word root for immovable or fixed:
    a. syn   b. ankyl
    c. stasis   d. spondyl

4. Noun ending:
    a. -ia   b. -ic
    c. -ous   d. -ed

5. Prefix for inward:
    a. exo-   b. meso-
    c. inner-   d. eso-

6. Suffix for split:
    a. -stasis   b. -schiz
    c. -schisis   d. -schist

7. Adjectival form for wrist bones:
    a. carpi   b. carpal
    c. carpus   d. metacarpal

8. Combining form for one of the pelvic bones:
    a. ischium   b. ileo
    c. ilio   d. ishci

9. Word root for walk:
    a. somn   b. duct
    c. kines   d. ambul

10. Suffix for control or stopping:
    a. -rrhexis   b. -stasis
    c. -schisis   d. -ectasis

11. Bony process at the end of the sternum:
    a. amnion   b. acromion
    c. xiphoid   d. phalanx

12. Combining form for spine:
    a. rachi/o   b. spondyl
    c. myel/o   d. ischi/o

▶ REVIEW ACTIVITIES

Select and Construct

Select the correct word parts from the list below and construct medical terms that represent the given meaning.

acromi/o(on)	al	algia	ambul/o	ankylo	ar
arteri/o	ate	brachi/o(al)	bulism	calcane/o	carp(o)(al)
cephalic	cervic/o(al)	clavicul/o(ar)	condyl/o(ar)	cost/o(al)	dactylia
dynia	ectomy	femor/o	fungi	humer/o(al)	ischi/o
ism	itis	meta	myco	nam	noct/i
nyct/o	opia	palat/o	phasi/o(ia)	pub(o)(is)(ic)	rachi/o
scapul/o(ar)	schisis	schizo	som	stasis	stern/o(al)
tars/o	tomy	urano	uria	xiph/o(oid)	

1. breast bone pain _____

2. pertaining to the arm and head _____

3. control of fungal growth _____

4. including the ischium and pubis _____

5. excision of a rounded bony process _____

6. split spine (spina bifida) _____

7. cleft palate _____

8. pertaining to the cartilage end of the sternum and the ribs _____

9. the bones of the hand beyond the wrist _____

10. split speech (incomprehensible) _____

11. sleepwalking _____

12. night blindness _____

13. excessive urination at night _____

14. stiffened fingers _____

▶ REVIEW ACTIVITIES

Give the correct combining form and the adjectival form for each of the following bones.

		Combining Form	Adjectival Form
skull	1.		
first seven vertebrae	2.		
clavicle	3.		
scapula	4.		
acromion process	5.		
humerus	6.		
sternum	7.		
xiphoid process	8.		
ulna	9.		
radius	10.		
carpus	11.		
metacarpus	12.		
phalanx	13.		
ischium	14.		
ilium	15.		
pubis	16.		
femur	17.		
patella	18.		
tibia	19.		
fibula	20.		
tarsus	21.		
metatarsus	22.		
calcaneus	23.		
ribs	24.		
cartilage	25.		

▶ **REVIEW ACTIVITIES**

Define and Dissect
Give a brief definition and dissect each term listed into its word parts in the space provided on the right. Check your answers by referring to the frame listed in parentheses and your medical dictionary. Then, listen to the audiotapes to practice pronunciation.

1. noctambulism (14.5)

    _____ / _____ / _____
    　　　rt　　　　　　rt　　　　　suffix

    _____
    　　　　　　　definition

2. nyctalopia (14.11)

    _____ / ____ / _____
    　　　rt　　　　rt　　　suffix

    _____

3. somnambulism (14.6)

    _____ / _____ / _____
    　　　rt　　　　　　rt　　　　　suffix

    _____

4. ankylodactylia (14.20)

    _____ / ____ / _____ / ____
    　　rt　　　v　　　　rt　　　　suffix

    _____

5. nycturia (14.15)

    _____ / ____ / ____
    　　　rt　　　rt　　suffix

    _____

6. enterostasis (14.25)

    _____ / ____ / _____
    　　rt　　　v　　　suffix

    _____

7. schizophrenia (14.28)

    _____ / _____ / ____
    　　pre　　　　rt　　　suffix

    _____

8. schistosomiasis (14.33)

    _____ / _____ / _____
    　　pre　　　　rt　　　suffix

    _____

9. palatoschisis (14.31)

    _____ / ____ / _____
    　　rt　　　v　　　suffix

    _____

10. calcaneodynia (14.66)

    _____ / ____ / _____
    　　rt　　　v　　　suffix

    _____

11. carpometacarpal (14.39)

    _____ / ____ / _____ / _____ / ____
    　　rt　　v　　　pre　　　　rt　　　suffix

    _____

12. ischioneuralgia (14.73)

    _____ / ____ / ____ / _____
    　　rt　　　v　　rt　　　suffix

    _____

▶ REVIEW ACTIVITIES

13. sternopericardial (14.79)   _____ / ___ / _____ / _____ / _____
                                     rt   v   pre   rt   suffix

14. acromiohumeral (14.50)   _____ / ___ / _____ / _____
                                     rt   v   rt   suffix

15. epicondyle (14.61)   _____ / _____
                                     pre   rt/suffix

16. ganglion (14.83)   _____ / _____
                                     rt   suffix

17. xiphocostal (14.82)   _____ / ___ / _____ / _____
                                     rt   v   rt   suffix

18. laminectomy (14.107)   _____ / _____
                                     rt   suffix

19. diskectomy (14.108)   _____ / _____
                                     rt   suffix

20. fungistasis (14.23)   _____ / ___ / _____
                                     rt   v   suffix

21. rachischisis (14.92)   _____ / _____
                                     rt   suffix

22. antipsychotic (14.29)   _____ / _____ / _____
                                     pre   rt   suffix

23. metatarsal (14.42)   _____ / _____ / _____
                                     pre   rt   suffix

24. radioulnar (14.55)   _____ / ___ / _____ / _____
                                     rt   v   rt   suffix

25. pubofemoral (14.77)   _____ / ___ / _____ / _____
                                     rt   v   rt   suffix

26. cervicobrachial (14.100)   _____ / ___ / _____ / _____
                                     rt   v   rt   suffix

▶ REVIEW ACTIVITIES

Abbreviation Matching
Match the following abbreviations with their definition.

_____ 1. ORTH

_____ 2. qn

_____ 3. hs

_____ 4. AMB

_____ 5. LP

_____ 6. L_1

_____ 7. Fx

_____ 8. T_3

a. ambulance
b. first thoracic vertebra
c. fracture
d. orthodontist
e. bedtime
f. every night
g. ambulate
h. first lumbar vertebra
i. twice a night
j. long-playing record
k. lumbar puncture
l. orthopedist
m. third thoracic vertebra

Abbreviation Fill-ins
Fill in the blanks with the correct abbreviation.

9. third cervical vertebra _____

10. fracture of both bones _____

11. registered occupational therapist _____

12. American Occupational Therapy Association _____

13. right _____

14. years old _____

15. open reduction with internal fixation _____

▶ CASE STUDIES

Write the term next to its meaning given below. Then, draw slashes to analyze the word parts. Note the use of medical abbreviations. Look these up in your dictionary or find them in Appendix B. If you have any questions about the answers, refer to your medical dictionary or check with your instructor for the answers in Appendix A.

CASE STUDY 14-1
OPERATIVE REPORT

Pt: **M**, 15 **y/o**

Dx: **Fx lateral** condyle, **rt** elbow

Procedure: Open **reduction** and **internal fixation** of fracture. Carl Cracken was **anesthetized** the skin was prepped with Betadine, **sterile** drapes were applied, and the **pneumatic** tourniquet inflated around the right arm. An **incision** was made around the area of the lateral **epicondyle** through a Steri-drape, and this was carried through **subcutaneous** tissue, and the fracture site was easily exposed. **Inspection** revealed the fragment to be rotated in two planes about 90 degrees. It was possible to **manually** reduce this quite easily, and then judicious manipulation resulted in an almost **anatomic** reduction. This was fixed with two pins driven across the **humerus**. These pins were cut off below skin level. The wound was closed with some plain catgut subcutaneously and 5-0 Nylon in the skin. Dressings were applied to Mr. Cracken and the tourniquet released. A long arm cast was applied.

1. looking   _____
2. using the hands   _____
3. toward the side   _____
4. cut into   _____
5. free of microorganisms   _____
6. below the skin   _____
7. pertaining to body structures _____
8. inside   _____
9. broken, fractured   _____
10. uses air   _____
11. made to have no sensation   _____
12. surgery to restore position   _____
13. hold in place   _____
14. upon the condyle   _____
15. upper arm bone   _____
16. male   _____
17. years old   _____
18. right   _____

► CROSSWORD PUZZLE

Check your answers by going back through the frames or checking the solutions in Appendix C.

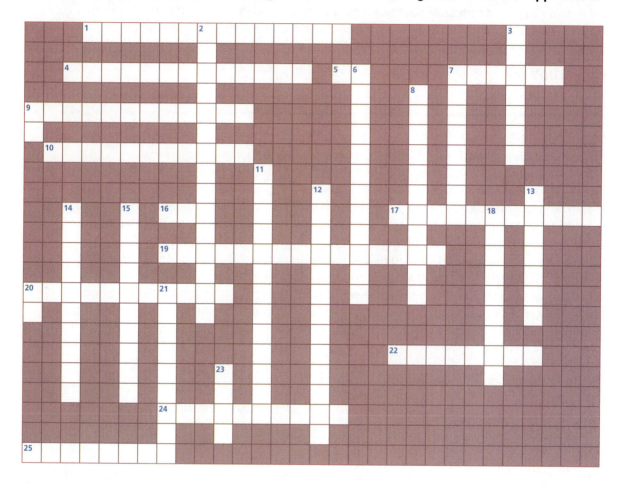

Across

1. including the upper arm bone and the shoulder blades
4. severe mental disorder with hallucinations
5. every night (abbreviation)
7. _____ tunnel syndrome
9. synonym for spina bifida cystica
10. excision of herniated lamina of a disk
16. podiatrist (abbreviation)
17. foot bones beyond the tarsals
19. muscle from upper arm to radius bone
20. synonym for mycostasis
22. group of nerve cell bodies
24. night blindness
25. walk (verb)

Down

2. sleeping sickness caused by a liver fluke
3. process at the end of the sternum
6. sleepwalking
7. plural for heel bone
8. physician specialist in skeletal disorders
9. right (abbreviation)
11. pertaining to neck and face
12. cleft palate
13. bone you sit on
14. pain in the breast bone
15. stop blood flow
18. condition of stiffening
20. fracture (abbreviation)
21. vehicle for emergency transport
23. orthopedist (abbreviation)

GLOSSARY

acromioclavicular	joint between the collar bone and the acromion process
acromiohumeral	joint between the acromion process and the humerus
acromion	the bony projection on the scapula at the humeroscapular joint
ambulance	vehicle used to transport patients
ambulatory	able to walk, walking (ambulate)
ankyloblepharon	stiffened adhered eyelids
ankylocheilia	stiffened lips
ankylodactylia	stiff immovable fingers and toes
ankyloglossia	tongue tied (stiff tongue)
ankylophobia	abnormal fear of ankylosis
ankyloproctia	closure (immobility) of the anus and rectum
ankylosis	condition of stiffening, loss of mobility
arteriostasis	control of arterial flow
brachial	pertaining to the arm
brachiocephalic	pertaining to the arm and head
brachioradialis	muscle that extends from the upper arm to the radius bone
calcaneodynia	heel pain (calcanealgia)
calcaneum, calcanean, calcaneus	heel bone
carpi, carpus, carpal	wrist bones
cervical	pertaining to the neck and neck of the uterus
cervicectomy	excision of the cervix of the uterus
cervicitis	inflammation of the cervix of the uterus
cervicobrachial	pertaining to the neck and arm
cervicofacial	pertaining to the neck and the face
cholestasis	control of flow of bile
condyle, condylar	a rounded process on a bone end
condylectomy	excision of a condyle
condyloid	resembling a condyle
diskectomy	excision of herniated inter-vertebral disk (discectomy)
enterostasis	control of intestine flow
epicondyle	upon a condyle
femur, femoral	the long thigh bone of the leg
fungistasis	control or stop growth of a fungus (mycostasis)
ganglion	a collection of nerve cell bodies
hemostasis	control of blood flow (hematostasis)
humeroradial	pertaining to the humerus and the radius
humeroscapular	pertaining to the humerus and the scapula
humeroulnar	pertaining to the humerus and the ulna
ileum	third part of the small intestine
ilium	upper pelvic bone

GLOSSARY			
ischiocele	herniation through the ischial bone	rachiometer	instrument to measure spinal curvature
ischioneuralgia	pain in the nerves near the ischium (sciatica)	rachioplegia	spinal paralysis
ischiopubic	pertaining to the ischium and the pubis	rachischisis	split spine (spina bifida cystica)
ischiorectal	pertaining to the ischium and the rectum	rachitis	inflammation of the spine (spondylitis)
laminectomy	excision of the lamina of the vertebral posterior arch	radioulnar	pertaining to the radius and the ulna
metacarpi	hand bones distal to the carpi	scapula	shoulder blade
metatarsals	foot bones distal to the tarsals	schistoglossia	split tongue (fissure)
noctambulism	sleepwalking (somnambulism)	schistosomiasis	infestation with *Schistosoma* (*mansoni, japonicum, haematobium*) flukes
nyctalbuminuria	excretion of albumin in urine at night	schizonychia	split finger or toe nails
nyctalgia	pain during the night	schizophasia	split speech (incomprehensible)
nyctalopia	night blindness	schizophrenia	severe mental disorder in which thinking, emotions, and behavior are disturbed (includes paranoia, hallucination, delusion, persecution, and jealousy)
nyctophobia	abnormal fear of the night (noctiphobia)		
nycturia	excessive urination during the night (nocturia)	sternalgia	sternal pain (sternodynia)
palatoschisis	cleft palate (uranoschisis)	sternopericardial	pertaining to the sternum and the pericardium
phlebostasis	control of venous flow	tarsi, tarsus, tarsal	bones of the ankle (not including the tibia)
pubofemoral	pertaining to the pubic bone and the femur	viscerostasis	control of an organ
pyostasis	control of pus formation	xiphocostal	pertaining to the xiphoid process and the ribs
rachialgia	spinal pain (rachiodynia)	xiphoid (process)	cartilage bony projection on the distal end of the sternum

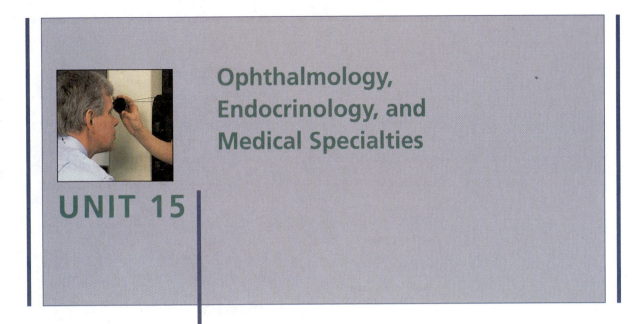

Ophthalmology, Endocrinology, and Medical Specialties

UNIT 15

15.1
ophthalm/o is used in words to mean eye. Ophthalm/itis means

inflammation of the eye
*_____.
pertaining to the eye
Ophthalm/ic means *_____.
NOTE: Ocular also means pertaining to the eye.

15.2
Ophthalm/algia and ophthalm/o/dynia both mean
pain in the eye
*_____.

✔ SPELL CHECK

15.3
Watch your spelling on this one. Before building words with this root, be sure you have the phth order of ophthalm/o straight. Pronounce it: off **thalm´** ō.

15.4
Build words meaning
    herniation of an eye (abnormal protrusion)
ophthalm/o/ptosis or
    _____ /_____ /_____;
off thal´ mop tō´ sis
    instrument for measuring the eye (curvature of the cornea)
exophthalmos
    _____ /_____ /_____.
eks of thal´ mōs
ophthalm/o/meter
of´ thal **mom´** ə ter

455

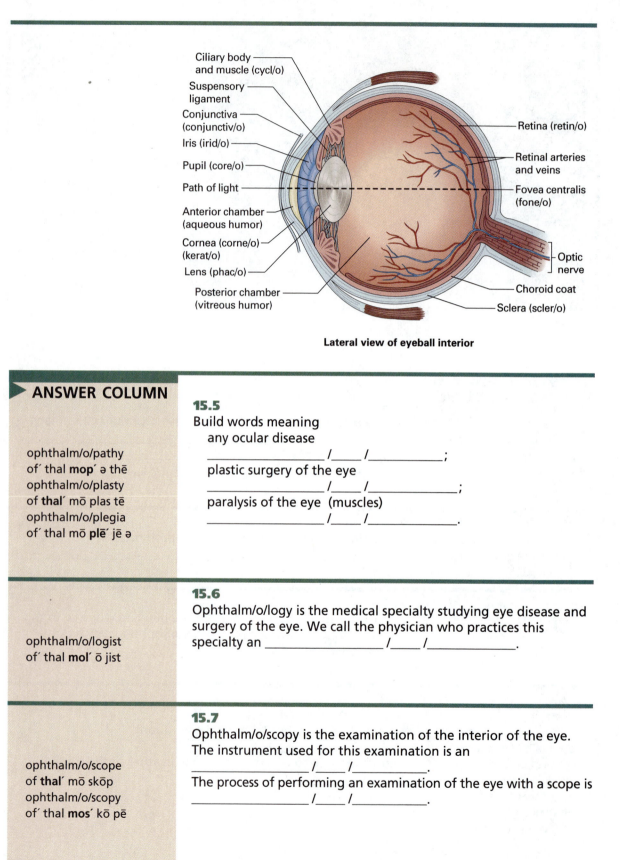

Ciliary body
and muscle (cycl/o)

Suspensory
ligament

Conjunctiva
(conjunctiv/o)

Iris (irid/o)

Pupil (core/o)

Path of light

Anterior chamber
(aqueous humor)

Cornea (corne/o)
(kerat/o)

Lens (phac/o)

Posterior chamber
(vitreous humor)

Retina (retin/o)

Retinal arteries
and veins

Fovea centralis
(fone/o)

Optic
nerve

Choroid coat

Sclera (scler/o)

Lateral view of eyeball interior

ANSWER COLUMN	
ophthalm/o/pathy of´ thal **mop** ə thē ophthalm/o/plasty of **thal**´ mō plas tē ophthalm/o/plegia of´ thal mō **plē**´ jē ə	**15.5** Build words meaning any ocular disease _____ /____ /_____; plastic surgery of the eye _____ /____ /_____; paralysis of the eye (muscles) _____ /____ /_____.
ophthalm/o/logist of´ thal **mol**´ ō jist	**15.6** Ophthalm/o/logy is the medical specialty studying eye disease and surgery of the eye. We call the physician who practices this specialty an _____ /____ /_____.
ophthalm/o/scope of **thal**´ mō skōp ophthalm/o/scopy of´ thal **mos**´ kō pē	**15.7** Ophthalm/o/scopy is the examination of the interior of the eye. The instrument used for this examination is an _____ /____ /_____. The process of performing an examination of the eye with a scope is _____ /____ /_____.

ANSWER COLUMN

The table below analyzes word parts pertaining to the eye and vision:

Word Part	Use
op/ia	suffix for vision
opt/ic	adjective—pertaining to vision
opt/o	combining form for vision
ophthalm/o	combining form for eye
ophthalm/ic	adjective—pertaining to eye

15.8

opt/o/metrist
op′ **tom′** ə trist
opt/ic
op′ tik
opt/o/metry
op **tom′** e trē

opt/o refers to vision. Use **opt/o** to build words meaning
   one who measures visual acuity
   _____ /_____ /_____;
   the cranial nerve for vision (adjective)
   _____ /_____;
   the measurement of vision (practice assessing vision disorders)
   _____ /_____ /_____.

NOTE: In some areas optometrists are licensed to treat eye disease and prescribe medications.

Professional Profiles ◀◀◀◀◀◀◀◀◀◀◀◀◀◀◀◀◀◀◀◀◀◀◀◀◀◀◀

Certified ophthalmic assistants (COAs), technicians (COTs) and **medical technologists (COMTs)** play an important role in assisting ophthalmologists by assessing visual acuity, performing diagnostic tests (e.g., glaucoma screening), asssisting with minor and major ophthalmic surgical procedures, and providing patient education. The Joint Commission on Allied Health Personnel in Ophthalmology (JCAHPO) is the certifying agency for ophthalmic medical personnel.

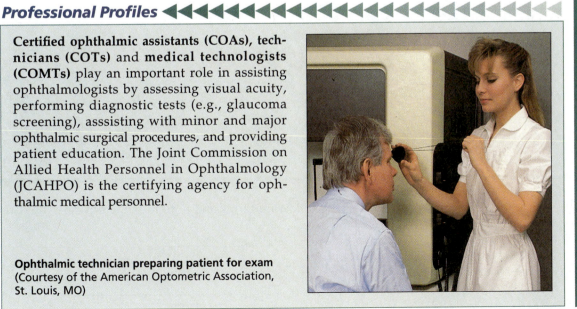

Ophthalmic technician preparing patient for exam
(Courtesy of the American Optometric Association, St. Louis, MO)

ANSWER COLUMN

eee TAKE A CLOSER LOOK

15.9
Notice the difference between the following:

ophthalmologist—physician (MD or DO) specialist in treating diseases of the eye and performing surgery.

optometrist—licensed practitioner (OD) limited to eye examinations and prescribing corrective lenses.

Both are called doctor, having received doctorate degrees from medical or optometry schools.

Ophthalm/ic
of **thal**′ mik

15.10
A special technician that assists ophthalmologists with eye exams and helps fit corrective lenses is called a certified _____ /_____ technician (COT).

xanth/opia
zan **thō**′ pē ə
chlor/opia
klor **ō**′ pē ə
erythr/opia
er i **thrō**′ pē ə

15.11
Recall the color word roots. **-opia** is a suffix denoting vision. Cyan/opia is a defect in vision that causes objects to appear blue. Form words meaning
yellow vision
_____ /_____;
green vision
_____ /_____;
red vision
_____ /_____.

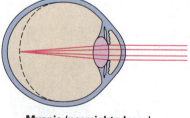 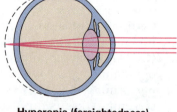

Myopia (nearsightedness)
Light rays focus in front of the retina

Hyperopia (farsightedness)
Light rays focus beyond the retina

nearsightedness
farsightedness
loss of accommodation
double vision

15.12
Look up the following terms and note the type of vision they are describing:
my/opia _____;
hyper/opia _____;
presby/opia * _____;
dipl/opia * _____.

▶ **ANSWER COLUMN**	
heart double double	**15.13** **diplo-** means double. Diplo/cardia means having a double _____. Diplo/genesis means production of _____ parts or _____ substances.
dipl/opia dip lō′ pē ə	**15.14** **-opia** is an involved form that we can use as a suffix. **-opia** means vision. Build a word meaning double vision: _____ / _____.
diplopia	**15.15** There are many kinds of diplopia. Crossed eyes causes one kind of _____.
diplopia	**15.16** Whenever both eyes fail to record the same image on the brain, _____ occurs.
-opia	**15.17** If you can see close objects but not distant ones, you may have my/opia or close vision. Presby/opia is experienced by older people as a loss of accommodation by the lens. The word literally means old vision. In each of these terms the suffix for vision is _____.
both	**15.18** **ambi-** means both or both sides. Ambi/later/al means pertaining to _____ sides.
both	**15.19** An ambi/dextr/ous person can work well with _____ hands.
ambi/opia am bē ō′ pē ə	**15.20** A word that means both eyes (ou—both eyes) form separate images (vision) is _____ / _____. **NOTE:** ambiopia is a term not commonly used in optometry.
dipl/opia (You pronounce)	**15.21** **dipl-** and **diplo-** are prefixes meaning double. The result of separate vision from both eyes is a double image or double vision. Medically, double vision can be expressed as _____ / _____. **NOTE:** **diplo-** and **ambi-** are combining forms used as prefixes.

ANSWER COLUMN	
	15.22
my/opia	Hyper/opia means farsightedness (able to focus on objects at a distance). The opposite of hyperopia is nearsightedness, or
mī ō´ pē ə	_____ /_____.

15.23
Look up ambivalence in any dictionary. Read its meaning. Analyze this word and the word ambivalent:

ambi/valence
am **biv**´ ə ləns
ambi/valent
am **biv**´ ə lənt

_____ /_____;
_____ /_____.

15.24
Recall that a diplo/bacillus is a bacillus that occurs in pairs. A coccus that grows in pairs is a _____ /_____.

diplo/coccus
dip lō **kok**´ əs

TAKE A CLOSER LOOK

15.25
Light travels through the lens of the eye, it is refracted, and an image is focused on the retina. **-opter** is a suffix meaning visible. A di/opter (Greek: *dia*, meaning through, and *optos*, meaning that which sees) is a unit of measurement of refraction in the eye.

15.26
Glasses or contact lenses are used to correct myopia, hyperopia, or presbyopia. A prescription written for corrective lenses that reads OS +1 D means left eye one _____ /_____.

di/opter
di´ op ter

15.27
A micr/o/scope is an instrument for examining something small. An instrument for examining through is a _____ /_____.

dia/scope
di´ ə skōp

15.28
A diascope is a glass plate held against the skin. The skin is looked at through the diascope to see superficial lesions (erythematous and others). The word part for through is _____.

dia-

WORD ORIGIN

15.29
Tropia is from the Greek *tropē* meaning turning. In ophthalmology, when the eyes appear to be turned in an abnormal position while open it is referred to as a strabismus or squint. The medical terms used indicating the eye position include exo/tropia, eso/tropia, hyper/tropia, hypo/tropia, and cyclo/tropia.

ANSWER COLUMN	
	15.30 exo- means outward. eso- means toward. hypo- means downward. hyper- means upward. From what you have just learned, build words that mean 　　eyes pointing outward 　　_____ /_____; 　　eyes pointing inward 　　_____ /_____; 　　eyes pointing upward 　　_____ /_____; 　　eyes pointing downward 　　_____ /_____; Good!

exo/tropia
eks ō **trō´** pē ə
eso/tropia
es ō **trō´** pē ə
hyper/tropia
hī per **trō´** pē ə
hypo/tropia
hī pō **trō´** pē ə

15.31
Write the abnormal direction of the eye positions indicated below:
　　hypertropia _____;
　　hypotropia _____;
　　esotropia _____; and
　　exotropia _____.

upward
downward
inward
outward

15.32
Hyper/tropia results when an eye muscle moves one eye upward. When one eye turns downward, we call it _____ /_____.

hypo/tropia
hī pō **trō´** pē ə

15.33
Another term for exotropia, esotropia, hypertropia, and hypotropia is _____.

strabismus
stra **bis´** mus
or squint

15.34
phor(ia) means to carry or bear. Dys/phoria means a feeling of depression—you carry with you an ill (bad) feeling. The word that means feeling of well-being is _____ /_____.

eu/phoria
yōō **fôr´** ē ə

15.35
When your diet is good, you have enough rest, and the world is a wonderful place in which to be, you are enjoying the state of
_____.

euphoria

ANSWER COLUMN	
	15.36 A phor/opt/er is an instrument used to determine the prescription strength needed for corrective lenses. An optometrist may use a
phor/opt/er for **op´** ter phor/o/meter fôr **om´** ə tər di/opter dī **op´** ter	_____ /_____ /____. The instrument that measures the tone and pull of the eye-moving (bearing) muscles is a _____ /____ /_____. The unit measure for vision is the ____ /_____.
	15.37
blephar/o	Blephar/o/ptosis means prolapse of an eyelid. The combining form for eyelid is _____ /____.
	15.38
eyelid eyelid	Edema is swelling due to fluid retention. Blepharedema means swelling of the _____. **blephar/o** seen anywhere makes you think of the _____.
🏛 WORD ORIGIN	**15.39** The word edema is related to the name of the Greek tragic hero Oedipus the king. Oedipus comes from the Greek verb *oidein* (to become swollen) and literally translated means swollen foot. After a bizarre series of events Oedipus kills his father and marries his own mother. Freud named his Oedipus complex theory after this story. The "oe" in Oedipus was later changed to "e" and the modern English medical term became edema. Edema/tous is the adjectival form.
	15.40 Blephar/edema means swelling of the eyelid. Build words that mean inflammation of an eyelid
blephar/itis blef´ ə **rī´** tis blephar/otomy blef´ ə **rot´** ə mē	_____ /_____; incision of an eyelid _____ /_____.
	15.41 Build words that mean excision of lesions on the eyelid

blephar/ectomy
blef´ ər **ek´** tō mē
blephar/o/plasty
blef´ ə rō plas tē
blephar/o/spasm
blef´ ə rō spaz əm
blephar/o/ptosis
blef´ ər op **tō´** sis
blephar/o/rrhaphy
blef´ ər **or´** ə fē
	_____ /_____;
	  surgical repair of an eyelid
	_____ /____ /_____;
	  twitching of an eyelid
	_____ /____ /_____;
	  prolapse of an eyelid (droopy eyelid)
	_____ /____ /_____;
	  suture of the eyelid
	_____ /____ /_____.

ANSWER COLUMN

15.42
The conjunctiva is the membrane that lines the eyelids (palpebral conjunctiva) and the sclera (ocular conjunctiva). Look up conjunctivitis in your dictionary. There are over 30 types of inflammation of the conjunctiva or

conjunctiv/itis
kon junk´ ti **vī´** tis

_____ /_____ .

15.43
Look up cornea in your dictionary. Look at the words in your dictionary that begin with corne. A combining form for cornea is

corne/o

_____ /_____. Look at the illustration of the eye on page 456. Write the meaning and analyze by drawing the slashes for the following terms:
corneal

corne/al
kôr´ nē əl
corne/o/ir/itis
kôr´ nē ō ī **rī´** tis
corne/o/scler/al
kôr´ nē ō **sklir´** əl

_____ /_____ , _____;
                          meaning
corneoiritis
_____ /_____ /_____ /_____ , _____;
                                      meaning
corneoscleral
_____ /_____ /_____ /_____ , _____.
                                       meaning

15.44
From the preceding frame identify two word roots that mean iris and sclera. They are _____ and _____.

ir
scler

15.45
Now, locate the lens. **phac/o** is the combining form for the crystalline lens of the eye. Recall the **-cele** is used for herniation or dislocation. Build a word that means dislocation of the lens:

phac/o/cele
fā´ kō sēl

_____ /_____ /_____.

🏛 *WORD ORIGIN*

15.46
The lens is shaped like a lentil. In Greek, *phacos* means lentil. Lentils have a biconvex shape just like the crystalline lens of the eye.

phac/o/emulsification
fā´ kō ēm ul´ si fi **kā´** shun

15.47
Cataracts are opacities of the lens of the eye. Cataracts can be treated with an ultrasonic device to emulsify the lens for removal. This procedure is called _____ /_____ /emulsification.

▶ **ANSWER COLUMN**

sclera
sklir´ ə
scler/o/sis
condition of hardness

15.48
Look up the first word in your dictionary beginning with scler.
It is _____. Read about the sclera. Does the word root
plus the Greek word *scleras*, meaning hard, from which it is
derived, suggest an already familiar combining form to you?
It is _____ /_____ /_____, which means
* _____.
(Remember: sclerosis.)

scler/al
sklir´ əl
scler/ectomy
skli **rek´** tə mē
scler/o/stomy
skli **ros´** tə mē
scler/itis
sklir ī´ tis

15.49
The sclera of the eye is the white, "hard" outer coat of the eye.
Build words meaning
    pertaining to the sclera (adjective)
    _____ /_____;
    excision of the sclera (or part)
    _____ /_____;
    formation of an opening into the sclera
    _____ /_____ /_____;
    inflammation of the sclera
    _____ /_____ /_____.

iris
ī´ ris

15.50
Look at the diagram of the eye on page 456. The colored part of
the eye is the _____.

15.51
Look up iris in your dictionary. **ir** and **irid** are word roots for the
iris. **ir/o** and **irid/o** are both combining forms for iris. **ir** has limited
use, usually with **-itis**, indicating inflammation of the iris. Also,
look up the plural form of iris.

ir/itis

corne/o/ir/itis

scler/o/ir/itis
(You pronounce)

15.52
With the information in Frame 15.51 and the word root you found,
build words meaning
    inflammation of the iris
    _____ /_____;
    inflammation of the cornea and iris
    _____ /_____ /_____ /_____;
    inflammation of the sclera and iris
    _____ /_____ /_____ /_____.

ir/ides
ir´ i dēz, ī´ ri dēz
irid/o

15.53
You may have found in your dictionary the plural of iris.
It is _____ /_____.
The combining form for iris is _____ /_____.

ANSWER COLUMN	

15.54
Using **irid/o**, build words meaning
  protrusion of the iris (dislocation)
  _____ /_____ /_____;
  pain in the iris
  _____ /_____;
  excision of part or all of the iris
  _____ /_____.

irid/o/cele
i **rid**′ ō sēl, ī **rid**′ ō sel
irid/algia
ir′ i **dal**′ jē ə, ī ri **dal**′ jē ə
irid/ectomy
ir′ i **dek**′ tə mē,
ī′ ri **dek**′ tə mē

15.55
Build words meaning (you insert the slashes):
  prolapse of the iris
  _____;
  softening of the iris
  _____;
  rupture of the iris
  _____.

irid/o/ptosis
ī′ rid op **tō**′ sis
irid/o/malacia
ī′ rid ō mal **ā**′ shə
irid/o/rrhexis
ī′ rid ō **rek**′ sis

15.56
There are two words to express paralysis of the iris. They are
_____ /_____ /_____ and
_____ /_____ /_____.

irid/o/plegia
irid/o/paralysis
(You pronounce)

15.57
The following forms make you think of:
  ir _____;
  irid/o _____;
  scler/o _____;
  corne/o _____.

iris
iris
sclera (hard)
cornea

15.58
Look up retina in your dictionary. Read about the retina. Look at the words beginning with **retin** in your dictionary. The combining form for words about the retina is _____ /____.

retin/o

15.59
Build words meaning
  pertaining to the retina
  _____ /_____;
  inflammation of the retina
  _____ /_____;
  fixation of a detached retina (repair)
  _____ /_____ /_____.

retin/al
ret′ i nəl
retin/itis
ret i **nī**′ tis
retin/o/pexy or
ret′ i nō pek sē
retin/o/plasty
ret′ i nō **plas**′ tē

ANSWER COLUMN

retin/o/scope
ret′ i nō skōp
retin/o/scopy
ret i **nos**′ kə pē

15.60
The instrument used to examine the refractive error of the eye (retina) is the _____ /_____ /_____. The process of using a retinoscope is _____ /_____ /_____.
NOTE: The actual proper term for retinoscopy is "skiascopy." Look it up!

INFORMATION FRAME

15.61
Glaucoma is disease of the eye in which the intraocular pressure is increased. If glaucoma is not treated, the person will become blind. There are three basic types of glaucoma: open angle, angle closure, and congenital.

glaucoma
glou **cō**′ ma

15.62
One part of a complete eye exam includes checking the intraocular pressure. This is done to look for signs of
_____.

INFORMATION FRAME

15.63
The pupil in the eye is the opening in the iris through which light passes. Identify the pupil in the illustration of the eye on page 456. The word root for pupil is **cor**.

cor/ectopia
kôr′ ek **tō**′ pē ə
cor/e/lysis
kôr′ **el**′ ə sis
cor/ectasia (is)
kôr′ ek **tā**′ zhə
anis/o/coria
an ī′ sō **kôr**′ ē ə

15.64
One combining form for pupil is **cor/e**. Build words meaning
   pupil out of place
   _____ /_____;
   destruction of the pupil
   _____ /_____ /_____;
   dilatation (stretching) of the pupil
   _____ /_____;
   unequal pupil size
   _____ /_____ /_____.

core/o/meter or
pupil/o/meter
core/o/metry or
pupil/o/metry
core/o/plasty
(You pronounce)

15.65
core/o is used also as a combining form for pupil. Using **core/o**, build words meaning
   instrument for measuring the pupil
   _____ /_____ /_____;
   measurement of the pupil
   _____ /_____ /_____;
   plastic surgery of the pupil
   _____ /_____ /_____.

▶ **ANSWER COLUMN**

cor

15.66
Whether **cor/e** or **core/o** is used, the word root for pupil of the eye is _____.

---

corne

15.67
You have already learned one word root for cornea. It is _____. Another word root for cornea is **kerat** and it is the more commonly used form.
(Think of kerats [carrots] and corn.)

---

kerat
kerat/o

15.68
The word root most commonly used for cornea is _____. The combining form is _____ /_____.

---

kerat/ectasia (is)
ker ə tek tā´ zhə
kerat/o/cele
ker´ ə tō sēl
kerat/o/plasty
ker´ ə tō plas tē

15.69
Using **kerat/o**, build words meaning
  forward bulging (dilatation) of the cornea
  _____ /_____;
  herniation of the cornea (protrusion of the cornea)
  _____ /_____ /_____;
  plastic operation of the cornea (corneal transplant)
  _____ /_____ /_____.

---

kerat/o/tomy

kerat/o/rrhexis

kerat/o/scler/itis
(You pronounce)

15.70
Again using **kerat/o**, build words meaning
  incision of the cornea
  _____ /_____ /_____;
  corneal rupture
  _____ /_____ /_____;
  inflammation of cornea and sclera
  _____ /_____ /_____ /_____.

---

kerat/o/tomy

15.71
Making small incisions into trhe cornea to improve vision for those with myopia is called radial _____ /_____ /_____.

 TAKE A
eee CLOSER LOOK

15.72
The combining form for ciliary body is **cycl/o**. Look up the ciliary body in your dictionary or an anatomy book and understand what it is. Turn to **cycl/o** words in your dictionary. *Cyclos* is Greek for circle. The ciliary body encircles the inside of the iris.

▶ **ANSWER COLUMN**

15.73
Find words meaning
  paralysis of the ciliary body (noun)

cycl/o/plegia
sī klō **plē**′ jē ə
cycl/o/pleg/ic
sī klō **plē**′ jik
cycl/o/keratitis
sī klō ker ə **tī**′ tis

_____ /_____ /_____;
  paralysis of the ciliary body (adjective)
_____ /_____ /_____ /_____;
  ciliary body and cornea inflammation
_____ /_____ /_____.

15.74
The following forms make you think of:

iris
retina
pupil
pupil
cornea
cornea
ciliary body

   irid/o _____;
   retin/o _____;
   cor/e _____;
   core/o _____;
   kerat/o _____;
   corne/o _____;
   cycl/o _____.

15.75
Look up lacrim/al in your dictionary. Lacrimal is a word
that means pertaining to _____.
Lacrim/ation is _____.

tears
tearing

15.76
The gland that secretes tears is the _____ /_____ gland.

lacrim/al
lak′ ri məl

15.77
The sac that collects lacrimal fluid is the _____ sac.

lacrimal

15.78
Lacrimal fluid is drained away by means of the
nas/o/_____ /_____ duct.

nas/o/lacrim/al
nā zō **lak**′ ri məl

15.79
Lacrimal fluid keeps the surface of the eye moistened. It is
continually forming and being drained. When there is more
formed than can be drained through a duct, you say the person is
* _____.

crying or tearing

15.80
Lacrimation means crying. Excessive lacrimation is called
dacry/o/rrhea. This word gives you another word root for tear. It is
_____, and the suffix for flow is _____.

dacry
-rrhea

ANSWER COLUMN

lacrimation
lak ri **ma**´ shun
dacry/o/rrhea
da´krē ō **rē**´ ə

15.81
Flow of tears is either _____ or
_____ /_____ /_____.

dacry/o/cyst/itis
dak´ rē ō sis **tī**´ tis
tear sac inflammation
dacry/o/aden/algia
dak´ rē ō ad´ ə **nal**´ jē ə
pain in a tear gland
dacry/oma
dak´ rē **ō**´ mə
tumor of the tear duct
  or gland

15.82
Analyze (you draw the slashes and define):
   dacryocystitis
   _____,
   * _____;
   dacryoadenalgia
   _____,
   * _____;
   dacryoma
   _____,
   * _____.

dacry/o/py/o/rrhea
discharge of pus from
  tear gland
dacry/o/cyst/o/cele
hernia of the tear sac

dacry/o/lith
stone in the tear sac
(You pronounce)

15.83
Define and draw the slashes:
   dacryopyorrhea
   _____,
   * _____;
   dacryocystocele
   _____,
   * _____;
   dacryolith
   _____,
   * _____.

excessive flow of tears

prolapse of the tear sac

an instrument for cutting
  (incising) the tear sac

15.84
If necessary you may use your dictionary to complete the
following:
   dacryorrhea means
   * _____;
   dacryocystoptosis means
   * _____;
   a dacryocystotome is
   * _____.

nails

15.85
Look in your dictionary for words beginning with **onych**. These
words refer to the _____.

► **ANSWER COLUMN**

15.86

By studying words beginning with **onych**, you can find its combining form. The combining form that refers to nail is

onych/o   _____ /_____.

✅ *SPELL CHECK*

15.87

Watch your spelling and pronunciation. The y is pronounced as a short "i" sound and the "ch" like a "k": o-n-y-c-h.

15.88

Build words meaning
  resembling a fingernail

onych/oid   _____ /_____;
on´ i koid
  tumor of the nail (or nail bed)
onych/oma
on i **kō´** mə   _____ /_____;
  any nail condition
onych/osis
on i **kō´** sis   _____ /_____.

15.89

Build words meaning
  softening of the nails

onych/o/malac/ia   _____ /_____ /_____ /____;
on´ i kō ma **lā´** shə
  fungus infection (condition) of the nails
onych/o/myc/osis
on´ i kō mī **kō´** sis   _____ /_____ /_____ /_____;
  nail biting (eating)
onych/o/phagia
on´ i kō **fā´** jē ə   _____ /_____ /_____.

15.90

Recall that **crypt** means hidden. Onych/o/crypt/osis means literally
hidden nail or condition   *_____.
  of nail being hidden

15.91

Look up onychocryptosis (on´ i kō krip **tō´** sis) in your dictionary. It
ingrown nail (usually a   refers to an *_____.
  toenail)

15.92

Par/onych/ia is a condition of infection in the tissues around the
nail. If the cuticle around the nail is infected, this is called
par/onych/ia   _____ /_____ /_____, also known as a "run around." To see
par´ ō **nik´** ē ə   this condition look at the pictures on page 471.

15.93

trich/o is used in words to mean hair. A trich/o/genous substance
hair   promotes the growth of _____.

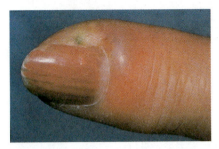

Paronychia, infection of tissues around the nail

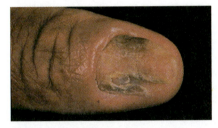

Onychomycosis, caused by parasitic fungus

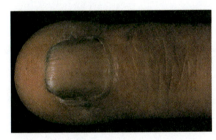

Onychocryptosis, or ingrown nail

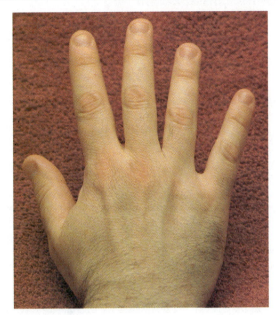

Onychophagy, or bitten nails

hair

15.94
Lith/iasis is the formation of calculi. Trich/iasis is the formation of _____ (in the wrong places).

15.95
Using **trich/o**, build words meaning
    hairy tongue (noun)

trich/o/glossia
trik´ ō **glos**´ ē ə
trich/oid
trik´ oid
trich/o/phobia
trik´ ō **fō**´ bē ə
trich/o/pathy
trik **op**´ ə thē

    _____ /_____ /_____;
    resembling hair
    _____ /_____;
    abnormal fear of hair
    _____ /_____ /_____;
    any hair disease
    _____ /_____ /_____.

▶ **ANSWER COLUMN**

eat or swallow eating or swallowing	**15.96** Recall that **phag/o** means *_____, and phagia is a condition of *_____.
eats (or ingests) eating (or ingesting)	**15.97** A phag/o/cyte is a cell that _____ microorganisms. Phag/o/cyt/osis is the process of the cells _____ microorganisms.
phag/o/cyte phag/o/cyt/osis (You pronounce)	**15.98** A cell that eats cells is a _____ /____ /_____. The process is _____ /____ /_____ /_____.
the ingestion of cells by phagocytes or phagocytosis	**15.99** Cyt/o/phagy is another way of saying *_____ _____.
cyt/o/meter sī **tom**´ ə tər cyt/o/metry sī **tom**´ ə trē	**15.100** Recall that an instrument for measuring (counting) cells is a _____ /____ /_____, and the process of measuring (counting) cells is _____ /____ /_____.
cyt/o/stasis sī **tos**´ tə sis cyt/o/scopy sī **tos**´ kə pē	**15.101** Stopping or controlling cells is called _____ /____ /_____. Examination of cells is _____ /____ /_____.
micr/o/phage **mī**´ krō fāj	**15.102** A large phagocyte is called a macr/o/phage. A small phagocyte is called a _____ /____ /_____.

ANSWER COLUMN

trich/o/phagy (ia)
tri **kof**´ ə jē
aer/o/phagy (ia)
air **of**´ ə jē

15.103
Onych/o/phagy (onychophagia) is nail biting. A word that means hair swallowing is _____ /_____ /_____.
Air swallowing is
_____ /_____ /_____.

---

endo/crine
en´ dō krin

15.104
Recall the prefix endo- meaning inside. Endo/crine literally means to secrete inside. Hormones are secreted from the _____ /_____ glands.

---

endo/crin/ology
en´ dō krin **o**´ lō jē
endo/crin/o/logist
en´ dō krin **ol**´ ō jist

15.105
The medical specialty studying the endocrine system is called _____ /_____ /_____.
The specialist (physician) in the study of the endocrine system is called an _____ /_____ /_____ /_____.

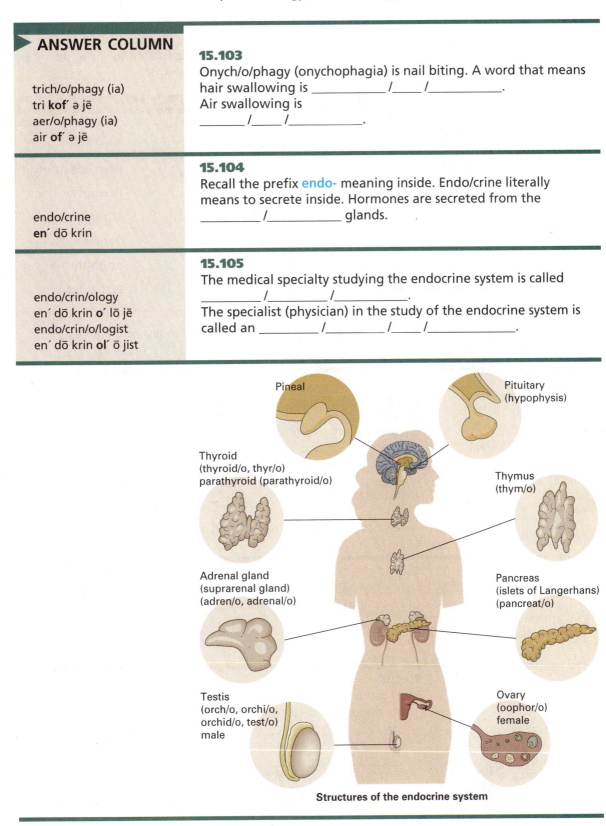

Pineal

Pituitary
(hypophysis)

Thyroid
(thyroid/o, thyr/o)
parathyroid (parathyroid/o)

Thymus
(thym/o)

Adrenal gland
(suprarenal gland)
(adren/o, adrenal/o)

Pancreas
(islets of Langerhans)
(pancreat/o)

Testis
(orch/o, orchi/o,
orchid/o, test/o)
male

Ovary
(oophor/o)
female

Structures of the endocrine system

▶ **ANSWER COLUMN**

The following table analyzes word parts related to the endocrine system. Refer to the illustration on page 473.

Combining Form	Meaning	Example
thyroid/o, thyr/o	thyroid gland	thyroidectomy
thym/o	thymus gland	thymosin
adren/o	adrenal gland	adrenalin
pancreat/o	pancreas	pancreatitis
oophor/o	ovary	oophoroma
testic/, orchid/o, orchi/o	testis	testicular

Review the male and female reproductive systems, Frames 5.33–5.116.

---

adrenal gland (adrenal cortex)

thyroid gland

testes

15.106
Analyzing the following hormones, name the gland by which they are produced:
　　adren/o/corticoid (cortisone)
　　* _____;
　　thyr/o/xine, or thyr/o/xin
　　* _____;
　　test/o/sterone
　　_____.
See how much you have learned about word building!

---

hypo/thyroid/ism
hī pō **thī**́ roid izm

15.107
Hyper/thyroid/ism is an overactive thyroid. An underactive (slow-acting) thyroid condition is called
_____ /_____ /_____.

---

adren/o/pathy
ad′ rēn **op**′ ath ē
adren/o/megaly
ad′ rēn ō **meg**′ əl ē
adren/o/lysis
ad′ rēn **ol**′ ə sis

15.108
Build terms meaning
　　any disease condition of the adrenal glands
　　_____ /____ /_____;
　　enlargement of the adrenal glands
　　_____ /____ /_____;
　　destruction of adrenal tissue
　　_____ /____ /_____.

> **ANSWER COLUMN**

15.109
The adrenal glands are also called the supra/renal glands because they are above the kidneys. Epi/nephr/ine is a hormone produced by the supra/renal glands. Define these two terms:
supra/renal

above the kidneys (adrenal)
a hormone produced upon the kidney

*_____;

epi/nephr/ine

*_____.

15.110
There are many hormones produced by the pituitary gland. Look up pituitary in your dictionary and read about its function. The pituitary gland (hypophysis) has front and back lobes. These are called the _____ lobe and the _____ lobe.

anterior
posterior

15.111
For another review recall that **-emia** is a suffix that means

condition of the blood or in the blood

*_____.

15.112
Isch/emia (is kē′ mē ə) is a condition in which blood flow is interrupted. Blood cancer (sign: abnormally increased leukocyte count) is called _____ /_____.

leuk/emia
l$\overline{oo}$ **kē**′ mē ə

15.113
A transient isch/emic attack (TIA) is a temporary interruption of _____ flow, usually occurring in the brain.

blood

15.114
Build words meaning
   reduction in red blood cells
     _____ /_____;
   too much blood (in one part)
     _____ /_____;
   urine constituents in the blood
     _____ /_____.

an/emia
e **nē**′ mē ə
hyper/emia
hī pər **ē**′ mē ə
ur/emia
y$\overline{oo}$ **rē**′ mē ə

ANSWER COLUMN	

	15.115
	-emia is used as a suffix meaning in the blood. **hemat/o** is a combining form used as a prefix meaning blood. Build words meaning
	    blood in the urine
	    _____ /_____ /____;
	    urine in the blood
	    ____ /_____.

hemat/ur/ia hēm at **yōō**′ rē ə ur/emia yōō **rē**′ mē ə	
	15.116 You now know many prefixes, suffixes, and combining forms. You even know how to find combining forms and form singular and plural forms of a word. You also know several ways to find combining forms in your dictionary.
	15.117 To prove it again, look up trauma in your dictionary. It means a * _____.
wound or injury	

Professional Profiles ◀◀◀◀◀◀◀◀◀◀◀◀◀◀◀◀◀◀◀◀◀◀◀◀◀◀◀◀◀◀◀◀◀

Emergency medical technicians (EMTs) provide basic emergency medical care including first aid, CPR, immobilizing injuries, extricating accident victims from unsafe environments, and providing transportation. They may work directly in the field or in emergency departments. **Paramedics (EMT-Ps)** provide advanced life support such as using monitors and defibrillators, administering intravenous medications, as well as basic emergency care. Licensure requirements vary greatly throughout North America, and education ranges from private short course instruction to college-based programs offering associate degrees.

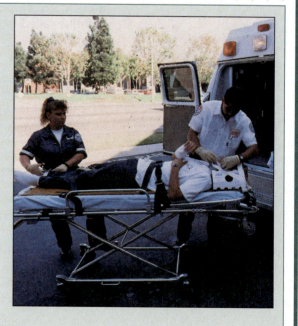

Emergency medical personnel aiding patient

ANSWER COLUMN

traumat/o	**15.118** Look at the next several words involving trauma. The combining form for trauma is _____ /_____.
traumat/o/logy trô mə **tol´** ə jē traumat/ic trô **ma´** tik	**15.119** The study of caring for wounds is called _____ /_____ /_____. Pertaining to wounds is _____ /_____.
wounds or injuries trauma	**15.120** A trauma center may provide twenty-four-hour care for treatment of *_____. Physicians can specialize in treatment of emergency cases including _____.

Ɛeee *TAKE A CLOSER LOOK*

15.121
A trauma can produce many injuries. Look up the following in the dictionary and write their definitions:
abrasion *_____;
contusion *_____;
evulsion *_____;
puncture *_____;
fracture *_____;
laceration *_____.
They are all types of wounds. Getting wounded is traumat/ic.

As a final review, notice that each of these medical specialties uses medical terminology. Use your knowledge of word-building systems to fill in the blanks in the following table. Check your answers on the next page.

Specialty	Specialist	Limits of Field
pathology	_____	diseases—nature and causes
_____	dermatologist	_____
neurology	_____	nervous system diseases
_____	gynecologist	female diseases
urology	_____	male diseases and all urinary diseases
_____	endocrinologist	glands of internal secretion
oncology	_____	neoplasms (new growths)
_____	_____	heart
ophthalmology	_____	eye
_____	otorhinolaryngologist	_____
obstetrics	_____	pregnancy, childbirth, and puerperium
_____	geriatrician	old age
pediatrics	_____	children
_____	orthopedist	bones and muscles
psychiatry	_____	mental disorders
_____	audiologist	hearing function
radiology	_____	diagnostic imaging therapeutic x-ray
_____	chiropractor	_____
_____	podiatrist	diseases of the foot

Specialty	Specialist	Limits of Field
	pathologist (15.122)	
dermatology (15.123)		skin (15.124)
	neurologist (15.125)	
gynecology (15.126)		
	urologist (15.127)	
endocrinology (15.128)		
	oncologist (15.129)	
cardiology (15.130)	cardiologist (15.131)	
	ophthalmologist (15.132)	
otorhinolaryngology (15.133)		ear-nose-throat (15.134)
	obstetrician (15.135)	
geriatrics (15.136)		
	pediatrician (15.137)	
orthopedics (15.138)		
	psychiatrist (15.139)	
audiology (15.140)		
	radiologist (15.141)	
chiropractic (15.142)		manipulation therapy (15.143)
podiatry (15.144)		

15.145
Great!
See, you really are competent in the study of systematic medical terminology.

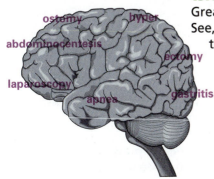

Abbreviation	Meaning
ACTH	adrenocorticotropic hormone
AOA	American Optometric Association
COA	certified ophthalmic assistant
COMT	certified ophthalmic medical technologist
COT	certified ophthalmic technician
d	diopter
EMT	emergency medical technician
EMT-P	EMT—paramedic
ENT	ear, nose, throat specialist
FSH	follicle-stimulating hormone
Fx	fracture
HCG	human chorionic gonadotropin
L&A	light and accommodation
Laser	light amplification by stimulated emission of radiation
mg	milligram (0.001 gram)
mm	millimeter (0.001 meter)
OAG	open-angle glaucoma
OB	obstetrician, obstetrics
od	right eye (oculus dexter)
OD	doctor of optometry
os	left eye (oculus sinister)
ou	both eyes (oculus uterque)
PERRLA	pupils equal, round, reactive to light and accommodation
T_3, T_4	triiodothyronine, tetraiodothyronine (thyroid function tests)
TIA	transient ischemic attack
TSH	thyroid-stimulating hormone

Now, work the last review activities on the next few pages and listen to the audiotapes that accompany *Medical Terminology: A Programmed Text,* 8th Edition, and practice your pronunciation.

Additional practice exercises for this unit are available on the Student Practice disk found in the back of the textbook.

Congratulations on your completion of this programmed study of medical terminology! May what you have learned in this course of study sustain you throughout your experiences in the health care field, and do not forget to celebrate your success!

▶ **REVIEW ACTIVITIES**

Circle and Correct
Circle the correct answer for each question. Then, check your answers in Appendix A.

1. Prefix meaning inward:
   a. inter-   b. exo-
   c. infra-   d. eso-

2. Suffix for vision:
   a. -ophthalmic   b. -metry
   c. -opia   d. -ophthic

3. Combining form for yellow:
   a. jaundice   b. xantho
   c. chloro   d. yello

4. Which of the following means nearsightedness?
   a. myopia   b. hyperopia
   c. presbyopia   d. exophoria

5. Combining form for eye:
   a. optalmo   b. opthalmo
   c. optic   d. ophthalmo

6. Word root for lens:
   a. lens   b. phac
   c. kerat   d. corne

7. Combining form for nail:
   a. onycho   b. omphalo
   c. optic   d. onchyo

8. Word root for suprarenal glands:
   a. aden   b. glandul
   c. genit   d. adren

9. Prefix meaning overactive:
   a. hyper-   b. ultra-
   c. supra-   d. meta-

10. Combining form for eyelid:
    a. maculo   b. cyclo
    c. lacrimo   d. blepharo

11. Which of the following does not have to do with tearing?
    a. lacrimation   b. cycloplegia
    c. dacryorrhea   d. dacryocystitis

12. Word root for hair:
    a. omphal   b. trich
    c. cyclo   d. onycho

13. Combining form for double:
    a. onycho   b. bi
    c. diplo   d. di

14. One combining form for cornea:
    a. kerato   b. irido
    c. cyclo   d. coreo

▶ REVIEW ACTIVITIES

Select and Construct

Select the correct word parts from the list below and construct medical terms that represent the given meaning.

adren	al	aniso	blephar	cardia
cele	cor(ne)(ia)	cyclo	dacry/o	diplo
disk	ectas(ia)(is)	ectomy	emia	emulsification
epi	eso	hyper	hypo	in(e)
ir	irid/o	itis	kerat (core)	lacrim
lamin/o	(o)logy	lysis	malacia	megaly
metry	my	myco	naso	nephrine
onych/o	oophoro	ophthalmo	opia	opt(ic)(o)
orchid	osis	otomy	pathy	phac/o
phobia	phoria	plasty	plegia	ptosis
retin(o)	rrhea	rrhexia	scope	thym/o
thyro(oid)	tomy	traumato	trich/o	

1. specialty measuring vision (OD) _____

2. paralysis of the ciliary body _____

3. softening of the nails _____

4. inflammation of the iris _____

5. excessive flow of tears _____

6. removal of the lens through a destruction procedure _____

7. hormone produced by the glands above the kidneys _____

8. farsightedness _____

9. instrument to examine the retina _____

10. study of wounds _____

11. surgical repair of the eye _____

12. dilatation of the pupil _____

13. prolapse of the eyelid _____

14. incision into the cornea _____

15. enlargement of the thyroid _____

16. unequal pupil size _____

17. inward crossed eyes _____

▶ **REVIEW ACTIVITIES**

Define and Dissect
Give a brief definition and dissect each term listed into its word parts in the space provided on the right. Check your answers by referring to the frame listed in parentheses and your medical dictionary. Then, listen to the audiotapes to practice pronunciation.

1. exotropia (15.30)

   _____ / _____
     pre   rt/suffix

   _____
              definition

2. phoropter (15.36)

   _____ / _____ / _____
      rt   rt   suffix

3. paronychia (15.92)

   _____ / _____ / _____
      pre   rt   suffix

4. ophthalmologist (15.6)

   _____ / _____ / _____
          rt   v   suffix

5. myopia (15.12)

   _____ / _____
      rt   suffix

6. optometrist (15.8)

   _____ / _____ / _____
      rt   v   rt/suffix

7. blepharoplasty (15.41)

   _____ / _____ / _____
          rt   v   suffix

8. corneoiritis (15.43)

   _____ / _____ / _____ / _____
         rt   v   rt   suffix

9. phacocele (15.45)

   _____ / _____ / _____
        rt   v   suffix

10. retinoscopy (15.60)

    _____ / _____ / _____
          rt   v   suffix

11. corelysis (15.64)

    _____ / _____ / _____
       rt   v   suffix

12. keratoscleritis (15.70)

    _____ / _____ / _____ / _____
         rt   v   rt   suffix

13. nasolacrimal (15.78)

    _____ / _____ / _____ / _____
       rt   v   rt   suffix

14. dacryocystocele (15.83)

    _____ / _____ / _____ / _____ / _____
          rt   v   rt   v   suffix

▶ **REVIEW ACTIVITIES**

15. onychophagia (15.89) _____ / ____ / _____
                                                       rt   v   suffix

16. trichopathy (15.95) _____ / ____ / _____
                                                       rt   v   suffix

17. phagocytosis (15.98) _____ / ____ / _____ / _____
                  rt   v   rt   suffix

18. endocrinologist (15.105) _____ / _____ / ____ / _____
                  pre   rt   v   suffix

19. adrenocorticoid (15.106) _____ / ____ / _____
                  rt   v   rt/suffix

20. hypothyroidism (15.107) _____ / _____ / _____
                  pre   rt   suffix

21. adrenomegaly (15.108) _____ / ____ / _____
                  rt   v   suffix

22. uremia (15.114) ____ / _____
                  rt   rt/suffix

23. pathologist (15.122) _____ / ____ / _____
                  rt   v   suffix

24. oncology (15.129) _____ / ____ / _____
                  rt   v   suffix

25. otorhinolaryngologist (15.133) ____ / ____ / _____ / ____ / _____ / ____ / _____
         rt   v   rt   v   rt   v   suffix

26. orthopedist (15.138) _____ / ____ / _____ / _____
                  rt   v   rt   suffix

27. radiology (15.141) _____ / ____ / _____
                  rt   v   suffix

28. chiropractor (15.142) _____ / ____ / _____
                  rt   v   rt/suffix

29. podiatry (15.144) _____ / _____
                  rt   suffix

30. audiology (15.140) _____ / ____ / _____
                  rt   v   suffix

▶ **REVIEW ACTIVITIES**

Abbreviation Matching

Match the following abbreviations with their definition.

_____	1. COT
_____	2. TIA
_____	3. od
_____	4. TSH
_____	5. PERRLA
_____	6. ENT
_____	7. OB
_____	8. OD
_____	9. Fx
_____	10. OAG

a. otorhinolaryngologist

b. both eyes

c. living and well

d. fracture

e. light and accommodation

f. thyroid-stimulating hormone

g. right eye

h. certified occupational therapy assistant

i. doctor of optometry

j. fasting sugar height

k. left ear

l. open-angle glaucoma

m. obstetrician

n. certified ophthalmic technician

o. follicle-stimulating hormone

p. pupils equal, round, reactive to light and accommodation

q. acute glaucoma

r. transient ischemic attack

Abbreviation Fill-ins

Fill in the blanks with the correct abbreviation.

11. American Optometric Association _____

12. emergency medical technician _____

13. follicle-stimulating hormone _____

14. thyroid function tests _____

15. both eyes _____

16. light and accommodation _____

▶ **CASE STUDIES**

Write the term next to its meaning given below. Then, draw slashes to analyze the word parts. Note the use of medical abbreviations. Look these up in your dictionary or find them in Appendix B. If you have any questions about the answers, refer to your medical dictionary or check with your instructor for the answers in Appendix A.

CASE STUDY 15-1
PHACOEMULSIFICATION

Surgeon: P.H. Ernest, M.D.

Preoperative and postoperative diagnoses

1. **cataract o.d.**, with low **corneal** endothelial cell count.
2. **myopia o.d.**

Operation performed: **phacoemulsification** of right eye with insertion of foldable **intraocular** lens of 22 power.

Summary: 2% Xylocaine and Wydase administered by peribulbar injection. A Honan balloon was placed on the eye for 20 minutes at 5-minute intervals. Betadine drops were instilled into the cul-de-sac and cornea. A temporal approach was made. A **paracentesis** incision was made and Viscoelastic was used to replace the aqueous. At the limbus, a temporally approached 3.2-mm incision and then dissection into the cornea was made with crescent blade. A 2.3-mm **keratome** was used to make an internal corneal cut through Descemet's membrane creating a square wound. Under Viscoelastic, multiple sphincterotomies were performed. A 360-degree **capsulorrhexis** was performed. Hydrocortical cleavage and hydrodelineation was performed. Using phacoemulsification, the nucleus was sculpted into perpendicular grooves. Using an Ernest nuclear cracker, the nucleus was cracked into four quadrants. The epinucleus and any residual cortex was removed using pulsed phaco, irrigation, and aspiration. Under Viscoelastic, a foldable intraocular lens was inserted, and positioned within the capsular bag. All Viscoelastic was removed both anterior and posterior from the intraocular lens using irrigation and aspiration. 500-cc balanced salt, 20-mg Vancomycin and 10-mg Tobramicin was instilled. The wound was tested to ensure no wound leaks. Maxitrol ointment and a shield was applied over the eye to ensure no inadvertent corneal **abrasion**. The patient was sent to the recovery room in good condition.

1. breakup of the lens _____
2. scrape wound _____
3. rupture of the capsule _____
4. within the eye _____
5. instrument used to cut thin slices of the cornea _____
6. nearsightedness _____
7. cloudy lesion on the lens _____
8. upon the nucleus _____
9. pertaining to the cornea _____
10. puncture for the removal of fluid _____
11. abbreviation, right eye _____

▶ CROSSWORD PUZZLE

Check your answers by going back through the frames or checking the solutions in Appendix C.

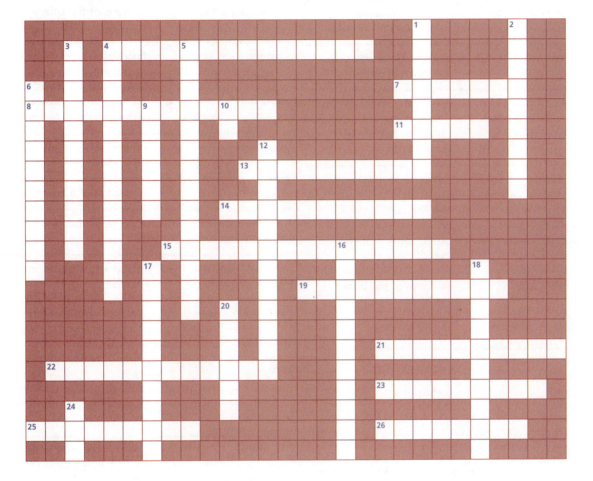

Across

4. instrument to look into the eye
7. measurement for lens prescription
8. study of hormones and glands
11. pertaining to vision
13. seeing red
14. synonym for dacryorrhea
15. hormone from the adrenal cortex
19. adrenal medulla hormone
21. tear duct stone
22. swollen eyelid
23. cross-eyed
25. bruise
26. wound with a flap

Down

1. synonym for diplopia
2. thyroid hormone
3. prolapsed iris
4. soft nails
5. slow thyroid
6. fix the retina
9. inflamed iris
10. optometrist (abbreviation)
12. hair eating
16. hair disease
17. pertaining to the eye
18. unequal pupils
20. white of the eye
24. otorhinolaryngologist (abbreviation)

► GLOSSARY

abrasion	scrape
adrenocorticoid	hormone manufactured in the adrenal cortex
adrenolysis	destruction of the adrenal glands
adrenomegaly	enlarged adrenal glands
ambivalence	unable to decide, wavering on both sides
anisocoria	pupils of unequal size
blepharedema	swelling of the eyelid
blepharoplasty	plastic surgery of the eyelid
blepharoptosis	prolapse of the upper eyelid (drooping)
blepharorrhaphy	suturing of the eyelid
blepharospasm	twitching eyelid
chloropia	seeing green
contusion	bruise
corectasia	dilation of the pupil
corectopia	displaced pupil
corelysis	destruction of the pupil
coreometer	instrument used to measure pupil size
coreoplasty	plastic surgery of the pupil
corneitis	inflammation of the cornea (keratitis)
corneoiritis	inflammation of the cornea and the iris
corneoscheral	pertaining to the cornea and the schlera

cyclokeratitis	inflammation of the ciliary body and the cornea
cycloplegia	paralysis of the ciliary body
cytophagy	destruction of other cells by phagocytes (cyto-phagia, phagocytosis)
dacryoadenalgia	pain in the tear gland
dacryocystitis	inflammation of the tear sac
dacryocystocele	herniation of a tear sac
dacryocystoptosis	prolapse of the tear sac
dacryocystotome	instrument for incision of a tear sac
dacryolith	calculus in the tear duct or sac
dacryoma	tumor of the lacrimal tissue
dacryopyorrhea	discharge of pus from the tear gland
diascope	a glass plate used to look through to examine the skin
diopter	measurement unit of refraction
diplopia	double vision (ambiopia)
endocrine	glands that secrete hormones
endocrinologist	specialist in the study of the endocrine system and treatment of disorders
endocrinology	the science studying the endocrine system

▶ GLOSSARY

epinephrine	hormone produced by the adrenal medulla
erythropia	seeing red
esotropia	condition in which the eyes point inward (cross-eyed)
euphoria	feeling good
evulsion	a tearing away
exotropia	condition in which the eyes point outward
fracture	break
glaucoma	condition in which the intraocular aqueous humor pressure is high
hyperopia	farsightedness
hypertropia	condition in which the eyes point upward
hyperthyroidism	overactive thyroid condition
hypotropia	condition in which the eyes point downward
hypothyroidism	underactive thyroid condition
iridalgia	iris pain
iridectomy	excision of the iris
iridocele	herniation of the iris
iridomalacia	softening of the iris
iridoplegia	paralysis of the iris (iridoparalysis)
iridoptosis	prolapse of the iris
iridorrhexis	rupture of the iris

keratectasia	protrusion of a thin scarred cornea
keratorrhexis	rupture of the cornea
keratoschleritis	inflammation of the cornea and schlera
keratotomy	incision into the cornea
laceration	a cut (verb form: lacerate)
lacrimation	tearing (dacryorrhea)
macrophage	large phagocyte
microphage	small phagocyte
myopia	nearsightedness
nasolacrimal	pertaining to the nasal passages and the tear ducts
onychocryptosis	ingrown nail
onychoid	resembling a nail
onychoma	nail tumor
onychomalacia	softening of the nails
onychomycosis	fungus infection of the nail
onychophagia	nail biting
ophthalmalgia	eye pain (ophthalmodynia)
ophthalmic	pertaining to the eye
ophthalmocele	herniation of the eye
ophthalmologist	physician specialist in treatment of eye disease
ophthalmometer	instrument used to measure the eye
ophthalmopathy	any eye disease
ophthalmoplasty	surgical repair of the eye

▶ GLOSSARY

ophthalmoplegia	ocular muscle paralysis	puncture	make a hole
ophthalmoscope	instrument used to examine the interior of the eye	retinal	pertaining to the retina
ophthalmoscopy	process of using an ophthalmoscope	retinitis	inflammation of the retina
optic	pertaining to vision	retinopexy	fixation of a detached retina (retinoplasty)
optometrist	specialist assessing and treating visual acuity problems and other eye diseases (limited license)	retinoscope	instrument used to look at the retina
		sclerectomy	excision of the sclera
optometry	the measurement of vision and the practice performed by the optometrist	sclerostomy	make an opening in the schlera
paronychia	condition of infection around a nail	suprarenal	upon the kidney, refers to the adrenal glands
phacocele	dislocation of the lens of the eye	testosterone	hormone produced in the testes (androgen)
		thyroxine	thyroid hormone
phacoemulsification	procedure to disintegrate cataracts	traumatology	the study of wound treatment
phagocyte	cell that eats cells (macrophage, leukocyte)	trichoglossia	condition of hair growth on the tongue
		trichoid	resembling hair
phorometer	instrument used to measure ocular muscle movement	trichopathy	any hair disease
		trichophagia	condition in which the person bites on or eats hair
phoropter	instrument used to measure prescription strength for lenses	trichophobia	fear of hair growth (women: on the face) or touching it
presbyopia	old eye, loss of accommodation	xanthopia	see yellow

► **ANSWERS**

Section B

Circle and Correct
1. d   2. a   3. d   4. b   5. c   6. c   7. b   8. d

Form the Plural
1. bursae   2. cocci   3. ova   4. sarcomata
5. protozoa   6. crises   7. appendices

Unit 1

Circle and Correct
1. b   2. d   3. b or d   4. c   5. c   6. d   7. b   8. a   9. b   10. c
11. a   12. d   13. d   14. c   15. b

Select and Construct
1. acroparalysis   2. dermatitis   3. cyanoderma
4. dermopathy (dermatopathy)   5. erythrocyte   6. melanoblast
7. thrombocytopenia   8. gastromegaly (megalogastria)   9. megalomania
10. electrocardiograph   11. duodenotomy   12. cardiac
13. echography (sonography)   14. echocardiogram   15. radiographer
16. leukocytosis   17. acromegaly   18. tomogram
19. xanthosis   20. cytology

Abbreviation Matching
1. l   2. k   3. d   4. b   5. h   6. g   7. m   8. n   9. i   10. c

Abbreviation Fill-in
11. CBC   12. WBC, RBC   13. MRI, XR   14. RT(R)   15. DMS, ECHO
16. CCU, EKG, ECHO   17. CPK, LDH

Case Study
1. acute   2. coronary   3. echocardiogram
4. substernal   5. telemetry   6. arteriosclerosis
7. angiography   8. cardiopulmonary   9. ambulance
10. etiology   11. electrocardogram   12. x-ray

Unit 2

Circle and Correct
1. a   2. c   3. b   4. a   5. c   6. c   7. b   8. b   9. d   10. b
11. c   12. a   13. c   14. b   15. d

Select and Construct
1. encephalocele   2. electroencephalograph   3. cranioplasty
4. cerebrospinal   5. adenocarcinoma   6. mucoid
7. lipoma   8. craniomalacia   9. cerebrotomy

▶ ANSWERS

10. meningitis   11. oncologist   12. sarcoma
13. lymphadenoma   14. hypertrophy   15. hypotension
16–20. Your own answers

Abbreviation Matching
1. d   2. l   3. g   4. c   5. n   6. k   7. h   8. i   9. m   10. b

Abbreviation Fill-in
11. MLT   12. BP, mm Hg, HCVD   13. TIA, CVA   14. BCC

Case Study
1. D&C   2. endocervical   3. poikilocytotic
4. dysplasia   5. atypia   6. grav IV, para IV
7. carcinoma   8. colposcopy   9. conization
10. gynecology   11. Pap   12. biopsies

Unit 3

Circle and Correct
1. c   2. d   3. a   4. b   5. c   6. a   7. d   8. b   9. c   10. d
11. d   12. b   13. c   14. a   15. d

Select and Construct
1. osteomalacia   2. abduction   3. hydrocyst
4. hydrocephalic   5. suprapubic   6. intercostal
7. abdominocentesis   8. arthroscopy   9. aberrant
10. orthodontist   11. tendinitis (tendonitis)   12. pelvimeter
13. cephalopelvic   14. orthopedist   15. osteosarcoma
16–20. your own answers

Abbreviation Matching
1. d   2. n   3. h   4. p   5. r   6. b   7. m   8. k   9. o   10. c

Abbreviation Fill-in
11. DTS   12. RUQ   13. OMT   14. DDS   15. ORTHO

Case Study
1. inflammation   2. arthroscope   3. mediolateral   4. menisectomy
5. chondromalacia   6. arthritis   7. arthroscopic   8. patella
9. orthopedic   10. medial   11. pyorrhea   12. incision
13. arthrotomy   14. arthroplasty

Unit 4

Circle and Correct
1. b   2. a   3. d   4. b   5. b   6. a   7. d   8. c   9. d   10. a   11. b
12. d   13. b   14. a   15. c   16. c   17. c   18. a   19. d   20. b   21. b   22. a

▶ ANSWERS

Select and Construct
1. bradycardia
2. tachyphagia
3. staphylitis (uvulitis)
4. cholelithiasis
5. otodynia (otalgia)
6. audiometry
7. dyspepsia
8. pyogenic
9. rhinorrhea
10. tympanogram
11. tympanites
12. cholecystogram
13. apnea
14. diathermy
15. polydipsia
16. synergy (synergistic)
17. microcephalus
18. macrocyte
19. prodromal
20. hypothermia

Mix and Match
1. f   2. d   3. a   4. c   5. b   6. e   7. g   8. h

Abbreviation Matching
1. r   2. l   3. f   4. a   5. q   6. p   7. d   8. s   9. n   10. o   11. i   12. m

Case Study
1. ductal
2. edematous
3. gallbladder
4. cholelith
5. cholangiogram
6. cm
7. epigastric
8. RUQ
9. cholecystectomy
10. ultrasound
11. T, °F

Unit 5

Circle and Correct
1. b   2. c   3. d   4. b   5. a   6. d   7. b   8. b   9. c   10. a
11. c   12. a   13. b   14. c   15. c   16. d   17. b   18. d

Select and Construct
1. pyelonephritis
2. ureterorrhaphy
3. cystoscopy
4. nephroptosis
5. renogram
6. cystopexy
7. urthrorrhagia
8. nephrolysis
9. cystostomy
10. endometritis
11. hysteroptosis (metroptosis)
12. cryptorchidism
13. prostatectomy
14. gynecologist
15. oogenesis
16. balanorrhea
17. colpalgia (colpodynia)
18. hysteroscope
19. urologist
20. hysterosalpingogram
21. orchidopexy (orchiopexy)
22. colposcopy

Abbreviation Matching
1. q   2. s   3. g   4. h   5. i   6. m   7. o   8. p   9. n   10. b
11. e   12. l   13. a   14. d

Abbreviation Fill-in
15. MD   16. PSA   17. TSE   18. AID   19. ESRD   20. Pap

Case Study
1. mg qid
2. benign
3. pathology
4. hyperplasia
5. prostatitis
6. chronic
7. H&P
8. hydronephrosis
9. TUR
10. hematuria
11. afebrile
12. cystoclysis
13. catheter
14. postoperative
15. transurethral

▶ **ANSWERS**

Unit 6

Circle and Correct
1. d   2. c   3. b   4. b   5. c   6. d   7. a   8. b   9. c   10. d   11. d   12. c

Select and Construct
1. stomatomycosis
2. sublingual (hypoglossal, subglassal)
3. cheiloplasty
4. gingivitis
5. enterorrhagia
6. esophagogastroduodenoscopy
7. enteroptosis
8. rectoclysis
9. proctoplegia
10. pancreatolith
11. splenomegaly
12. gastrectasia
13. sigmoidoscope
14. hepatitis
15. rectocele
16. esophagogastric (gastroesophageal)
17. cholangiopancreatography
18. colorectal

Abbreviation Matching
1. f   2. k   3. i   4. j   5. g   6. h   7. o   8. q   9. r   10. e   11. a

Suffix Matching
1. j   2. e   3. a   4. f   5. h   6. c

Case Study
1. anterior
2. vomiting
3. hemorrhage
4. nasogastric
5. endoscope
6. mucosal
7. aspirate
8. isotonic
9. ulcer
10. gastointestinal
11. melenic
12. hypotensive
13. duodenal
14. thrombi
15. EGD

Unit 7

Circle and Correct
1. c   2. a   3. d   4. a   5. c   6. a   7. b   8. b   9. a   10. d
11. c   12. d   13. d   14. c   15. c   16. a   17. a

Select and Construct
1. arteriosclerosis
2. phlebectasia
3. enterorrhexis
4. angiogram (angiograph)
5. esthesiometer
6. anesthesiologist
7. analgesic
8. parahepatitis
9. aphonia
10. myograph
11. dyskinesia
12. audiometer
13. dysphasia
14. paraplegia
15. fibromyoma
16. atherosclerosis
17. angioplasty
18. thrombosis
19. myospasm
20. fibroneuroma
21. thrombophlebitis
22. neurologist
23. cardiomyopathy

Abbreviation Matching
1. k   2. t   3. l   4. j   5. g   6. e   7. p   8. f   9. d   10. r

Abbreviation Fill-in
11. HDL   12. MI   13. PT   14. CABG   15. IV
16. BK   17. MD   18. TENS

▶ **ANSWERS**

Case Study
1. appendectomy
2. hemoglobin
3. cc
4. lb, oz
5. admission
6. C-section
7. bilateral
8. salpingectomy
9. myomectomy
10. leiomyomata
11. neonate
12. gm

Unit 8

Circle and Correct
1. b   2. d   3. a   4. b   5. c   6. b   7. d   8. b   9. d   10. d
11. c   12. a   13. c   14. a   15. c   16. b   17. c   18. a   19. d   20. c   21. b

Select and Construct—Part I
1. myeloblast
2. neuropathy
3. dialysis
4. lithotripsy
5. chondrodysplasia
6. psychotropic
7. pharmacology
8. procephalic
9. diagnosis
10. psychomotor
11. hyperplasia
12. myelodysplasia

13–16. Your own answers

Select and Construct—Part II
1. anteroposterior
2. cephalocaudal
3. anterolateral
4. dyspepsia
5. euphoria
6. chromophilic
7. hemostasis
8. pseudotuberculosis
9. aerobic
10. parietal pleura
11. visceral peritoneum
12. omphalorrhea
13. euthanasia
14. dysmenorrhea
15. eupnea

Diagram Labels
1. cephalic (cephalad)
2. superior (hyper, super, supra)
3. inferior (hypo, sub, infra)
4. anterior, ventral (pre, pro, ante)
5. circum
6. posterior, dorsal (retro, post)
7. abduct (lateral)
8. adduct (medial)
9. distal
10. proximal
11. sagittal

Abbreviation Matching
1. h   2. b   3. k   4. d   5. m   6. n   7. f   8. l   9. c   10. q

Abbreviation Fill-in
11. LOA
12. STD
13. RPR (VDRL)
14. LAT
15. LMP
16. Bx
17. TB

Case Study
1. hypothyroidism
2. incontinence
3. psychiatric
4. obsessive compulsive disorder
5. UTI
6. EST
7. diarrhea
8. BP, P, R
9. Ua c̄ C+S
10. paranoia

▶ **ANSWERS**

Unit 9

Circle and Correct
1. b   2. d   3. a   4. b   5. d   6. b   7. a   8. b   9. d   10. c

Count with Prefixes
1. nulli, nulligravida
2. primi, primipara
3. mono, monocyte
4. bi, bifurcate (bifurcation)
5. tri, trilateral
6. quad, quadriplegia
7. quint, quintuplets
8. sexti, sextigravida
9. septi, septipara
10. octo, octogenarian
11. noni, nonigravida
12. deca, decaliter
13. centi, centimeter
14. kilo, kilocalorie
15. multi, multiglandular

Select and Construct
1. laparoscope
2. endogenous
3. pyrosis
4. hyperhidrosis (hidrosis, hidrorrhea)
5. mesentery
6. retroperitoneal
7. glycolysis
8. endocardial
9. ectopic
10. paracystitis
11. anteflexion
12. retroversion
13. endoscope
14. hyperglycemia
15. glucolipid (glycolipid)
16. decagram
17. millimeter

Abbreviation Matching—Part I
1. e   2. i   3. h   4. c   5. b   6. a   7. k   8. l

Abbreviation Matching—Part II
1. g   2. d   3. j   4. k   5. h   6. a   7. l   8. b

Abbreviations—Weights and Measures
1. kg
2. oz
3. cc
4. MHz
5. t, tsp
6. lb, #
7. dr
8. iss, 1.5, 1½

Case Study
1. catheterization
2. apnea
3. IDDM
4. URI
5. narcolepsy
6. CPAP
7. hypoventilation
8. syndrome
9. symptoms
10. U
11. hypoglycemic
12. analgesic
13. cephalalgia
14. dyspnea
15. ventilatory

Unit 10

Prefix and Word
1. ab, abduct
2. de, descending
3. ex, excise
4. iso, isotonic
5. aniso, anisocytosis
6. dia, diathermy
7. per, percussion
8. peri, pericardium
9. circum, circumduction
10. sub, sublingual (or subglossal) (hypo, hypoglossal)

Select and Construct
1. excretion
2. abort
3. narcolepsy
4. mastocarcinoma
5. abrade
6. perihepatitis
7. narcotic
8. decalcification

▶ ANSWERS

9. isotonic   10. circumcision   11. ablation   12. percussion

13. anisocytosis   14. ablactation   15. dehydration   16. perfusion

17–20. You own answers

Abbreviation Matching
1. g   2. h   3. m   4. i   5. f   6. j   7. c   8. b

Abbreviation Fill-in
9. q4h   10. D/W   11. NS   12. qid   13. †   14. Dx

Case Study
1. subcuticular   2. anesthesia   3. multifocal

4. carcinoma in situ   5. dissected   6. axillary

7. hemostasis   8. mastectomy   9. mammogram

10. sterile   11. retraction   12. microcalcifications

13. biopsy

Unit 11

Select and Construct
1. antibiotic (antiseptic)   2. contraceptive   3. homosexual

4. anisocytosis   5. sympodia   6. substernal (infrasternal)

7. mammography   8. ultrasonographer (sonographer)   9. epidural

10. extracytosis   11. trilateral   12. metastasis

13–16. Your own answers

Prefix and Word
1. homo, homosexual   2. hetero, heterogeneous   3. sym, sympodia

4. super, superficial   5. supra, suprarenal   6. a/an, amenorrhea

7. a/an, anesthesia   8. epi, epigastric   9. extra, extracellular

10. infra, infrasternal   11. meta, metacarpals   12. ultra, ultrasound (ultrasonic)

13. bi, bilateral   14. anti, antiarthritic   15. contra, contraindicated

16. trans, transurethral

Abbreviation Matching
1. g   2. f   3. i   4. h   5. a   6. j   7. l   8. c

Abbreviation Fill-in
9. AAMA   10. s̄   11. inf   12. XM

Case Study
1. subdural   2. anesthesiologist   3. incision

4. hemostasis   5. subcutaneous   6. pericramium

7. retracted   8. perforator   9. dura mater

10. transferred   11. hemiparesis

▶ **ANSWERS**

Unit 12

Prefix and Word
1. ex, exhale
2. in, incise
3. in, incompetent
4. mal, malnutrition
5. tri, trigeminal
6. bi, bifocal
7. uni, unilateral
8. semi, semiconscious
9. hemi, hemiatrophy
10. con, congenital
11. dis, disinfectant
12. post, postmastectomy
13. pre, presurgical
14. pre, prefrontal
15. retro, retroesophageal
16. ante, antefebrile
17. intra, intradermal
18. inter, intercellular
19. sub, subcutaneous

Select and Construct
1. antenatal (prenatal)
2. postpartum
3. hemicardia
4. semicomatose
5. unicellular
6. uninuclear
7. precancerous
8. inject
9. incontinent
10. insane
11. malformation
12. malaria
13–18. Your own answers

Abbreviation Matching
1. g   2. f   3. i   4. c   5. h   6. k   7. l   8. b

Abbreviation Fill-in
9. exc   10. AIH   11. ID   12. iii   13. am   14. inf

Case Study
1. bilateral
2. endometriomata
3. incised
4. transversely
5. visceroperitoneum
6. preoperative
7. dissection
8. posterior
9. intracystic
10. appendectomy
11. salpingo-oophorectomy
12. adhesions
13. postoperative
14. dissection

Unit 13

Circle and Correct
1. c   2. c   3. a   4. d   5. a   6. b   7. c   8. a   9. d   10. a   11. d

Select and Construct
1. pulmonary (pulmonic)
2. pneumonomelanosis
3. dermatomycosis (mycodermatitis)
4. embolus (embolism)
5. mycology
6. nasomental
7. pharyngoscope
8. pleurocentesis
9. dextropedal
10. sinistromanual
11. pediatrician
12. histolysis
13. bronchitis
14. laryngalgia (laryngodynia)
15. phrenoplegia
16. bronchiectasis (bronchodilatation)
17. psychiatrist
18. tracheostomy
19. chiropractor

▶ ANSWERS

Abbreviation Matching
1. f   2. n   3. a   4. l   5. m   6. k   7. h   8. j   9. c   10. p

Abbreviation Fill-in
11. PE   12. PFT   13. CO_2 14. R   15. COPD   16. RRA

Matching
1. e   2. d   3. a   4. f   5. c   6. b

Case Study
1. bronchitis   2. pulse   3. tachypnea   4. intravenous
5. oximetry   6. O_2 7. %   8. respiratory
9. asthmaticus   10. viral

Unit 14

Circle and Correct
1. c   2. d   3. b   4. a   5. d   6. c   7. b   8. c   9. d   10. b   11. c   12. a

Select and Construct
1. sternalgia (sternodynia)   2. brachiocephalic   3. mycostasis (fungistasis)
4. ischiopubic   5. condylectomy   6. rachischisis
7. palatoschisis (uranoschisis) 8. xiphocarpal   9. metacarpals
10. schizophasia   11. somnabulism (noctambulism)   12. nyctalopia
13. nycturia (nocturia)   14. ankylodactylia   15–20. Your own answers

Skeletal Combining Forms and Adjectival Forms
1. cranio, cranial   2. cervico, cervical   3. cleido, clavicular
4. scapulo, scapular   5. acromio, acromial   6. humero, humeral
7. sterno, sternal   8. xipho, xiphoid   9. ulno, ulnar
10. radio, radial   11. carpo, carpal   12. metacarpo, metacarpal
13. phalango, phalangeal   14. ischio, ischial   15. ilio, ilial
16. pubo, pubic   17. femoro, femoral   18. patello, patellar
19. tibio, tibial   20. fibulo, fibular   21. tarso, tarsal
22. metatarso, metatarsal   23. calcaneo, calcaneal   24. costo, costal
25. chondro, chondral

Abbreviation Matching
1. l   2. f   3. e   4. g   5. k   6. h   7. c   8. m

Abbreviation Fill-in
9. C_3 10. FxBB   11. OT(R), OTR   12. AOTA   13. R
14. y/o (yrs)   15. ORIF

Case Study
1. inspection   2. manually   3. lateral   4. incision
5. sterile   6. subcutaneous   7. anatomic   8. internal
9. Fx   10. aerobic   11. anesthetized   12. fixation

▶ **ANSWERS**

13. reduction   14. epicondyle   15. humerus   16. M
17. y/o   18. rt

Unit 15

Circle and Correct
1. d   2. c   3. b   4. a   5. d   6. b   7. a   8. d   9. a   10. d
11. b   12. b   13. c   14. a

Select and Construct
1. optometry   2. cycloplegia   3. onychomalacia
4. iritis   5. dacryorrhea   6. phacoemulsification
7. adrenalin (epinephrine) 8. hyperopia   9. retinoscope
10. traumatology   11. ophthalmoplasty   12. corectasis (corectasia)
13. blepharoptosis   14. keratotomy   15. thyromegaly
16. anisocoria   17. esophoria   18–20. Your own answers

Abbreviation Matching
1. n   2. r   3. g   4. f   5. p   6. a   7. m   8. i   9. d   10. l

Abbreviation Fill-in
11. AOA   12. EMT   13. FSH   14. T3, T4   15. ou   16. L&A

Case Study
1. phacoemulsification   2. abrasion   3. capsulorrhexis
4. intraocular   5. keratome   6. myopia
7. cataract   8. epinucleus   9. corneal
10. paracentesis   11. OD

► ABBREVIATIONS

The following lists of abbreviations are grouped by topic. To assist you in learning, they are arranged in columns. Column 1 lists the abbreviation, column 2 the meaning, and column 3 is left blank as a work space. Study the abbreviation and its meaning. Then, cover the abbreviation and read the meaning. Write the abbreviation correctly in the blank. You may use the same method to learn the meanings by covering the meaning and reading the abbreviation. Write the meaning correctly on a separate piece of paper. Abbreviations that correspond to word parts presented in the frames are also listed at the end of each unit.

WEIGHTS AND MEASURES

Metric:

kg	kilogram(s) [1000 g]	_____
hg	hectogram [100 g]	_____
dag	decagram [10 g]	_____
gm or g	gram	_____
dg	decigram [0.1 g]	_____
cg	centigram [0.01 g]	_____
mg	milligram [0.001 g]	_____
mcg, μg	microgram [0.001 mg]	_____

Standard:

lb, #	pound	_____
oz, $\overline{3}$	ounce	_____
dr, 3	dram	_____
gr	grain	_____

Volume:

cu mm	cubic millimeter [mm^3]	_____
cc	cubic centimeter [cm^3]	_____
cu m	cubic meter [m^3]	_____
cu in	cubic inch [in^3]	_____
cu ft	cubic foot [ft^3]	_____
cu yd	cubic yard [yd^3]	_____

Apothecary:

$\overline{i}, \overline{ii}, \overline{iii}$	one, two, three	_____
$\overline{iv}, \overline{v}$, etc.	four, five, etc.	_____
$\overline{iss}$	one and one half	_____

► ABREVIATIONS

Lengths:

in, "	inch [2.54 cm]	_____
ft, '	foot [12 in]	_____
yd	yard [36 in]	_____
µm	micrometer [0.000001 m]	_____
mm	millimeter [0.001 m]	_____
cm	centimeter [0.01 m]	_____
m	meter	_____
km	kilometer [1000 m]	_____

Liquid Volume:

t, tsp	teaspoon	_____
T, Tbsp	tablespoon	_____
c	cup	_____
m, min	minim	_____
ml	milliliter [0.001 L]	_____
cc	cubic centimeter [1 ml]	_____
cl	centiliter [0.01 L]	_____
dl	deciliter [0.1 L]	_____
L	liter [1000 ml]	_____
dal	decaliter [10 L]	_____
hl	hectoliter [100 L]	_____
fl dr, fl ʒ	fluid dram [60 min]	_____
fl oz, fl ʒ	fluid ounce [8 fl dr]	_____
pt	pint [16 oz]	_____
qt	quart [32 oz]	_____
gal, °	gallon [4 qt]	_____
gt	drop [1 min]	_____
gtt	drops	_____

Miscellaneous:

at wt	atomic weight	_____
C, kcal	calorie	_____
c, Ci	curie	_____
ht	height	_____
mA	milliampere	_____
mEq	milliequivalent	_____
MHz	megahertz	_____
mg%	milligram percent	_____
mw	molecular weight	_____
IU	international units	_____

► ABBREVIATIONS

U	units	_____
°C	degrees Celsius	_____
°F	degrees Fahrenheit	_____

CHEMICAL SYMBOLS

Al	aluminum	_____
Ar	argon	_____
As	arsenic	_____
Ba	barium	_____
B	boron	_____
Br	bromine	_____
Ca	calcium (Ca^{2+} ion)	_____
Cd	cadmium	_____
C	carbon	_____
CO_2	carbon dioxide	_____
pCO_2	partial pressure carbon dioxide	_____
Cl	chlorine (Cl^- ion)	_____
Cr	chromium	_____
Co	cobalt	_____
Cu	copper (Cu^{++} ion)	_____
F	fluorine	_____
$C_6H_{12}O_6$	glucose	_____
He	helium	_____
H	hydrogen	_____
H_2O	water	_____
I	iodine [I^{131} radioactive]	_____
Fe	iron [ferrum—Latin]	_____
K	potassium [kalium—Latin]	_____
Kr	krypton	_____
Pb	lead [plumbum—Latin]	_____
Li	lithium	_____
Mg	magnesium	_____
Mn	manganese	_____
Hg	mercury [hydrargyrum—Latin]	_____
Ne	neon	_____
N	nitrogen	_____
O	oxygen [O_2]	_____
P	phosphorus	_____
pO_2	partial pressure oxygen	_____

► ABREVIATIONS

Ra	radium	
Se	selenium	
Si	silicon	
Ag	silver [argentum—Latin]	
AgNO$_3$	silver nitrate	
Au	gold	
Na	sodium [natrium—Latin]	
NaCl	sodium chloride	
S	sulfur	
U	uranium	
Zn	zinc	

DIAGNOSES

ABE	acute bacterial endocarditis	
ACVD	acute cardiovascular disease	
AF (Afib)	atrial fibrillation	
AI	aortic insufficiency	
AID	acute infectious disease	
	artificial insemination donor	
AIDS	acquired immunodeficiency syndrome	
AIH	artificial insemination husband	
ALL	acute lymphocytic leukemia	
ALS	amyotrophic lateral sclerosis	
AMI	acute myocardial infarction	
AML	acute myelocytic leukemia	
AOD	arterial occlusive disease	
ARC	AIDS related complex (conditions)	
ARD	acute respiratory disease	
ARF	acute respiratory failure	
	acute renal failure	
	acute rheumatic fever	
ARV	AIDS related virus	
AS	aortic stenosis	
	arteriosclerosis	
	left ear (auris sinistra)	
ASCVD	arteriosclerotic cardiovascular disease	
ASHD	arteriosclerotic heart disease	
AV, A-V	arteriovenous, atrioventricular	
BCC	basal cell carcinoma	

▶ **ABBREVIATIONS**

BO	body odor	
BPH	benign prostatic hyperplasia (hypertrophy)	
Ca, CA	cancer	
CAD	coronary artery disease	
CD	childhood disease	
CE	cardiac enlargement	
CF	cystic fibrosis	
CHD	congestive heart disease	
	congenital hip dislocation	
	congenital or coronary heart disease	
CHF	congestive heart failure	
CIS	carcinoma in situ	
CLD	chronic liver disease	
	chronic lung disease	
COLD	chronic obstructive lung disease	
COPD	chronic obstructive pulmonary disease	
CP	cerebral palsy	
	cor pulmonale	
CPD	cephalopelvic disproportion	
CRF	chronic renal failure	
CT	carpal tunnel (syndrome)	
	coronary thrombosis	
CVA	cerebrovascular accident (stroke)	
CVD	cardiovascular disease	
DNA	do not resuscitate	
DOA	dead on arrival	
DRG	diagnostic related group	
DTs	delirium tremens	
Dx	diagnosis	
ESRD	end stage renal disease (failure)	
FAS	fetal alcohol syndrome	
FB	foreign body	
FOD	free of disease	
FTND	full term normal delivery	
FTT	failure to thrive	
FUO	fever of unknown origin	
Fx	fracture	
FxBB	fracture both bones	

506

▶ ABREVIATIONS

GERD	gastroesophageal reflux disease	
GNID	gram-negative intracellular diplococci	
Grav 1/ab 1	one pregnancy/one abortion	
HA	headache	
	hearing aid	
	hemolytic anemia	
	hepatitis A	
HAA	hepatitis associated antigen	
HC	Huntington's chorea	
HCVD	hypertensive cardiovascular disease	
HD	Hodgkin's disease	
HDN	hemolytic disease of newborn	
HF	heart failure	
HH	hiatal hernia	
	hard of hearing	
HIV	human immunodeficiency virus	
HLV	herpes-like virus	
HPV	human papilloma virus	
HSV	herpes simplex virus	
HTLV/III	human T-cell lymphotropic virus/three	
HTN	hypertension	
Hx	history	
IDDM	insulin-dependent diabetes mellitus	
IHD	ischemic heart disease	
IM	infectious mononucleosis	
LAV	lymphadenopathy-associated virus	
LE	lupus erythematosus	
LGB	Landry-Guillain-Barré syndrome	
LOA	left occiput anterior	
MBD	minimal brain dysfunction	
MD	manic depression	
	muscular dystrophy	
	myocardial disease	
met., metas., mets.	metastasis	
MI	myocardial infarction	
Mono	mononucleosis	
MP	metacarpophalangeal (joint)	

MS	mitral stenosis
	multiple sclerosis
MVP	mitral valve prolapse
NIDDM	noninsulin-dependent diabetes mellitus
NMT	nebulizing mist treatment
OA	osteoarthritis
OAG	open angle glaucoma
OM	otitis media
PAC	premature atrial contraction
PAR	perennial allergic rhinitis
	postanesthesia recovery
para	paraplegic
para (I,II…)	live births (one, two…)
PAT	paroxysmal atrial tachycardia
PCD	polycystic disease
PD	Parkinson's disease
	pulmonary disease
PE	pulmonary edema
	pulmonary embolism
PERRLA	pupils equal, round, reactive to light and accommodation
PID	pelvic inflammatory disease
PKU	phenylketonuria
PMS	premenstrual syndrome
PND	paroxysmal nocturnal dyspnea
	postnasal drip
preg	pregnant
PVC	premature ventricular contraction
Px	prognosis
RA	rheumatoid arthritis
ROP	right occiput posterior
S-C disease	sickle cell hemoglobin-c disease
schiz	schizophrenia
SIDS	sudden infant death syndrome
staph	staphylococcus
STD	sexually transmitted disease
strep	streptococcus
Tb	tubercle bacillus

ABBREVIATIONS

► ABBREVIATIONS

TB	tuberculosis	_____
TCS	transcavital sonography	_____
Thal	Thalassemia	_____
TEE	transesophageal echocardiography	_____
TIA	transient ischemic attack	_____
TSD	Tay-Sachs disease	_____
TVS	transvaginal sonography	_____
URI	upper respiratory infection	_____
UTI	urinary tract infection	_____

PROCEDURES

AB	abortion	_____
A&P	auscultation and percussion	_____
ABG	arterial blood gas	_____
A, B, O, AB	blood typing groups	_____
ACT	activated clotting time—Lee-White	_____
ACTH	adrenocorticotropic hormone (test)	_____
AFB	acid fast bacillus	_____
AID	artificial insemination donor	_____
AIH	artificial insemination husband	_____
ANA	antinuclear antibodies (RIA)	_____
BaEn, BE	barium enema	_____
BP	blood pressure	_____
BUN	blood urea nitrogen	_____
Bx	biopsy	_____
CABG	coronary artery bypass graft	_____
CAD	computer aided design	_____
CAT	computerized axial tomography scan	_____
Cath	catheter	_____
CBC	complete blood count	_____
CAPD	continuous ambulatory peritoneal dialysis	_____
CH, Chol	cholesterol	_____
CPAP	continuous positive airway pressure	_____
CPK	creatine phosphokinase	_____
CPR	cardiopulmonary resuscitation	_____
C&S	culture and sensitivity	_____
C-section	Cesarean section	_____
CSF	cerebrospinal fluid	_____
CT	computerized tomography (scan)	_____

► **ABBREVIATIONS**

CXR	chest x-ray	
Cysto	cystoscopy	
D&C	dilation and curettage	
Del	delivery	
DHT	dihydrotestosterone	
DNA	deoxyribonucleic acid	
DPT	diphtheria-pertussis-tetanus (vaccine)	
ECG, EKG	electrocardiogram	
ECHO	echocardiogram	
ECT	electroconvulsive therapy	
EEG	electroencephalogram	
EGD	esophagogastroduodenoscopy	
EMG	electromyogram	
ERCP	endoscopic retrograde cholangiopancreatography	
ERG	electroretinogram	
ESR	erythrocyte sedimentation rate (sed. rate)	
ESWL	extracorporeal shockwave lithotripsy	
exam	examination	
exc	excise	
FBS	fasting blood sugar	
FME	full mouth extraction	
FSH	follicle stimulating hormone	
GA	gastric analysis	
GTT	glucose tolerance test	
GxT	graded exercise test	
HA	hearing aid	
HAA	hepatitis associated antigen (test)	
HAI	hemagglutination inhibition— rubella test	
Hb, Hgb	hemoglobin	
HBV	hepatitis B vaccine	
HCG (hcg)	human chorionic gonadotropin	
Hct	hematocrit	
HDL	high density lipoprotein	
Hib	*Hemophilus influenzae* vaccine	
H&P	history and physical	
HGH	human growth hormone	

ABREVIATIONS

HSG	hysterosalpingogram	_____
Hx	history	_____
IABP	intra-aortic balloon pump	_____
ICAT	indirect Coomb's test	_____
ICSH	interstitial cell stimulating hormone	_____
I&D	incision and drainage	_____
Ig	immunoglobulin, gamma (A, E, D, G, or M)	_____
inf	infusion	_____
instill	instillation (drops)	_____
IPPB	intermittent positive pressure breathing	_____
IUD	intrauterine device	_____
IVC	intravenous catheter	_____
	intravenous cholangiogram	_____
IVP	intravenous pyelogram	_____
KUB	kidney-ureter-bladder (x-ray)	_____
lab	laboratory	_____
LAVH	laparoscopically assisted vaginal hysterectomy	_____
LASER	light amplification by stimulated emission of radiation	_____
LDH	lactose dehydrogenase	_____
LDL	low density lipoprotein	_____
LH	luteinizing hormone	_____
LP	lumbar puncture	_____
MASER	microwave amplification by stimulated emission of radiation	_____
MFT	muscle function test	_____
MMRV	measles, mumps, rubella vaccine	_____
MRI	magnetic resonance imaging	_____
OC	office call	_____
OMT	osteopathic manipulative therapy	_____
O&P	ova and parasites test	_____
OPG	oculoplethysmography	_____
OPV	oral polio vaccine	_____
P&A	percussion and auscultation	_____
Pap	Papanicolaou test (smear)	_____
PAP	pulmonary artery pressure	_____
PBI	protein bound iodine	_____

▶ **ABBREVIATIONS**

PCTA	percutaneous transluminal angioplasty	
PCV	packed cell volume	
PE	physical examination	
PET	positron emission tomography	
PFT	pulmonary function test	
pH	hydrogen ion concentration, acid/base	
PSA	prostate specific antigen	
PT, protime	prothrombin time	
PTCA, PTA	percutaneous transluminal coronary angioplasty	
PTT	partial thromboplastin time	
2hr pc	two hour postcibal blood glucose	
2hr pg	two hour postglucose blood glucose	
2hr pp	two hour postprandial blood glucose	
P+V	pyloroplasty and vagotomy	
RATx	radiation therapy	
RBC	red blood cell (count)	
RIA	radioimmunoassay	
RPG	retrograde pyelogram	
RPR	syphilis test (also: DRT, VDRL, STS)	
Rx	take, prescribe	
SALT (old SGPT)	serum alanine aminotransferase	
SAST (old SGOT)	serum aspartate aminotransferase	
SOP	standard operating procedure	
sp gr	specific gravity (urine)	
T3	thyroid test (triiodothyronine)	
T4	thyroid test (tetraiodothyronine)	
T, temp	temperature	
TAH	total abdominal hysterectomy	
Td	tetanus	
TENS	transcutaneous electrical nerve stimulation	
TSE	testicular self-exam	
TSH	thyroid stimulating hormone	
TUR (TURP)	transurethral resection (of the prostate)	
Tx	treatment, traction, transplant	
UA	urinalysis	

► ABREVIATIONS

UV	ultraviolet (light)
WBC	white blood cell (count)
VCG	vectorcardiogram
VDRL	Venereal Disease Research Laboratory (syphilis test)
XM	cross match for blood (type and cross match)
XR	x-ray
YAG	yttrium-aluminum-garnet (laser)
V, Y, W, Z, -plasty	various types of plastic surgery

HEALTH PROFESSIONS AND GROUPS

AA	Alcoholics Anonymous
AAFP	American Academy of Family Physicians
AAMA	American Association of Medical Assistants
AAMT	American Association of Medical Transcriptionists
AANA	American Association of Nurse Anesthetists
AAP	American Academy of Pediatrics
AAPA	American Academy of Physician Assistants
ACOA	Adult Children of Alcoholics
ACS	American Cancer Society
	American College of Surgeons
ADA	American Dental Association
	American Diabetes Association
ADA	American Dietetic Association
AEMT	Advanced Emergency Medical Technician (Paramedic)
AHA	American Heart Association
AHIMA	American Health Information Management Association
AL-Anon, Alateen	Families of Alcoholics Groups
AMA	American Medical Association
ANA	American Nurses' Association
ANA	American Neurologic Association
AOA	American Optometric Association
	American Osteopathic Association

▶ ABBREVIATIONS

APA	American Psychiatric Association	_____
APTA	American Physical Therapy Association	_____
ARDMS	American Registry of Diagnostic Medical Sonographers	_____
ARRT	American Registry of Radiologic Technologists	_____
ART	Accredited Records Technician	_____
ASCP	American Society of Clinical Pathologists	_____
BSN	Bachelors of Science in Nursing	_____
CDC	Centers for Disease Control	_____
CENA, CNA	Certified Nursing Assistant, Competency Eligible Nursing Assistant	_____
CHUC	Certified Health Unit Coordinator (Clerk)	_____
CLA	Certified Laboratory Assistant	_____
CMA	Certified Medical Assistant	_____
CMT	Certified Medical Transcriptionist	_____
COMA	Certified Ophthalmic Medical Assistant	_____
COMT	Certified Ophthalmic Medical Technician	_____
COTA	Certified Occupational Therapy Assistant	_____
CRNA	Certified Registered Nurse Anesthetist	_____
CRTT	Certified Respiratory Therapy Technician	_____
CST	Certified Surgical Technologist	_____
DC	Doctor of Chiropractic	_____
DDS	Doctor of Dental Surgery	_____
DO	Doctor of Osteopathy	_____
DPM	Doctor of Podiatric Medicine	_____
EENT	Eye, Ear, Nose, and Throat specialist	_____
EMT	Emergency Medical Technician	_____
EMT-P	Paramedic—EMT	_____
ENT	Ear, Nose, and Throat specialist	_____
FACP	Fellow of the American College of Physicians	_____
FACS	Fellow of the American College of Surgeons	_____

ABBREVIATIONS

▶ ABREVIATIONS

GYN	Gynecologist	_____
HMO	health maintenance organization	_____
ICU	intensive care unit	_____
LPN	Licensed Practical Nurse	_____
LVN	Licensed Vocational Nurse	_____
MD	Doctor of Medicine	_____
MLT	Medical Laboratory Technician	_____
MSN	Masters of Science in Nursing	_____
MT (ASCP)	Medical Technologist (American Society of Clinical Pathologists	_____
NAHUC	National Association of Health Unit Coordinators (Clerks)	_____
NANDA	North American Nursing Diagnosis Association	_____
NLN	National League for Nursing	_____
NP	Nurse Practitioner	_____
OA	Overeaters Anonymous	_____
OB	Obstetrician	_____
ORTH	Orthopedist	_____
OSHA	Occupational Safety and Health Administration	_____
OTR	Occupational Therapist Registered	_____
PA	Physician's Assistant	_____
Pharm D	Doctor of Pharmacy	_____
PT	Physical Therapy (Therapist)	_____
RD	Registered Dietician	_____
RDMS	Registered Diagnostic Medical Sonographer	_____
RN	Registered Nurse	_____
R.Ph	Registered Pharmacist	_____
RRA	Registered Records Administrator	_____
RRT	Registered Respiratory Therapist	_____
RT (R)	Radiologic Technologist (Registered)	_____
RT (N)	Radiologic Technologist (Nuclear)	_____
USP	United States Pharmacopeia	_____

CHARTING ABBREVIATIONS

aa	of each	_____
ac	before meals (ante cibum)	_____
AD	right ear (auris dextra)	_____

▶ **ABBREVIATIONS**

ADL	activities of daily living
ad lib	as desired (at liberty)
adm	admission
AE	above the elbow
AJ	ankle jerk
AK	above the knee
am	before noon (ante meridiem)
AMA	against medical advice
AMB	ambulate
ant	anterior
AP	anteroposterior
approx	approximately
ASAP	as soon as possible
AS or LE	left ear (auris sinistra)
AV	atrioventricular
BE	below the elbow
bid	twice a day (bis in die)
bin	twice a night (bis in nocte)
BK	below the knee
BM	bowel movement
BMR	basal metabolic rate
BP	blood pressure
BRP	bathroom privileges
$\bar{c}$, w/	with (Latin: cum)
C_1, C_2, C_3 ... C_7	cervical vertebrae first, second, third ... seventh
C	Centigrade, Celsius, or large calorie (kilocalorie)
cap(s)	capsules
CBR	complete bed rest
CC	chief complaint
CCU	cardiac care unit (coronary care unit)
c/o	complains of
cont	continue
D	diopter (ocular measurement)
dc	discontinue
DC	discharge from hospital
DNA	does not apply
DNR	do not resuscitate

ABBREVIATIONS

ABREVIATIONS

DNS	did not show	
Dr	doctor	
D/W	dextrose in water	
Dx	diagnosis	
EOM	extraocular movement	
ER	emergency room	
Ex	examination	
F	Fahrenheit	
FHS	fetal heart sounds	
FHT	fetal heart tones	
GB	gallbladder	
GI	gastrointestinal	
GU	genitourinary	
h, hr, °	hour	
hpf	high power field	
hs	hour of sleep, bedtime (hora somni)	
hypo	hypodermic injection	
ICU	intensive care unit	
IM	intramuscular	
I&O	intake and output	
i̇ss	one and one half	
IU	international units	
IV	intravenous	
L	left	
L_1, L_2, L_3 ... L_5	lumbar vertebrae first, second, third ... fifth	
L&A	light and accommodation	
LAT	lateral	
L&W	living and well	
LLQ	left lower quadrant	
LMP	last menstrual period	
LOA	left occipitoanterior	
LPF	low power field (10x)	
LUQ	left upper quadrant of abdomen	
MTD	right ear drum (membrana tympani dexter)	
MTS	left ear drum (membrana tympani sinister)	
neg	negative	

▶ ABBREVIATIONS

NG	nasogastric	
NPO	nothing by mouth	
NS	normal saline	
OD	right eye (oculus dexter)	
OP	outpatient	
OR	operating room	
OS or OL	left eye (oculus sinister, oculus laevus)	
OU	each eye (oculus uterque)	
	both eyes (oculi unitas)	
P	pulse	
PA	posteroanterior	
pc	after meals (post cibum)	
PDR	Physicians' Desk Reference	
PI	present illness	
po	by mouth (per os)	
PO	postoperative	
pm	afternoon or evening (post meridiem)	
prn	as needed or desired (pro re nata)	
q	every (quaque)	
qd	every day (quaque die)	
qh	every hour (quaque hora)	
q2h, q4h	every two hours, every four hours	
qid	four times a day (quater in die)	
qm	every morning (quaque mane)	
qn	every night (quaque nocte)	
R	right, respiration	
RBC	red blood cell, erythrocyte count	
Rh	blood factor, Rh+ or Rh-	
RLQ	right lower quadrant (abdomen)	
R/O	rule out	
ROM	range of motion	
RUQ	right upper quadrant (abdomen)	
s̄, w/o	without (sine)	
sc, subcu, sq, subq	subcutaneously (into fat layer)	
sed rate	sedimentation rate (erythrocyte)	
SOB	short of breath	
SOS	if necessary (si opus sit)	

ABBREVIATIONS

▶ ABREVIATIONS

s̈s, ½, .5	half (Latin: semis)
staph	staphylococcus
stat	immediately (statim)
strep	streptococcus
Sx	symptoms
T_1, T_2, T_3 … T_{12}	thoracic vertebrae: first, second, third… twelfth
T, temp	temperature
tab(s)	tablets
TC&DB	turn, cough, and deep breathe
tid	three times a day (ter in die)
tinct	tincture
TPN	total parenteral nutrition
trans	transverse
ULQ	upper left quadrant (abdomen)
ung	ointment (unguentum)
URQ	upper right quadrant (abdomen)
VS	vital signs
WBC	white blood cell, leukocyte count
wm, bm	white male, black male
wf, bf	white female, black female
x	times, power
−	negative
F, ♀	female
M, ♂	male
+/−	positive or negative
*	birth
†	death
p̄	after (post—Latin)
ā	before (ante—Latin)
#	pound, number
↑	increase
↓	decrease
>	greater than
<	less than

▶ PUZZLE SOLUTIONS

Unit 1

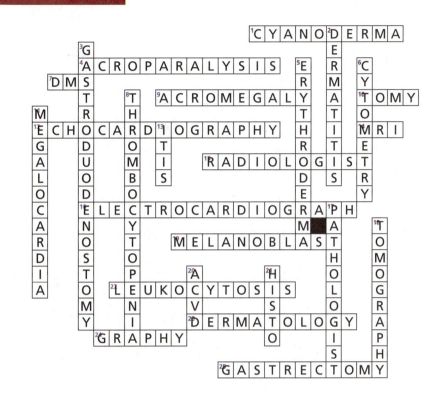

Unit 2

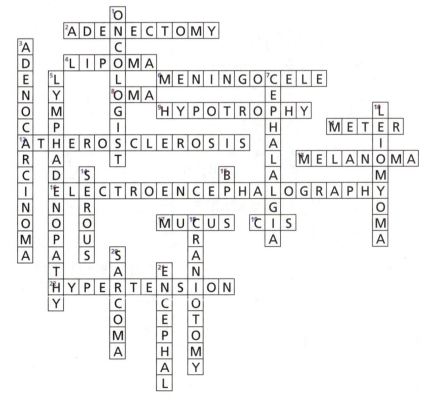

▶ PUZZLE SOLUTIONS

Unit 3

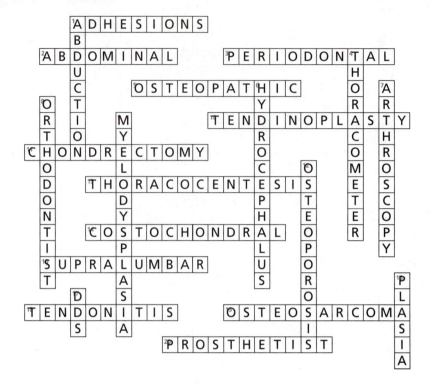

Unit 4

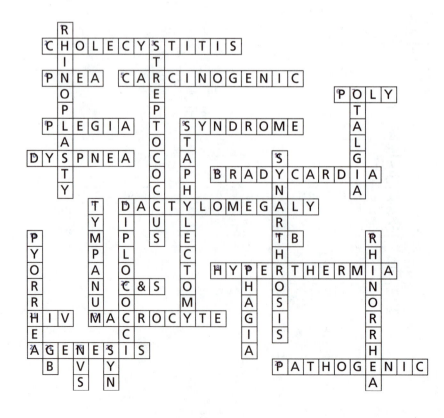

PUZZLE SOLUTIONS

Unit 5

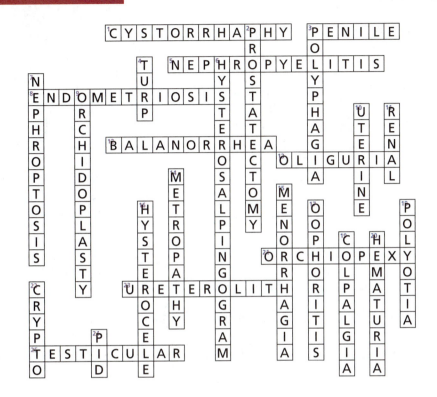

Unit 6

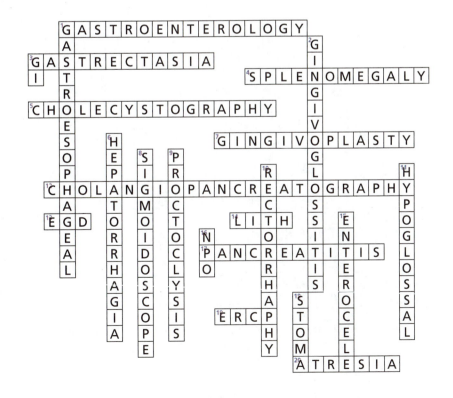

PUZZLE SOLUTIONS

Unit 7

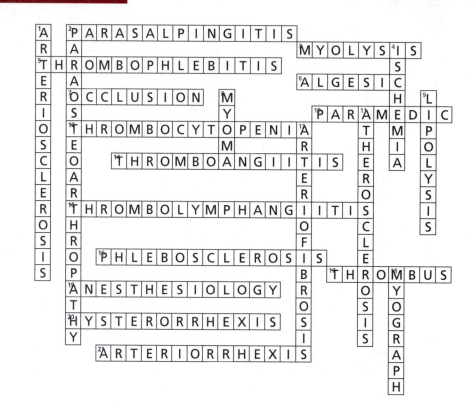

Unit 8

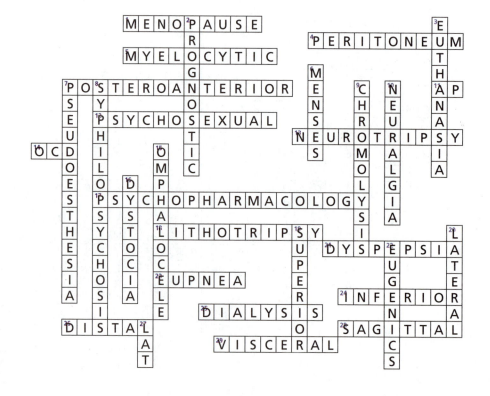

▶ PUZZLE SOLUTIONS

Unit 9

Unit 10

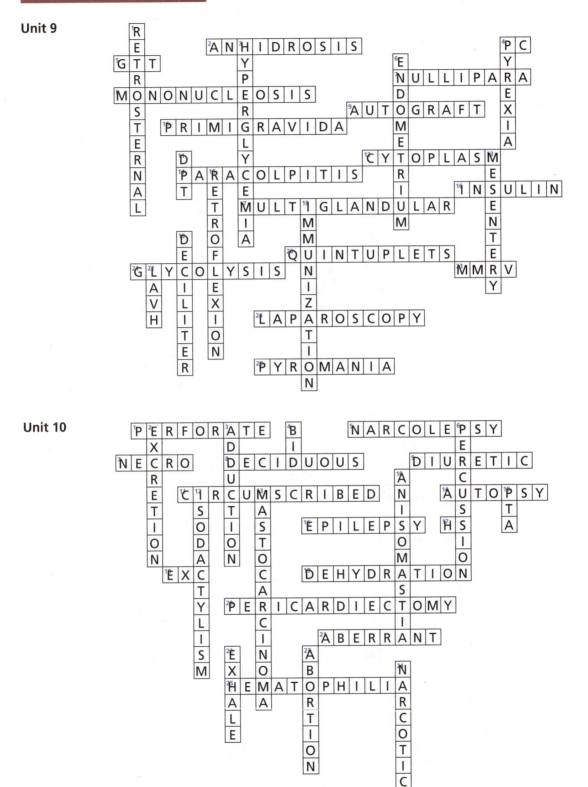

► **PUZZLE SOLUTIONS**

Unit 11

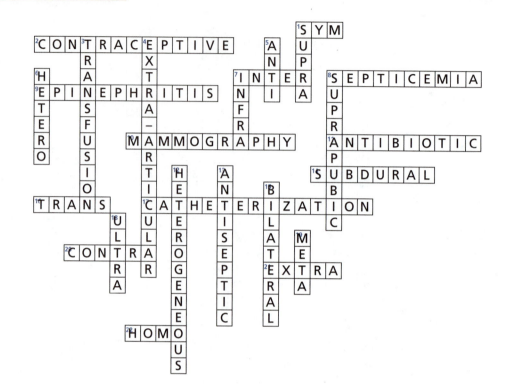

Unit 12

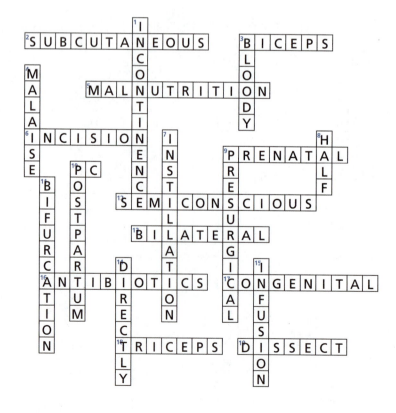

▶ **PUZZLE SOLUTIONS**

Unit 13

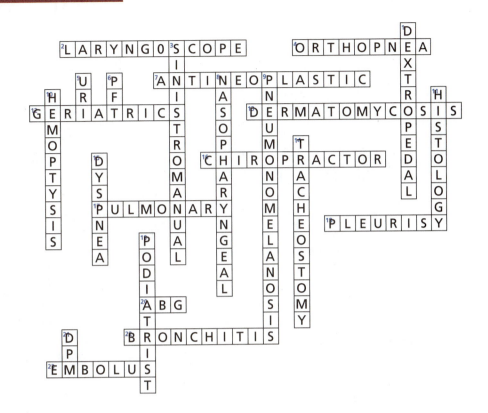

Unit 14

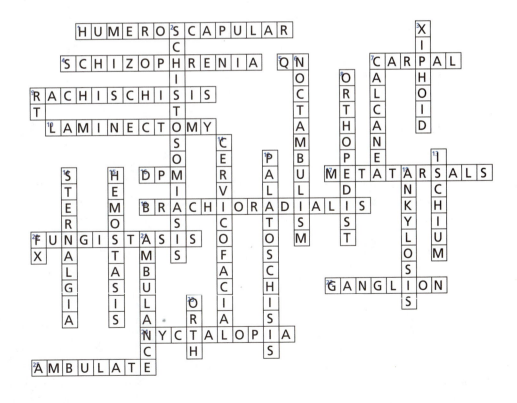

▶ PUZZLE SOLUTIONS

Unit 15

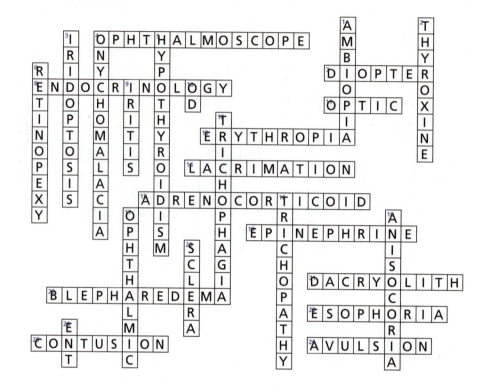

▶ ADDITIONAL WORD PARTS

Following are word parts in addition to those presented in your study of the frames. Use these lists, your knowledge of word building, and your medical dictionary to enrich your medical vocabulary.

1) pick a word part from the alphabetic list that interests you;
2) look for it in your medical dictionary;
3) find words that begin or end with this part and make a list;
4) write the meanings of the new words you discovered;
5) use the key in your dictionary to decipher the correct pronunciation, and practice saying the new words.

Word Part	Meaning	Example
acid/o	acid	acid/osis
acne	point	acne vulgaris
actin/o	ray (radiation)	actin/o/dermat/itis
acu	needle	acu/puncture
adenoid	resembling a gland	aden/oid/ectomy
adnex/al	adjacent, accessory	adnex/ectomy
albin/o	white	albin/ism
alkal/o	base	alkal/osis
all/o	other, different	all/o/pathy, all/ergy
ambly/o	dim, dull	ambly/opia
amyl/o	starch	amyl/ase
andr/o	man	andr/o/gen
aneurysm	abnormal dilation	aneurysm/o/rrhaphy
aort/o	aorta	aort/o/graphy
atel/o	imperfect, collapsed	atel/ectasis
bar/o	weight, heavy	bar/iatrics
bil/i	bile	bil/i/rubin
cac/o	bad, diseased	cac/hexia
cat/a	down, downward	cat/a/tonic
celi/o	abdominal region	celi/ac artery
cerumin	wax	cerumin/o/lysis
chalas/ia	relaxation	a/chalas/ia
chem/o	chemical, drug	chem/o/therapy
chron/o	time	chronological, chronic
chym/o	juice	ec/chym/o/sis
cirrhos	orange-yellow	cirrh/o/sis
clasia	breaking down	arthr/o/clasia
cleisis	closure, occlusion	colp/o/cleis/is
coll/o	glutinous, jellylike	coll/agen
cry/o	freezing	cry/o/surgery
decub/o	lying down	decubit/us ulcer
eczem/o	boil out	eczem/a
effer	to bring out	effer/ent
effus	to pour out	effus/ion
fec/a	feces	fec/a/lith
glomerul/o	glomerulus	glomerul/o/nephr/itis

528

▶ ADDITIONAL WORD PARTS

Word Part	Meaning	Example
gonad/o	ovaries, testes	gonad/o/tropin
halit/o	breath	halit/o/sis
kal/i	potassium	hyper/kal/emia
kary/o	nucleus	kary/o/type
ket/o	ketones	ket/o/sis
klept/o	stealing	klept/o/mania
kyph/o	humped	kyph/o/sis
lord/o	bending	lord/o/sis
mediastin/o	mediastinum	mediastin/al
morph/o	form	meso/morph/ic
muscul/o	muscle	muscul/o/skelet/al
natr/i	sodium	hyper/natr/emia
orexis	appetite	an/orex/ia
pach/y	thick	pach/y/dermat/ous
-poiesis	produce, form	hemat/o/poies/is
poikil/o	irregular shape	poikil/o/cyt/o/sis
prax/ia	action	a/prax/ia
prur/i	itch	prur/itis
pteryg/o	wing	pteryg/o/mandibul/ar
ptyal/o	saliva	ptyal/in
radicul/o	root	radicul/o/neur/itis
roentgen/o	x-ray	roentgen/o/graphy
scoli/o	lateral curve	scoli/o/sis
scot/o	darkness	scot/oma
seb/o	fatty, sebum	seb/o/rrhea
sial/o	saliva	sial/aden/itis
somat/o	body	psych/o/somat/ic
sphygm/o	pulse	sphygm/o/man/o/meter
sphyxis	pulse (related to O_2)	a/sphyxia
stere/o	solid, three-dimensional	stere/o/metry
steth/o	chest	steth/o/scope
sthenia	strength	my/e/sthen/ia
stigma	point	a/stigmat/ism
stigmat/o	mark, point	a/stigmat/ism
taxia	muscle coordination	a/tax/ia
tel/e	distant, far	tel/e/metry
terat/o	monster, wonder	terat/o/genic
tetra	four	tetra/cycline
thel/o	nipple	thel/o/rrhagia
tresia	perforation, closure	a/tres/ia
vagin/o	vagina	vagin/itis
varic/o	twisted vein	varic/o/sity
vulv/o	vulva	vulv/o/vagin/itis
xen/o	strange, foreign	xen/o/phob/ia
xer/o	dry	xer/o/derma

▶ GLOSSARY OF PROPER NAMES OF DISEASES AND PROCEDURES

Addison's disease	deficiency in adrenocortical hormones caused by a progressive destruction of the adrenal glands	Coomb's test	postnatal blood test of cord blood for antibodies against fetal blood type (Rh neg mother, Rh pos fetus)
Bartholin cyst	cyst of the gland located in the cleft between the labia minora and the hymenal ring that secretes mucous lubricant	Cullen's sign	bluish color encircling the umbilicus and indicative of blood in the peritoneal cavity
Bell's palsy	Idiopathic facial palsy of CN VII resulting in asymmetry of the palpebral fissures, nasolabial folds, mouth, and facial expression on the affected side	Cushing's syndrome	hypersecretion of the adrenal cortex causing excessive production of glucocorticoids. May be caused by a tumor.
Biot's respirations	irregularly irregular respiratory pattern caused by damage to the medulla	Down syndrome	extra chromosome (trisomy) of 21 or 22, variety of signs and symptoms including retardation, sloping forehead, flat nose or absent bridge, and generally dwarfed physique
Bouchard's node	bony enlargement of the proximal interphalangeal joint of the finger		
Braxton Hicks contractions	uterine contractions that are irregular and painless; also known as false labor	Electra complex	girl's sexual attraction toward their fathers and rivalry with their mothers
Brushfield's spots	small, white flecks located around the perimeter of the iris and associated with Down syndrome	Fallopian tubes	uterine tubes
		Giardia	genus of protozoan flagellate causing dysentery
Cesarean section	delivery of the fetus by abdominal surgery (hysterotomy)	Glasgow coma scale	international scale used in grading neurological response
Chadwick's sign	blue soft cervix occurring normally during pregnancy	Graafian follicle	mature vesicular follicle of the ovary, matures ovum and secretes estrogen and progesterone
Chandelier's sign	cervix motion tenderness on palpation	Grave's disease	disease characterized by hyperthyroidism, exophthalmic goiter, and thyromegaly, and dermopathy
Cheyne-Stokes respirations	crescendo/decrescendo respiratory pattern interspersed between periods of apnea		
Cooley's anemia	thalasemia major	Guillan-Barre syndrome	autoimmune inflammation causing destruction to the myelin sheath

▶ GLOSSARY OF PROPER NAMES OF DISEASES AND PROCEDURES

Harlequin color change	one half of the newborn's body is red or ruddy and the other half appears pale
Heberden's node	enlargement of the distal interphalangeal joint of the finger
HELLP syndrome	pregnancy-induced hypertension, hemolysis, elevated liver enzymes and low platelets
Hirsutism	excessive body hair
Hodgkin's disease	cancerous lympho-reticular tumor
Homan's sign	pain in the calf when the foot is dorsiflexed
Hornet's syndrome	paralysis of the cervical sympathetic nerve causing contracted pupil and blepharoptosis
Korotkoff sounds	sounds generated when the flow of blood through an artery is altered by the inflation of a blood pressure cuff around the extremity
Korsakoff's syndrome	polyneuritic psychosis caused by chronic alcoholism
Kussmaul's respirations	respirations characterized by extreme increased rate and depth, as in diabetic ketoacidosis
Lou Gehrig's disease	amyotrophic lateral sclerosis
Mantoux test	test for tuberculosis

McBurney's point	anatomic location that is approximately at the normal location of the appendix in the RLQ; point of increased tenderness in appendicitis
Mongolian spots	various irregularly sized areas of deep bluish pigmentation on the upper back, shoulders, buttocks, and lumbosacral area of newborns of African, Latino, and Asian descent
Mongolism	obsolete term for Down syndrome
Montgomery's tubercles	sebaceous and milk glands present on the areola that produce secretions during breastfeeding
Murphy's sign	abnormal finding elicited during abdominal palpation in the RUQ and revealing gallbladder inflammation, patient will abruptly stop inspiration and complain of a sharp pain
Nabothian cysts	small, round, yellow lesions on the cervical surface
Non-Hodgkin's lymphoma	lymphoma that arises directly from the thymus gland
Oedipus complex	boy's sexual attraction to their mothers and feelings of rivalry toward their fathers
Paget's disease	1. malignant neoplasm of the mammary ducts. 2. osteitis deformans

GLOSSARY

▶ GLOSSARY OF PROPER NAMES OF DISEASES AND PROCEDURES

Papanicolaou test	Pap smear, tissue slide examination to detect cervical cancer	Stensen's ducts	openings from the parotids glands
Parkinson's disease	chronic degenerative nerve disease character-ized by palsy, muscle stiffness and weakness, tremor, and fatigue and malaise	Tay-Sachs disease	autosomal recessive trait inherited causing lack of hexosaminase A, this disease is characterized by mental and physical re-tardation, blindness, con-vulsions, cephalomegaly, and death by age 4.
Persian Gulf syndrome	variety of symptoms experienced by veterans of the Persian Gulf war including respiratory, gastrointestinal, joint, and muscle discomforts, fatigue, and memory loss	Tourette's syndrome	symptoms include lack of muscle coordination, spasms, tics, grunts, barks, involuntary swearing, and coprolalia
Rosving's sign	technique to elicit referred pain indicative of peritoneal inflammation	Weber's test	tuning fork used to measure hearing loss and determine if it is con-ductive or sensoneural
Skene's glands	paraurethral glands	Wharton's ducts	openings to the submaxillary glands
Snellen chart	chart used for testing dis-tance vision using stand-ardized numbers and letters of various sizes		

Reference: Estes, *Health Assessment & Physical Examination.* Delmar 1997, and *Tabor's Cyclopedic Medical Dictionary,* 18th Ed. F. A. Davis 1993.

▶ INDEX OF WORD PARTS LEARNED

NOTE: Indexing is by frame number.

License Agreement for Delmar Publishers
an International Thomson Publishing company

Educational Software/Data

You the customer, and Delmar incur certain benefits, rights, and obligations to each other when you open this package and use the software/data it contains. BE SURE YOU READ THE LICENSE AGREEMENT CAREFULLY, SINCE BY USING THE SOFTWARE/DATA YOU INDICATE YOU HAVE READ, UNDERSTOOD, AND ACCEPTED THE TERMS OF THIS AGREEMENT.

Your rights:

1. You enjoy a non-exclusive license to use the enclosed software/data on a single microcomputer that is not part of a network or multi-machine system in consideration for payment of the required license fee, (which may be included in the purchase price of an accompanying print component), or receipt of this software/data, and your acceptance of the terms and conditions of this agreement.

2. You own the media on which the software/data is recorded, but you acknowledge that you do not own the software/data recorded on them. You also acknowledge that the software/data is furnished "as is," and contains copyrighted and/or proprietary and confidential information of Delmar Publishers or its licensors.

3. If you do not accept the terms of this license agreement you may return the media within 30 days. However, you may not use the software during this period.

There are limitations on your rights:

1. You may not copy or print the software/data for any reason whatsoever, except to install it on a hard drive on a single microcomputer and to make one archival copy, unless copying or printing is expressly permitted in writing or statements recorded on the diskette(s).

2. You may not revise, translate, convert, disassemble or otherwise reverse engineer the software/data except that you may add to or rearrange any data recorded on the media as part of the normal use of the software/data.

3. You may not sell, license, lease, rent, loan, or otherwise distribute or network the software/data except that you may give the software/data to a student or and instructor for use at school or, temporarily at home.

Should you fail to abide by the Copyright Law of the United States as it applies to this software/data your license to use it will become invalid. You agree to erase or otherwise destroy the software/data immediately after receiving note of Delmar Publishers' termination of this agreement for violation of its provisions.

Delmar Publishers gives you a LIMITED WARRANTY covering the enclosed software/data. The LIMITED WARRANTY can be found in this product and/or the instructor's manual that accompanies it.

This license is the entire agreement between you and Delmar Publishers interpreted and enforced under New York law.

Limited Warranty

Delmar Publishers warrants to the original licensee/ purchaser of this copy of microcomputer software/ data and the media on which it is recorded that the media will be free from defects in material and workmanship for ninety (90) days from the date of original purchase. All implied warranties are limited in duration to this ninety (90) day period. THEREAFTER, ANY IMPLIED WARRANTIES, INCLUDING IMPLIED WARRANTIES OF MERCHANTABILITY AND FITNESS FOR A PARTICULAR PURPOSE ARE EXCLUDED. THIS WARRANTY IS IN LIEU OF ALL OTHER WARRANTIES, WHETHER ORAL OR WRITTEN, EXPRESSED OR IMPLIED.

If you believe the media is defective, please return it during the ninety day period to the address shown below. A defective diskette will be replaced without charge provided that it has not been subjected to misuse or damage.

This warranty does not extend to the software or information recorded on the media. The software and information are provided "AS IS." Any statements made about the utility of the software or information are not to be considered as express or implied warranties. Delmar will not be liable for incidental or consequential damages of any kind incurred by you, the consumer, or any other user.

Some states do not allow the exclusion or limitation of incidental or consequential damages, or limitations on the duration of implied warranties, so the above limitation or exclusion may not apply to you. This warranty gives you specific legal rights, and you may also have other rights which vary from state to state. Address all correspondence to:

Delmar Publishers
3 Columbia Circle
P. O. Box 15015
Albany, NY 12212–5015